The Rat Electrocardiogram in Pharmacology and Toxicology

PROCEEDINGS OF AN INTERNATIONAL WORKSHOP HELD IN
HANNOVER, FEDERAL REPUBLIC OF GERMANY, JULY 1980
(AN OFFICIAL SATELLITE SYMPOSIUM OF THE SECOND
INTERNATIONAL CONGRESS ON TOXICOLOGY, BRUSSELS,
BELGIUM, JULY 1980)

Editors:

R. BUDDEN

Abt. Spezielle Pharmakologie, Sparte Pharma,
Kali-Chemic AG, D-3000 Hannover, FRG

D. K. DETWEILER

School of Veterinary Medicine, University of Pennsylvania,
Philadelphia, Pennsylvania 19104, USA

G. ZBINDEN

Institute of Toxicology,
Swiss Federal Institute of Technology and University of Zurich,
CH-8603 Schwerzenbach, Switzerland

PERGAMON PRESS

OXFORD · NEW YORK · TORONTO · SYDNEY · PARIS · FRANKFURT

U.K.	Pergamon Press Ltd., Headington Hill Hall, Oxford OX3 0BW, England
U.S.A.	Pergamon Press Inc., Maxwell House, Fairview Park, Elmsford, New York 10523, U.S.A.
CANADA	Pergamon Press Canada Ltd., Suite 104, 150 Consumers Road, Willowdale, Ontario M2J 1P9, Canada
AUSTRALIA	Pergamon Press (Aust.) Pty. Ltd., P.O. Box 544, Potts Point, N.S.W. 2011, Australia
FRANCE	Pergamon Press SARL, 24 rue des Ecoles, 75240 Paris, Cedex 05, France
FEDERAL REPUBLIC OF GERMANY	Pergamon Press GmbH, 6242 Kronberg-Taunus, Hammerweg 6, Federal Republic of Germany

First edition 1981

British Library Cataloguing in Publication Data
The rat electrocardiogram in pharmacology and toxicology.
1. Electrocardiography—Congresses
2. Rats—Physiology—Congresses   3. Laboratory animals—Congresses
I. Budden, R.   II. Detweiler, D. K.
III. Zbinden, G.   IV. International Congresses on Toxicology. *Satellite Symposium (2nd: 1980: Brussels)*
636′.932′320754   QP112.5.E4
ISBN 0-08-026867-6

Printed in Great Britain by A. Wheaton & Co. Ltd, Exeter

Preface

Many years ago, the rat ECG was regarded as something of a biological curiosity. Cardiovascular pharmacology was performed only in cats and dogs, and cardiovascular toxicology was not included in routine testing protocols. Only a few investigators have devoted their time and effort to the study of the rat's cardiovascular system. In the introduction to his paper on the rat ECG in toxicology (page 83), Detweiler pays tribute to these pioneers who have developed experimental techniques and who have accumulated considerable information on the rat ECG.

In recent years things have changed considerably. Rapid developments in instrumentation and miniaturization have greatly facilitated cardiovascular studies with small animals. The rat, which is the most frequently used laboratory animal in many areas of classical and biochemical pharmacology and chemotherapy, can now also be used for experiments on cardiovascular function that were formerly only possible in large animals.

The ECG, probably the most important diagnostic tool in clinical cardiology, was also introduced into the toxicological routine, first in chronic dog studies, more and more also in subacute and chronic experiments in rats. From the rapidly expanding literature on this subject it is evident that the rat ECG may be very useful for the discovery of cardiotoxic chemicals causing degenerative cardiomyopathies and ischemic lesions, as well as functional abnormalities, such as arrhythmias. A generally applicable standard technique, however, has not yet been developed, nor are all problems of nomenclature, interpretation, and evaluation solved. Many pharmacologists and toxicologists are still hesitant to incorporate the rat ECG in their daily routine. They are not convinced that the technique is simple, that it provides relevant and reproducible results, and that it will contribute significantly to the information package assembled for new drugs and other chemicals.

In order to dispel these doubts, a Workshop was organized in Hannover, FRG, in July 1980. During this meeting the use of the rat ECG in acute and chronic pharmacology and toxicology was discussed. The present book contains the main lectures given at the workshop and a selection of posters and demonstrations. From the proceedings of the workshop it becomes evident that monitoring of the rat ECG has gained a firm place in pharmacology and toxicology and that the techniques must be adapted to each experimental problem. One important advantage is the low cost of the animals. It permits the use of relatively large groups of experimental subjects. This, in turn, creates the problem of storage and evaluation of a mass of data. Thus, the use of computers for the evaluation of the rat ECG is becoming an almost inevitable necessity.

The Workshop on the Rat ECG was made possible thanks to the efforts of Dr. J. Fink and the staff of the Institute of Pharmacology, Toxicology, and Pharmacy, Tierärztliche Hochschule Hannover, and its director, Prof. Kämmerer. It was sponsored by the Section on Toxicology of the International Union of Pharmacology and the German Society of Pharmacology and received financial contributions from the Paul-Martini-Stiftung der Medizinisch-Pharmazeutischen Studiengesellschaft e.V.; Boehringer Mannheim GmbH; Byk-Gulden Lomberg Chemische Fabrik GmbH, Konstanz; Boehringer Ingelheim GmbH; Chemiewerk Homburg, Frankfurt am Main; Cilag AG, Schaffhausen; Giulini Pharma Hannover; Gödecke AG, Freiburg; Grünenthal GmbH, Stolberg; E. Merck, Darmstadt; Schering AG, Berlin; Temmler Werke, Marburg. The company Kali-Chemie AG not only provided financial support, but took charge of many of the organizational problems.

It is hoped that the publication of the Proceedings of the Workshop will encourage many colleagues to explore the use of the rat ECG for their specific goals in pharmacology and toxicology. It should also remind us of the great contributions in the area of electrocardiography in animals made by Professor H. Spörri, Zurich. The preparation of this publication coincides with the 70th birthday of this eminent physiologist, and it is with great admiration for the scientific work and leadership of Professor Spörri that we dedicate this book to him.

R. BUDDEN, *Hamburg*
D. K. DETWEILER, *Philadelphia, PA*
G. ZBINDEN, *Zurich*

Contents

List of Contributors   ix

The Normal Rat Electrocardiogram (ECG). P. Driscoll   1

The Electrocardiogram (ECG) of the Rat. B. E. Osborne   15

Relationship between the Scaler Electrocardiogram and Cellular
Electrophysiology of the Rat Heart. J. F. Spear   29

The Rat ECG in Acute Pharmacology and Toxicology. R. Budden,
G. Buschmann and U. G. Kühl   41

The Use of Electrocardiography in Toxicological Studies with Rats.
D. K. Detweiler   83

Spontaneous and Induced Arrhythmias in Rat Toxicity Studies. G.
Zbinden   117

Cardiac Arrhythmias Accompanying Sialodacryoadenitis in the Rat.
D. K. Detweiler, R. A. Saatman and P. J. De Baecke   129

Short Communications and Poster Demonstrations

Measurements of the Electrocardiogram of the Colworth Wistar Rat.
G. W. Cambridge, J. F. Parsons and R. Safford   135

Relationship between Arterial Pressure and ECG Wave Form in
Rats. Experiments carried out on Spontaneously Hypertensive (SHR)
and Normotensive (NR) Control Rats. G. V. Marchetti, E. Baldoli,
A. Nava, M. Capellini, G. Bianchi and G. F. Di Francesco   139

Comparison of ECG and Morphological Parameters in Male and
Female Spontaneously Hypertensive Rats (SHR). R. Müller-Peddinghaus, U. G. Kühl and G. Buschmann   145

Measurement of the Cardiodynamics, Hemodynamics and the ECG
in the Anesthetized Rat. Effects of Catecholamines (Dopamine and
Isoproterenol). G. Schroeder, B. Maass, D. Bartels and G. Mannesmann   155

Graphical Representation of the Time Evolution of ECG Data using
a Computer Data Storage and Plot Package. J. Elsner and R. Knutti   161

A New Method for the Evaluation of ECG and Blood Pressure
Parameters in Anesthetized Rats by On-line Biosignal Processing.
W. Schumacher, R. Budden, G. Buschmann and U. G. Kühl   171

Computer-assisted Analysis of Arrhythmias in the Rat. P. W. Macfarlane, K. A. Kane, M. Podolski and E. Winslow   179

Development of ECG Changes during the Infusion of Beta-blockers
in Anesthetized Rats. G. Buschmann, U. G. Kühl and R. Budden   185

Development of ECG and Blood Pressure Changes in Anesthetized
Rats during the Infusion of Antiarrhythmic Compounds. U. G. Kühl,
G. Buschmann and R. Budden   197
Computer Control of a Modified Langendorff Perfusion Apparatus
and Assessment of the Isolated Heart Viability by Fourier Analysis.
C. G. Adem, F. I. Chaudhry and J. B. Harness   209
The Effects of Antiadrenergic and Antihistaminic Drugs on ECG
Alterations induced by Anthracyclines in Rats. G. Soldani, M. del
Tacca, L. Giovannini and A. Bertelli   213
Drug-induced Alterations in Electrical, Mechanical and Biochemical
Activity of the Isolated Perfused Rat Heart. C. E. Aronson   217
The Surface ECG and Cardiac Histopathology during Chronic
Administration of Anthracycline Antitumor Agents in the Rat.
J. P. Buyniski and R. S. Hirth   231
The Anesthetized Rat as a Model for Investigating Early Post-liga-
tion Dysrhythmias. K. A. Kane, F. M. McDonald and J. R. Parratt   235
Ventricular Fibrillation following Coronary Artery Ligation in the
Rat. T. Abrahamsson and O. Almgren   239
ECG and Other Responses to Ligation of a Coronary Artery in the
Conscious Rat. K. M. Johnston, B. A. MacLeod and M. J. A. Walker   243
A Rapid *in vivo* Technique for the Screening of Potential Anti-
dysrhythmic Agents. P. G. Dolamore and P. R. Sawyer   253
Retardation of Aconitine-induced ECG-alterations in Rats as an
Indication of Membrane-stabilizing Drug Effects. G. Scholtysik   257
Bibliography of Papers on the Rat ECG   265

List of Contributors

T. ABRAHAMSSON, Department of Pharmacology, AB Hässle, Mölndal, Sweden.

C. G. ADEM, Postgraduate Schools of Chemical and Control Engineering, University of Bradford, Bradford, England.

O. ALMGREN, Department of Pharmacology, AB Hässle, Mölndal, Sweden.

C. E. ARONSON, Laboratories of Pharmacology and Toxicology, University of Pennsylvania, School of Veterinary Medicine, Philadelphia, Pa, U.S.A.

F. BALDOLI, Lepetit Research Laboratories, Milan, Italy.

D. BARTELS, Schering AG, Department of Cardiovascular Pharmacology, Berlin/Bergkamen, FRG.

A. BERTELLI, Department of Medical Pharmacology, University of Pisa, Pisa, Italy.

G. BIANCHI, Lepetit Research Laboratories, Milan, Italy.

R. BUDDEN, Chr. Fred Leuschner & Co., Laboratorium für Toxikologische und Pharmakologische Prüfungen, Löhndorf, Post Wankendorf, FRG.

G. BUSCHMANN, Department of Pharmacology, Kali-Chemie AG, Hannover, FRG.

J. P. BUYNISKI, Departments of Pharmacology and Toxicology, Bristol Laboratories, Syracuse, N.Y., U.S.A.

G. W. CAMBRIDGE, Physiology/Pharmacology Section, Environmental Safety Division, Unilever Research, Colworth Laboratory, Sharnbrook, Bedford, England.

M. CAPELLINI, Lepetit Research Laboratories, Milan, Italy.

F. I. CHAUDHRY, Postgraduate Schools of Chemical and Control Engineering, University of Bradford, Bradford, England.

P. J. DE BAECKE, Safety Evaluation Section, I.C.I. Americas Inc., Wilmington, Del., U.S.A.

M. DEL TACCA, Department of Medical Pharmacology, University of Pisa, Pisa, Italy.

D. K. DETWEILER, Comparative Cardiovascular Studies Unit, Department of Animal Biology, School of Veterinary Medicine, University of Pennsylvania, Philadelphia, Pennsylvania, U.S.A.

G. F. DI FRANCESCO, Lepetit Research Laboratories, Milan, Italy.

P. G. DOLAMORE, Department of Pharmacology, Glaxo Group Research Ltd., Greenford, Middlesex, England.

P. DRISCOLL, Institut für Verhaltenswissenschaft der ETH Zürich, Switzerland.

J. ELSNER, Institute of Toxicology, Swiss Federal Institute of Technology and University of Zürich, Schorenstrasse 16, 8603 Schwerzenbach, Switzerland.

L. GIOVANNINI, Department of Medical Pharmacology, University of Pisa, Pisa, Italy.

J. B. HARNESS, Postgraduate Schools of Chemical and Control Engineering, University of Bradford, Bradford, England.

R. S. HIRTH, Departments of Pharmacology and Toxicology, Bristol Laboratories, Syracuse, N.Y., U.S.A.

K. M. JOHNSTON, Department of Pharmacology, Faculty of Medicine, The University of British Columbia, Vancouver, B.C., Canada.

K. A. KANE, Department of Physiology and Pharmacology, University of Strathclyde, Glasgow, Scotland.

R. KNUTTI, Institute of Toxicology, Swiss Federal Institute of Technology and University of Zurich, Schorenstrasse 16, 8603 Schwerzenbach, Switzerland.

U. G. KÜHL, Department of Pharmacology, Kali-Chemie AG, Hannover, FRG.

B. MAASS, Schering AG, Department of Cardiovascular Pharmacology, Berlin/Bergkamen, FRG.

P. W. MACFARLANE, University Department of Medical Cardiology, Royal Infirmary, Glasgow, Scotland.

B. A. MACLEOD, Department of Pharmacology, Faculty of Medicine, The University of British Columbia, Vancouver, B.C., Canada.

G. MANNESMANN, Schering AG, Department of Cardiovascular Pharmacology, Berlin/Bergkamen, FRG.

G. V. MARCHETTI, Lepetit Research Laboratories, Milan, Italy.

F. M. MCDONALD, Department of Physiology and Pharmacology, University of Strathclyde, Glasgow, Scotland.

R. MÜLLER-PEDDINGHAUS, Department of Pharmacology, Kali-Chemie AG, Hannover, FRG.

A. NAVA, Lepetit Research Laboratories, Milan, Italy.

B. E. OSBORNE, Bio-Research Laboratories, Montreal, Canada.

J. R. PARRATT, Department of Physiology and Pharmacology, University of Strathclyde, Glasgow, Scotland.

J. F. PARSONS, Physiology/Pharmacology Section, Environmental Safety Division, Unilever Research, Colworth Laboratory, Sharnbrook, Bedford, England.

M. PODOLSKI, University Department of Medical Cardiology, Royal Infirmary, Glasgow, Scotland.

R. A. SAATMAN, Safety Evaluation Section, I.C.I. Americas Inc., Wilmington, Del., U.S.A.

R. SAFFORD, Physiology/Pharmacology Section, Environmental Safety Division, Uniliver Research, Colworth Laboratory, Sharnbrook, Bedford, England.

P. R. SAWYER, Department of Pharmacology, Glaxo Group Research Ltd., Greenford, Middlesex, England.

G. SCHOLTYSIK, Preclinical Research, Sandoz Ltd., Basle, Switzerland.

G. SCHROEDER, Schering AG, Department of Cardiovascular Pharmacology, Berlin/Bergkamen, FRG.

W. SCHUMACHER, Central EDP Department and Department of Pharmacology, Kali-Chemie AG, Hannover, FRG.

G. SOLDANI, Department of Medical Pharmacology, University of Pisa, Pisa, Italy.

J. F. SPEAR, Department of Animal Biology, School of Veterinary Medicine, University of Pennsylvania, Philadelphia, Pennsylvania, U.S.A.

M. J. A. WALKER, Department of Pharmacology, Faculty of Medicine, The University of British Columbia, Vancouver, B.C., Canada.

E. WINSLOW, Organon Laboratories Ltd., Newhouse, Lanarkshire, Scotland.

G. ZBINDEN, Institute of Toxicology, Swiss Federal Institute of Technology, and University of Zurich, Schorenstrasse 16, 8603 Schwerzenbach, Switzerland.

The Normal Rat Electrocardiogram (ECG)

P. DRISCOLL

ABSTRACT

The origins and nomenclature of the waves and intervals measured in the normal rat ECG are described, as are the genesis of, and types of leads required for, vector analysis (which is gradually becoming more widely used in studies concerned with the rat ECG). After consideration of the usual bipolar and unipolar leads utilized for ECG recordings in rats, the normal values, measurement parameters and peculiarities of the rat ECG are illustrated and discussed. This is done also in the light of certain variables found in the literature such as recording position, age, weight, sex and genetic background of the subjects. It is stressed that the use of anesthesia, e.g. pentobarbital, ether, urethane, or the non-use of anesthesia, e.g. restraint, telemetry, is perhaps the most important factor that could have a direct bearing on toxicological testing, as it pertains to the rat ECG. Finally, a consideration of computers in rat ECG studies, although their use has been limited to date, is made.

ECG recordings, as well as much of the modern-day nomenclature connected to them, were originally described by Einthoven (1903). Since then, numerous publications have appeared dealing with ECG recordings in man and many species of animals, including virtually every species of laboratory animal known which possesses a heart. The present paper deals almost exclusively with the rat ECG. Although a complete review of all studies which have dealt with the steadily expanding field of rat ECG research is probably overdue, the present paper is intended only as an introduction to the normal rat ECG, in the light of its present-day capabilities as a research tool, and readers are referred to other publications (e.g. Cooper, 1969; Heering, 1970) for a more thorough survey of many of the earlier papers in the field.

DEFINITION OF THE ECG

The ECG may be defined as the graphic record of the voltage produced by cardiac muscle cells during de- and repolarization plotted against time

* This paper is dedicated to Professor H. Spörri, on the occasion of his 70th birthday. The author gratefully acknowledges the encouragement and support of Professor K. Bättig in the undertaking of this project.

1

(Osborne, 1974). Depolarization implies that the electrons stream to the pole of lowest electron content in order to distribute the negative charge equally. The wave of depolarization and the restoration of potential, or repolarization, are the impulses recorded on the ECG. In the normal ECG, the wave of depolarization originates at the sino-auricular (SA) node, and travels through the atrial muscle (registered as the **P wave** in the ECG) to the atrioventricular (AV) node in the septum. From there, the wave of depolarization traverses the bundle branches (the P wave, plus the depolarization traversing the AV node and the bundles comprises the **PR interval** in the ECG) to the apex of the heart. The movement of the wave through the septum, to the epicardium up both lateral walls, and back to the base of the heart comprises the **QRS complex.** The **T wave** represents the repolarization of the ventricles. To summarize briefly, the P wave represents atrial excitation, the QRS complex represents ventricular excitation and the T wave represents ventricular recovery.

Before defining vectors, which have become increasingly utilized in recent years by investigators working with the rat ECG, a more complete description of the QRS complex is necessary. Beinfield and Lehr (1968a) have divided this electrical event into three periods according to the sequence and direction of ventricular depolarization. The first period is a brief episode of about 2.5 msec at the onset of QRS during which electrocardiographic manifestations of septal depolarization are directed to the right and superiorly. In the second phase, the summated depolarization forces originating in the ventricle are directed inferiorly and to the left. The QRS deflection of the greatest magnitude is inscribed regularly during this period. Finally, the terminal phase of ventricular depolarization occurs, in which a superior and rightward direction of depolarization is compatible with activation of the base of the heart.

DEFINITION OF VECTORS

Before covering the types of leads used in ECG recordings with the rat, it is desirable to complete the theoretical considerations of the QRS complex with an introduction to vector analysis. Although no references deal directly with this topic as it pertains to the rat, references do exist which approach vector analysis in relation to animals of similar comportment, as distinguished from man. The paper by Hamlin and Smith (1960), which also emphasizes the differences in the orientation of the heart between man and in that case, the dog, may be used as an adequate basis for these considerations. Since vectors deal with deflections generated by ventricular and interventricular septal excitation (the QRS complex), an understanding of this form of interpretation of the ECG can be brought about through an expanded commentary on the events described in the previous paragraph.

The three major vector quantities (dipoles) are represented by the following three fronts of activation:

(a) Activation of the septum (left to right and right to left). The left component is greater and earlier, so the ECG records it as such (left to right).

(b) Spread to the epicardial surfaces, also simultaneously through both ventricles. The ECG records this event as if the front were moving only from the left ventricular endocardium to the left ventricular epicardium, because the left ventricle is much thicker than the right ventricle.

(c) The termination of ventricular activation when the base of the heart is activated in an apicobasilar direction.

These three fronts of activation have magnitudes proportional to the muscle mass activated by each and directions according to their pathway through the heart. They are called, respectively, Vectors I, II and III. A single vector of appropriate magnitude, direction and sense (or polarity) is used to represent all of the complex electrical forces generated by the excitation of given volumes of muscle in given directions at a single instant. This may be along one or a combination of three axes: dorsoventral—Z axis, cephalocaudal—Y axis or sinistrodextral—X axis (Hamlin and Smith, 1960).

TYPES OF LEADS USED FOR ECG RECORDINGS AND VECTOR ANALYSIS

Before going into vectors in more detail, it is necessary to describe the various leads used in recording the rat ECG. These leads fall into one of two categories, bipolar or unipolar. A bipolar lead records all electrical events between the two electrode terminals by revealing the changes of one electrode over and above the changes affecting the other. By utilizing the limbs (extremities) to hold the electrodes, all leads are sufficiently distant from the heart so that none are disproportionately influenced. Lead I (right and left foreleg) may be roughly stated to lie in the axis of the horizontal heart, lead II (right foreleg and left hindleg) in line with the neutrally placed heart, and lead III (left foreleg and left hindleg) in line with the vertical heart. Leads I and III may be said to be vectors of lead II, so the waves seen in lead II should be a sum of the addition of the other two leads. Many of the earlier studies with rats involved the use of these bipolar leads only (e.g. Weiss *et al.*, 1938; Lombard, 1952; Heise and Kimbel, 1955; Normann *et al.*, 1961).

Unipolar leads consist of one inactive and one active electrode and are of several types. The various precordial leads, used most extensively in man, consist of active electrodes placed at several locations on the chest wall, in order to thoroughly and simultaneously explore the right and left ventricles and septum. The inactive electrode is placed on a limb. The closeness of the active electrode to the heart obviously results in the domination of that electrode over the distantly placed inactive electrode in the subsequent recordings (hence the descriptive terms "active" and "inactive". Although these leads (usually designated V_1 to V_6) have been often used by investigators working with rats (e.g. Hill *et al.*, 1960; Sambhi and White, 1960; Cooper, 1969; Dunn *et al.*, 1978; Baur and Pierach, 1979), most of these studies have also utilized the application of extremity leads on both a bipolar and a unipolar basis, and Yamori *et al.* (1976) have reported apparent difficulties encountered in applying the many leads involved in this type of lead system to rats, due to their movable skin.

A (bipolar) variation of the chest lead system, which has proven to be effective in rat ECG studies (although not applicable to vector analysis), was originally developed for the guinea pig by Spörri (1944), based on the Nehb leads for man, and later refined to 3 basic leads (designated D, A and J) by Jasiński and Grauwiler (1960). This system has been subsequently referred to as the Nehb–Spörri lead system and used in investigations with guinea pigs (Driscoll, 1976), cats (Beglinger *et al.*, 1977) and rats (Driscoll, 1979). Zbinden *et al.* (1978, 1980) and Zbinden and Rageth (1978) have used it in an abbreviated form (lead D only) in several toxicological and nutritional studies with rats. The electrode placements are on the left side of the thorax (apex of heart), the right scapula and over the lumbar vertebrae. The results with rats, in particular, have indicated the importance of using multiple lead systems in ECG studies. Driscoll (1979) has demonstrated several contrasts between this lead system and the lead system utilizing the extremities in the same study, including differences in the detection of changes in T wave amplitude resulting from pentobarbital injections, and in the detection of rat strain differences in S wave amplitude.

The most frequently used unipolar leads are designated aVL, aVR and aVF, these leads having the advantage that they may be recorded together with the bipolar extremity lead recordings, since they make use of the identical electrode placements. The active electrodes are on the left foreleg (aV"L"), right foreleg (aV"R") and one of the hindlegs (aV"F"—for "foot" in man). By convention, in all of the lead systems, the R wave is always positive, the Q (when present) and S waves always negative, and the T wave either positive or negative. The aVL, aVR and aVF leads have been used in numerous studies with rats, all of which have also included leads I, II and III (e.g. Beinfield and Lehr, 1956, 1968a, 1968b; Sambhi and White, 1960; Godwin and Fraser, 1965; Cooper, 1969; Heering, 1970; Wexler *et al.*, 1973; Dunn *et al.*, 1978; Driscoll, 1979; Baur and Pierach, 1979; Mulvaney and Sironde, 1979). An example of the normal rat ECG, representing lead II, is diagrammatically shown in Fig. 1. The reader is referred to the

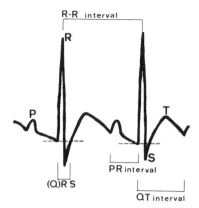

Fig. 1. Diagrammatic representation of 2 normal rat ECG cycles. Dashed lines represent the isoelectric baselines for each. The average value of several consecutive R–R intervals is normally used to establish the heart rate.

literature cited here for illustrations (when given) of the various other leads mentioned.

Returning now to vector analysis, Hamlin and Smith (1960) have stressed the importance of using correct leads to measure the forces on the three axes in animals. They recommended the use of lead I (positive pole on left foreleg, negative pole on right foreleg) to measure the X axis forces, in which leftward-directed forces cause a positive deflection, and leads aVF, II and III to determine Y axis forces, in which caudally-directed forces result in a positive deflection. "Lead V_{10}" (positive electrode on the thoracic vertebrae and negative electrode under the sternum) was recommended to determine Z axis forces, in which dorsally-directed forces result in a positive deflection. They went on to describe normal vector deflections for the dog, which may or may not provide a suitable reference for the normal rat. There have, however, been several studies which have investigated ventricular hypertrophy in hypertensive rats from the standpoint of changes in vector orientation and magnitude. The three which will be mentioned here are noteworthy partly due to the selection of leads which were used toward these ends.

As the results of the three reports are not in complete agreement with one another (which is not surprising, considering the outstanding differences in leads, equipment, type and depth of anesthesia, recording positions, and types of hypertensive rats used: i.e. spontaneous vs experimental hypertensive rats), the reader is referred to the respective publications for details concerning the findings of each. The first of these (Sambhi and White, 1960) made use of the three conventional bipolar leads (I, II and III), the three conventional unipolar leads (aVL, aVR and aVF) and three unipolar chest leads, uniquely designated V_A, V_B and V_C. Ether anesthesia was used, and the rats were placed on their backs (supine position). Of the other two studies, that of Dunn et al. (1978) was most similar to the first in regard to the leads used, those being the six standard leads (I, II, III, aVL, aVR and aVF), and three precordial leads corresponding to V_1, V_2 and V_5 in man. These rats were also anesthetized (lightly) with ether and positioned supinely.

In the third study of this type (Yamori et al., 1976), a most interesting and original lead system, called the Takayasu system, was described. This system consisted of two small electrodes (on the bridge of the nose and around the base of the tail), and four large electrodes (one on each side of the thorax, one over the thoracic vertebrae and one under the sternum). The rats were positioned ventrally (prone) and pentobarbital anesthesia was administered. The three axes were, in the opinion of the authors, most optimally delineated. They were, in a fashion similar to that of Hamlin and Smith (1960), designated as follows: X = left to right, Y = cranial to caudal and Z = ventral to dorsal. ECGs were also recorded, separately, before or after the recordings made for the vectorcardiograms, using extremity or chest leads for this purpose.

EVALUATION OF THE NORMAL RAT ECG

Before considering normal values for the rat ECG, some details regarding their determination must be looked at. First of all, the P, QRS and T deflections, in addition to the intervening segments in the rat ECG, usually do not share a common baseline. Any given wave may terminate at a level different from that at which it originated. To measure the magnitudes of the various deflections, therefore, a reference point for determination of the isoelectric baseline is a necessity. To this end, often the best reference point has been determined to be the point at which the PR interval terminates and the QRS complex begins, as this point is subject to the least variation and alteration by other electrical events which may occur during the cardiac cycle (Beinfield and Lehr, 1968b). Secondly, although the QRS complex is usually referred to as such, the Q wave is absent on most leads of the rat ECG. This phenomenon has often been noted in the literature (e.g. Lombard, 1952; Hill et al., 1960; Sambhi and White, 1960; Wexler et al., 1973), and is the reason for the term (Q)RS being sometimes used instead of the term QRS, or for the term PR being used in place of PQ, etc. Two other characteristic peculiarities of the rat ECG, also apparent in Fig. 1, are the lack of a definite ST segment and the occurrence of asymmetrical T waves, either or both of which have been noted and discussed by many of the authors cited here (Lombard, 1952; Heise and Kimbel, 1955; Beinfield and Lehr, 1956, 1968a; Grauwiler and Spörri, 1960; Sambhi and White, 1960; Cooper, 1969; Wexler *et al.*, 1973; Dunn *et al.*, 1978; Budden and Buschmann, 1979). According to Grauwiler and Spörri (1960), the lack of a definite ST segment was first noted by Schinzel, in Munich, in 1933. Infant rats, apparently, do show an ST segment, which begins to disappear at about 20 days of age. In any case, this situation in adult rats is also characteristic of several other species, such as the mouse, mole and kangaroo.

A composite of normal rat ECG values is shown in Table 1. These data, which represent some of the traditionally measured parameters of the rat ECG, show some of the variation between studies which is commonly seen in the literature, and which could be due to one or more of the variables which will be briefly described in the next two sections. Especially noteworthy are the consistent differences in the heart rate seen between anesthetized and non-anesthetized rats. Several measurement parameters which have been only recently applied to the rat ECG in toxicological investigations have not been included in Table 1. These are as follows:

(a) Ratio R:S = R voltage expressed as percent of R plus S (Zbinden *et al.*, 1978).

(b) QTc = QT corrected for heart rate = QT interval (sec)/$\sqrt{RR}$ interval (sec) (Zbinden and Rageth, 1978; Zbinden *et al.*, 1980).

(c) the measurement of the SαT segment — deepest point of S to apex of T, and of the QRαT interval and αTP segment.

The apex of T (αT) is used in these calculations in order to compensate for the difficulties usually encountered in determining the start and end of the T wave (Budden and Buschmann, 1979). In reference to (b) above, it should be mentioned here that Willard and Horvath (1959) have also reported a method for correcting QT values for heart rate.

FACTORS THAT MAY INFLUENCE THE NORMAL RAT ECG

In addition to the many types of leads used, differences in normal rat ECG measurements found in the literature may be due to such variables as the recording position, age, weight, sex or genetic background of the subjects. All of these will be briefly surveyed in this section. Further potential variables are differences in the equipment used (e.g. the gain and frequency responses of the amplifier, the frequency response of the recorder, etc.) and the paper (or film) speed of the recorder. The most important variable of all, in the opinion of this author, and that which probably directly affects all toxicological studies, is the presence or absence of anesthesia and, respectively, the type of anesthetic or form of restraint used. This last subject will be discussed separately, in the next section.

TABLE 1. NORMAL RAT ECG VALUES FROM SELECTED LITERATURE, INCLUDING MOST OF THE ROUTINELY-MEASURED ECG PARAMETERS. HEART RATE = BEATS/MIN, QRS, PR AND QT = MSEC, P, R AND T = MV

Reference	Anesthetic	Heart rate	QRS	PR	P	R	QT	T	Comments
Weiss et al. (1938)	none	500!							placed on back with feet tied
Lombard (1952)	pentobarbital	347 ± 31	23	42	0.083	0.363			lead II
Heise and Kimbel (1955)	barbiturate	275–400	21–30	25–44	0.12	0.71	64–106	0.12	lead II
Beinfield & Lehr (1956)	nembutal	270–380		40–50	0.05–0.1	0.3–0.9	50–70	0.05–0.1	lead II
Hill et al. (1960)	none	380–480							
Normann et al. (1961)	ether	388 (340–504)		60	0.03	0.163	54		lead II
Beinfield & Lehr (1968a,b)	light ether	240–444	15.1	49	0.08	0.775	78.7	0.145	lead II
Cooper (1969)	pentobarbital	350 (220–470)		50			90		
Heering (1970)	urethane	314 (222–415)	18	50			78	0.38	lead II
	none	464 (437–489)	20	46			57	0.22	lead II
Wexler et al. (1973)	barbiturate and ether	366		51		0.46	102.5	0.12	lead II
Zbinden and Rageth (1978)	urethane	326–371	15.3–16	44–52		0.7–0.76		0.24–0.28	lead D
Caprino et al. (1978)	pentobarbital	430		45	0.19	0.84		0.33	lead II
Mulvaney & Seronde (1979)	light ether		16.6–19.2	51–53		0.52–0.6	80–100	1.2–2.0	lead II
Driscoll (1979)	pentobarbital	250–390	15–18	52–57		0.74–1.1	46–56	0.12–0.22	lead D
	none	403–448							
Zbinden et al. (1980)	urethane	310–390							lead D
	none	440–480							lead D

In regard to equipment differences, it can safely be said that there are almost as many different recording devices, all with different specifications, as there are investigators working with the rat ECG! Most of this equipment, however, falls basically into one of two categories: direct-writing instruments producing recordings directly on paper, or instruments (e.g. string galvanometers, cathode-ray oscilloscopes, etc.) that record on film. Some studies, such as that of Baur and Pierach (1979), have used the approach of obtaining records through Polaroid photographs made directly from an oscilloscope. Most authors who have expressed a preference, however, have favored the direct-writing instruments (e.g. Godwin and Fraser, 1965; Osborne, 1974), partly due to their greater ease of operation and portability. In any case, many instruments of both types are currently available that have the characteristics necessary for the reliable recording of rat ECGs. The paper (or film) speed used in the non-computerized studies cited here varied from 3 cm/sec (Hill *et al.*, 1960) to 16 cm/sec (Grünberg and Hundt, 1958). The majority of studies, however, have used speeds of between 5 and 10 cm/sec, and it would appear as though 5 cm/sec is the allowable minimum for obtaining accurate measurements of the normal rat ECG time intervals.

Certain advantages for making ECG recordings with the rat in a ventral (prone) position have been claimed by Beinfield and Lehr (1956, 1968a), who have emphasized that that position is obviously more "physiologic" or natural for rats. Several of the publications cited here, however, including some recent ones, refer to using the supine position during recording of the ECG in that species. The different recording positions, especially in regard to unanesthetized rats, have undoubtedly led to differences in the ECGs recorded in some experiments (e.g. heart rates—see Weiss *et al.*, 1938), and may have been responsible for the differences in the spatial orientation of the heart vectors seen in the vector experiments cited earlier in this present paper. One study, however, has reported more marked differences between the right and left lateral positions, as compared to no particular differences between the ventral and supine positions (Grünberg and Hundt, 1958), and Osborne (1974) has suggested that the most important factor is to retain a constant position during recording.

Within-study heart rate differences have been reported depending upon the age (Beinfield and Lehr, 1968a; Wexler and Greenberg, 1974), weight (Beinfield and Lehr, 1968a), sex (Driscoll, 1979) and strain (Dunn *et al.*, 1978; Driscoll, 1979) of healthy, anesthetized rats. Within-study strain and sex differences, other than in the heart rate, have also been noted. Godwin and Fraser (1965) reported S wave amplitude differences between Wistar and Sprague–Dawley rats used at their laboratory under deep ether anesthesia, and Driscoll (1979) reported QT interval and S and T wave amplitude differences between Roman high- and low-avoidance rats, as well as

QT interval and S wave amplitude differences between males and females within the Roman low-avoidance strain, under pentobarbital anesthesia.

ANESTHESIA *VS* RESTRAINT

The problem of whether or not to use anesthesia in studies dealing with the effects of toxic substances on the rat ECG goes much deeper than the differences in heart rates consistently reported within or between studies using anesthetized and/or unanesthetized rats (see Table 1). Osborne (1974) has stated that anesthetics are precluded in these types of studies because of (a) possible synergism between the anesthetic used and the compound being tested, and (b) possible changes being produced in the ECG by the anesthetic agent itself. In regard to pentobarbital anesthesia, both Watanabe and Aviado (1975) and Driscoll (1979) have restated this opinion. In addition to demonstrating conclusively a pentobarbital-induced bradycardia, the latter study also showed that as the heart rate subsequently increased after a low point at 40 min after injection, the PR and QT intervals actually continued to lengthen progressively throughout the 2 hr duration of the experiment, accompanied by equally steady increases in the T wave amplitude. Jasiński and Grauwiler (1960) have shown, in the guinea pig, that the T wave effects induced by pentobarbital anesthesia may even last as long as 48 hr after the animal regains consciousness. The other two anesthetic agents most often used in rat ECG experiments are ether and urethane. Osborne (1974) has flatly come forward against the use of ether in this type of toxicology study with rats, claiming that ether anesthesia leads to arrhythmias and that a constant plane of anesthesia is too difficult to maintain. Beinfield and Lehr (1968a) have also reported transient changes in the ECG caused by ether anesthesia, notably in the nature of the T wave. The fewest problems seem to be encountered with urethane, although Heering (1970) has demonstrated a urethane-induced bradycardia, mediated through a lengthening of the PQ and QT intervals, as well as temporary deformations of the P wave caused by that substance. Zbinden *et al.* (1980) have also reported a significant slowing of the heart rate with urethane anesthesia in rats, and it is apparent from Table 1 that all three of the anesthetic agents in question affect the heart in this fashion.

The alternative to anesthesia in the rat, in studies concerned with the effects of toxic substances on the ECG, is some kind of restraint. The most acceptable method seems to be the utilization of hollow plastic cylinders, equipped with longitudinal slots along the sides to accommodate electrode wires (Osborne, 1974; Zbinden *et al.*, 1980). Although this method is undoubtedly stressful to some degree, it probably does not result in much more serious ECG changes than a moderate rise in the heart rate. The only alternative to anesthesia available which is truly stress-free is the use of telemetry (e.g. Bohus, 1974), but it is not yet possible to obtain much more than heart rate determinations with that method in the rat.

THE USE OF COMPUTERS

Several investigators have reported the use of partial automatization in the storage and retrieval of rat ECG recordings. Heering (1970) and Lehr and Werner (1974), the latter of which actually accomplished the feat with mice, have recorded and stored amplified signals on magnetic tape. These could be periodically recorded on paper or fed into a multi-channel computer for storage, and written out later when desirable. Heering (1970) produced computer-made curves which bridged over the very variable individual cycles of the rats, amply illustrated in his report. The various wave amplitudes and interval durations were measured by hand. More recently, Zbinden *et al.* (1978) have reported the storage of all rat ECG measurements in a PDP11 computer, with plotting being done with a printer-plotter, and Budden and Buschmann (1979) have reported the use of digital-to-analog computer reconstruction.

By far the most ambitious effort toward the full automatization of ECG recording in the rat has been that of Caprino *et al.* (1978). Their report describes the hardware (computer, magnetic tape recorder, console, analog-to-digital and digital-to-analog converters), software and input parameters of the LUCA system, in detail. Automatic ECG recordings (output values) are presented as a printout which identifies the following values for each wave: index (expressed as the peak height to base amplitude ratio in mV/sec), base (in sec), height (in mV), area (in mV.sec), time from the preceding QRS complex and the number of isotypical waves identified. A histogram is constructed for each ECG cycle from the input values, and a dynamic baseline is then calculated from the histogram by selecting that value corresponding to the maximum occurrence. The very brief resolution time (2 msec) of this system has enabled them to analyze very high rate ECGs such as those of the rat, and they maintain that quantitative instant-by-instant evaluation of changes in common parameters (e.g. height, duration, area) of each single ECG wave is theoretically possible. However, the system does not recognize waves with parameters with less than critically sensitive values, so some may be left out, and R wave detection being based on the deviation from the baseline (height) causes considerable difficulty, especially when filtering off high frequencies. In addition, several limitations of the system due to the variability and frequency of rat ECGs are described, such as failing to identify some waves or complexes and thus ignoring them completely, losing minimum derivative values (e.g. QRS complex) in the noise signal and incorrectly analyzing overlapping waves and complexes.

HEART SOUNDS AND A CONCLUSION

It should be mentioned, before closing, that the recording of heart sounds (the phonocardiogram), one of the most-closely related developments to the ECG and extensively used for diagnostic and experimental purposes in several of the larger animal species and man, has been almost completely ignored in the rat. Although relatively refined methods for measuring heart sounds have existed for many years (Hess, 1920), it may be assumed that the small heart volume and rapid heart rate of the rat has generally discouraged the utilization of this method with that laboratory animal species. Phonocardiograms in rats have, however, been occasionally recorded and briefly reported in the literature (e.g. Grünberg and Hundt, 1958; Grauwiler and Spörri, 1960; Heering, 1970). Hopefully, this potentially informative ECG method will become more useful in future toxicological experiments with rats, especially in the light of modern advances being made in amplification and recording techniques.

In conclusion, based on the literature cited in this paper, the author feels that the following points may be of particular relevance in regard to application of the rat ECG to toxicological research:

(a) The use of a suitable method of restraint is apparently preferable to the use of anesthesia in obtaining accurate ECG recordings.

(b) As many leads as possible should be utilized, particularly when vector analysis is included in the study.

(c) The ventral (prone) position is probably preferable for maintaining a natural orientation of the rat's heart during the recording session.

(d) Potential variables such as age, weight, sex and genetic background of the subjects should be appreciated when planning experiments and making across-study comparisons.

REFERENCES

Baur, H. R. and Pierach, C. A. (1979) Electrocardiographic changes after bilateral carotid sinus denervation in the rat. *Am. J. Physiol.* **237**, H475–H480.

Beglinger, R., Heller, A. and Lakatos, L. (1977) Elektrokardiogramme, Herzschlagfrequenz und Blutdruck der Hauskatze (Felis catus). *Zbl. Vet. Med.* **A24**, 252–257.

Beinfield, W. H. and Lehr, D. (1956) Advantages of ventral position in recording electrocardiogram of the rat. *J. Appl. Physiol.* **9**, 153–156.

Beinfield, W. H. and Lehr, D. (1968a) QRS–T variations in the rat electrocardiogram. *Am. J. Physiol.* **214**, 197–204.

Beinfield, W. H. and Lehr, D. (1968b) P–R interval of the rat electrocardiogram. *Am. J. Physiol.* **214**, 205–211.

Bohus, B. (1974) Telemetered heart rate responses of the rat during free and learned behavior. *Biotelemetry* 1, 193–201.

Budden, R. and Buschmann, G. (1979) Cardiovascular pharmacology: electrocardiographic studies. In: *Pharmacological Methods in Toxicology* (G. Zbinden and F. Gross, ed.), pp. 77–80. Pergamon, Oxford.

Caprino, L., Borrelli, F., Falchetti, R., Biader, U. and Franchina, V. (1978) A new computerized system for automatic ECG analysis: an application to hypoxic rat ECGs. *Comput. Biomed. Res.* 11, 195–207.

Cooper, D. K. C. (1969) Electrocardiographic studies in the rat in physiological and pathological states. *Cardiovasc. Res.* 3, 419–425.

Driscoll, P. (1976) Inhalation of smoke from high- and low-nicotine cigarettes by guinea pigs: behavioral and ECG effects. In: *Adverse Effects of Environmental Chemicals and Psychotropic Drugs* (M. Horvath, ed.), Vol. II, pp. 241–256. Elsevier, Amsterdam.

Driscoll, P. (1979) The electrocardiogram of Roman high- and low-avoidance rats under pentobarbital sodium anesthesia. *Arzneim. Forsch./Drug Res.* 29, 897–900.

Dunn, F. G., Pfeffer, M. A. and Frohlich, E. D. (1978) ECG alterations with progressive left ventricular hypertrophy in spontaneous hypertension. *Clin. Exp. Hypertension* 1, 67–86.

Einthoven, W. (1903) Die galvanometrische Registrirung des menschlichen Elektrokardiogramms, zugleich eine Beurtseilung der Anwendung des Capillar-Elektrometers in der Physiologie. *Pflügers Arch. Ges. Physiol.* 99, 472–480.

Godwin, K. O. and Fraser, F. J. (1965) Simultaneous recording of ECG's from disease-free rats, using a cathode-ray oscilloscope and a direct-writing instrument. *Q. J. Exp. Physiol.* 50, 277–281.

Grauwiler, J. and Spörri, H. (1960) Fehlen der ST-Strecke im Elektrokardiogramm von verschiedenen Säugetierarten. *Helv. Physiol. Acta* 18, C77–C78.

Grünberg, H. and Hundt, H.-J. (1958) Ueber Typenwechsel im Elektrokardiogramm der Ratte bedingt durch die Körperhaltung. *Z. Kreislaufforsch.* 47, 874–877.

Hamlin, R. L. and Smith, C. R. (1960) Anatomical and physiologic basis for interpretation of the electrocardiogram. *Am. J. Vet. Res.* 21, 701–708.

Heering, H. (1970) Das Elektrokardiogramm der wachen und narkotisierten Ratte. *Arch. Int. Pharmacodyn.* 185, 308–328.

Heise, E. and Kimbel, K. H. (1955) Das normale Elektrokardiogramm der Ratte. *Z. Kreislaufforsch.* 44, 212–221.

Hess, W. R. (1920) Die graphische Aufzeichnung der Herztöne nach neuer Methode. *Pflügers Arch. Ges. Physiol.* 180, 35–60.

Hill, R., Howard, A. N. and Gresham, G. A. (1960) The electrocardiographic appearances of myocardial infarction in the rat. *Br. J. Exp. Pathol.* 41, 633–637.

Jasiński, B. and Grauwiler J. (1960) Veränderungen im Elektrokardiogramm des Meerschweinchens wahrend der Barbiturat-Narkose. *Cardiologia* 37, 23–32.

Lehr, E. and Werner, G. (1974) Eine Methode für die quantitative Analyse des Herzrhythmus zum Nachweis vegetativer Reaktionen auf Neuropharmaka. *Arzneim. Forsch./Drug Res.* 24, 1844–1847.

Lombard, E. A. (1952) Electrocardiograms of small mammals. *Am. J. Physiol.* 171, 189–193.

Mulvaney, D. A. and Seronde, J. (1979) Electrocardiographic changes in vitamin B_1, deficient rats. *Cardiovasc. Res.* 13, 506–513.

Normann, S. J., Priest, R. E. and Benditt, E. P. (1961) Electrocardiogram in the normal rat and its alteration with experimental coronary occlusion. *Circul. Res.* 9, 282–287.

Osborne, B. E. (1974) Uses and applications of electrocardiography in toxicology. In: *Experimental Model Systems in Toxicology and Their Significance in Man*, Vol. XV, pp. 85–97. Excerpta Medica, Amsterdam.

Sambhi, M. P. and White, F. N. (1960) The electrocardiogram of the normal and hypertensive rat. *Circul. Res.* 8, 129–134.

Spörri, H. (1944) *Der Einfluss der Tuberkulose auf das Elektrokardiogramm, Untersuchungen an Meerschweinchen und Rindern*. Habilitationsschrift, Vet. Med. Fac., Univ., Zürich, 1944 and *Arch. Wiss. Prakt. Tierheilk.* 79, 1–57.

Watanabe, T. and Aviado, D. M. (1975) Toxicity of aerosol propellants in the respiratory and circulatory systems. VII. Influence of pulmonary emphysema and anesthesia in the rat. *Toxicology* **3**, 225–240.

Weiss, S., Haynes, F. W. and Zoll, P. M. (1938) Electrocardiographic manifestations and the cardiac effect of drugs on vitamin B_1 deficiency in rats. *Am. Heart J.* **15**, 206–220.

Wexler, B. C. and Greenberg, B. P. (1974) Effect of exercise on myocardial infarction in young *vs.* old male rats: electrocardiographic changes. *Am. Heart J.* **88**, 343–350.

Wexler, B. C., Willen, D. and Greenberg, B. P. (1973) Electrocardiographic differences between non-arteriosclerotic and arteriosclerotic rats. *Atherosclerosis* **18**, 129–140.

Willard, P. W. and Horvath, S. M. (1959) Electrocardiographic studies on rats before and after cardiac arrest induced by hypothermia and asphyxia. *Am. J. Physiol.* **196**, 711–714.

Yamori, Y., Ohtaka, M. and Nara, Y. (1976) Vectorcardiographic study on left ventricular hypertrophy in spontaneously hypertensive rats. *Japan. Circul. J.* **40**, 1315–1329.

Zbinden, G. and Rageth, B. (1978) Early changes of cardiac function in rats on a high-fat diet. *Food Cosmet. Toxicol.* **16**, 123–127.

Zbinden, G., Bachmann, E., Holderegger, C. and Elsner, J. (1978) Cardiotoxicity of tricyclic antidepressants and neuroleptic drugs. In: *Proc. 1st Int. Cong. Toxicol,* pp. 285–308. Academic, New York.

Zbinden, G., Kleinert, R. and Rageth, B. (1980) Assessment of emetine cardiotoxicity in a subacute toxicity experiment in rats. *J. Cardiovasc. Pharmacol.* **2**, 155–164.

The Electrocardiogram (ECG) of the Rat

B. E. OSBORNE

ABSTRACT

A restraining apparatus facilitating recording of the rat ECG was developed and used to obtain baseline ECG data on 200 male and 200 female animals ranging from 1–24 months of age. Such data revealed (a) no obvious sex related differences, (b) increases in age were associated with decreases in heart rate and increases in P–R and Q–T intervals, (c) ECG waveform amplitudes which were extremely variable (probably related to the poor frequency response of the electrocardiograph used), (d) ECG abnormalities (sinus arrhythmia, bradycardia, ectopic beats, partial A–V block, etc.) in two-year-old animals.

Anesthetization of rats with tribromoethyl alcohol produced no obvious ECG changes except bradycardia. When using the rat restraining tube, only minor changes were seen subsequent to 90° alterations in body positions. Pregnancy produced no consistent changes in lead II, except for reduced R wave amplitude, the latter being probably a result of displacement of the heart by the growing fetuses.

The intravenous ED_{50} of epinephrine-induced extrasystoles, increased during pregnancy. The bradycardia and duration of T wave elevation subsequent to an intravenous dose of vasopressin was less in pregnant animals. Such results suggest that, in the rat, pregnancy influences the animal's response to these agents.

It is concluded that ECG recording and evaluation can be successfully performed in the conscious rats and thus assist in cardiovascular studies in this species.

Much of the author's work on the rat ECG was undertaken some five years ago during an investigation into the uses and applications of electrocardiography in toxicology. During the course of this research, the opportunity was taken initially to design apparatus for recording the rat ECG and then to use it to make such recordings on over 400 animals. As a result, a not inconsiderable amount of data on the parameters of the rat ECG was produced. Subsequently, investigations were made into the effects of age, sex and pregnancy on the ECG of this species. For these investigations, a Devices C1 Hot Stylus, single channel recorder whose frequency response was relatively low (40 Hz) was used. This machine dictated that recording of the rat ECG was undertaken using a maximum paper speed of 50 mm/s and a standardization of 2 cm per millivolt. Nowadays, much more sensitive and accurate ECG recorders are available, of course, for obtaining the rat ECG. The main objective of this work was to determine a simple recording technique which could be used repeatedly

15

and easily during the course of toxicity studies in rodents and then, establish ranges of normality for the rat ECG.

Examination of the literature[1–16,18,20,21] revealed that much of the early work on the ECG of the normal rat was performed on animals which were either lightly or completely anaesthetized. In those instances where the animals were conscious, the number of rats used was relatively small (up to 60). In one case, the workers did not standardize their records and such valid comparisons with their findings could not be made.

Similar examination into methods of restraint revealed that several devices have been produced specifically for rats. Many of these facilitate collection of blood specimens or the administration of intravenous injections, etc. To restrain rats for ECG recording, Ensor[5] attached tapes to the four limbs of the animal which itself was then gently stretched, abdomen down, on a cork board and held there by placing pins through the tapes into the board. A two-fingered clamp on the neck prevented the rat from turning its head and nibbling on the electrodes. Hill *et al.*[9] secured rats in a clamp while Hundley *et al.*[10] hand-held the rat in a normal prone position, interference from the handler being prevented by using rubber gloves. Weiss *et al*[21] obtained their recordings with the animal placed supine on a board to which its feet were then tied.

In the first instance, the author considered measurement of the rat ECG lead II using a recording board. This consisted of a wooden block board into which were embedded three nickel-plate electrodes (human size, approximately two inches long and one inch wide). The terminals of these electrodes were connected to the ECG machine. In practice, using a rubber-gloved hand, the rat was placed lightly on a saline-soaked sponge to wet its feet. It was then transferred to the recording board and held in its natural prone position such that its left forelimb and left and right hindlimbs were placed on the relevant ECG electrodes. The heart's changing electrical potentials were thus conducted via the animal's saline-coated feet to the electrocardiograph. This method proved impractical, the animal feeling less and less inclined to stand still as recording time increased. Furthermore, it was found that traces of saline on the rat abdomen could cause short circuiting between the electrodes and thus render ECG recording impossible. Attempting to hold the animal down more firmly usually worsened the situation. Such problems were considered sufficient to render this method of recording impractical.

An alternative apparatus was therefore developed and subsequently described by the author[17]. Illustrated in Figs. 1 and 2, it consists of a perspex tube approximately eight inches long and three inches wide. It is sealed at one end by a removable aluminum nose cone. Along each side of the perspex tube is a wide U-shaped slot. These slots permit accurate placement of the ECG electrodes on the animal's shoulders and thighs. At

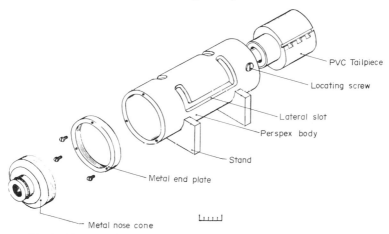

Fig. 1. Diagram of rat-restraining apparatus. (Scale line represents 50 mm)

the opposite end of the tube, a small screw is inserted into the side such that it projects slightly into the inside of the tube. This screw is used in locating the tailpiece. The tailpiece itself is a large plastic stopper which in practice works on the same principle as a bottle cork. It incorporates a quick release mechanism which consists of a series of slots on part of the

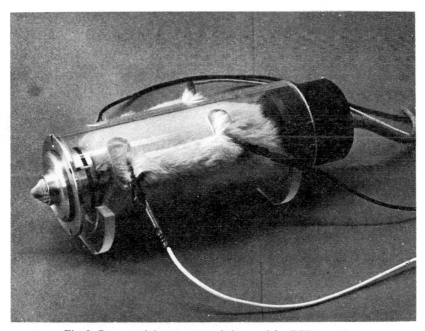

Fig. 2. Rat restraining apparatus being used for ECG recording.

circumference of the tailpiece all of which meet along the longitudinal groove of the same width. By locating the longitudinal groove of the tail-piece opposite the screw projecting into the interior of the perspex tube, the tailpiece can be inserted into the tube for any desired distance.

A 15° clockwise rotation of the tailpiece will then permit the projecting screw in the side of the perspex body to locate in one of the tailpiece slots and thus lock it into position. It can be seen from Fig. 2 that the tailpiece itself has a hollow core. This is not essential for recording the ECG but was included in the design to allow the rat's tail to project from the end of the restraining tube and thus permit intravenous injections into the tail while simultaneously recording its ECG. Two perspex feet enable the apparatus to rest steadily on a flat surface.

In practice, the rat is introduced into the tube until its nose projects from the center of the nosepiece, thus allowing it to breathe freely. Once the rat is positioned in the tube, the tailpiece can be inserted and locked into a position which will produce comfortable restraint of the animal in a pos-ition which allows little forward, backward or lateral movement. Appli-cation of electrode-jelly to the shoulders and thighs via the U-shaped slot on each side of the tube can then be followed by attachment of alligator-clip electrodes, and subsequently, a recording made of the animal's ECG. Reversal of the assembly procedure permits removal of the animal when required. This method is relatively simple, efficient and rapid and permits rat ECG recording by one person. While placement of electrodes on limb extremities is the normal procedure, the alternative siting of the electrodes on the shoulders and thighs is considered clinically sound and, provided that the same method of recording is used on all occasions, satisfactory, and comparable ECG's can be obtained. The ECG is recorded with the rat in a prone or ventral position which, according to Beinfield and Lehr[1], appears to produce definite advantages over the dorsal or supine position.

In order to accommodate body weight increases with age, it was found necessary to design restraining tubes of three different sizes to allow for animals ranging from 100 g to 900 g body weight.

Using such a rat-restraining tube, ECG lead II was recorded on a total of 400 animals namely, 20 male and 20 female Sprague–Dawley rats of either 1, 2, 3, 4, 5, 6, 9, 12, 18 or 24 months of age. ECG measurements (rate, duration and amplitude) were then made on these recordings and the results are presented in Table 1. It can be seen that increasing age produces the expected decrease in heart rate, a mean heart rate of animals of one month of age being 501 beats/min as compared to a mean heart rate of 402 beats/min in two-year-old rats. As a direct result of this lowering of heart rate, increases in the duration of P–R, QRS and Q–T intervals occur. Not surprisingly, such increases are statistically significant ($p < 0.05$). As far as amplitude measurements are concerned, it can be seen there is considerable

TABLE 1. VARIATION OF THE ECG PARAMETERS OF THE RAT WITH AGE

Age group (wk)	Heart rate (beats/min)	Duration (sec)			QTc	Amplitude (mm)*			
		P–R	QRS	Q–T		P†	R†	S†	T†
Males									
1–4	496 ± 126	0.041 ± 0.006	0.017 ± 0.005	0.060 ± 0.010	0.175 ± 0.048	0.455 ± 0.374	1.695 ± 1.284		0.925 ± 0.881
5–8	468 ± 99	0.039 ± 0.007	0.020 ± 0.004	0.064 ± 0.017	0.183 ± 0.048	0.720 ± 0.482	1.365 ± 1.503	0.175 ± 1.409	1.795 ± 2.226
9–12	499 ± 116	0.038 ± 0.008	0.020 ± 0.004	0.064 ± 0.014	0.182 ± 0.059	1.060 ± 0.801	1.820 ± 2.428	0.625 ± 2.489	1.920 ± 2.188
13–16	463 ± 68	0.046 ± 0.011	0.018 ± 0.009	0.064 ± 0.011	0.177 ± 0.030	0.530 ± 0.119	1.840 ± 1.029		1.195 ± 0.553
17–20	448 ± 138	0.042 ± 0.013	0.019 ± 0.006	0.058 ± 0.007	0.164 ± 0.030	0.921 ± 0.733	2.858 ± 1.654		2.274 ± 1.637
21–24	462 ± 52	0.047 ± 0.010	0.019 ± 0.006	0.064 ± 0.010	0.180 ± 0.032	0.715 ± 0.461	2.265 ± 1.071		1.315 ± 0.604
37–40	450 ± 88	0.046 ± 0.011	0.020 ± 0.004	0.066 ± 0.010	0.183 ± 0.032	0.530 ± 0.255	1.970 ± 1.451	0.025 ± 0.234	1.015 ± 0.759
48–52	421 ± 123	0.048 ± 0.013	0.020 ± 0.0	0.071 ± 0.018	0.187 ± 0.034	0.485 ± 0.313	1.670 ± 1.274		1.190 ± 0.698
75–78	438 ± 72	0.050 ± 0.015	0.020 ± 0.0	0.070 ± 0.017	0.188 ± 0.039	0.620 ± 0.356	1.635 ± 1.453	0.050 ± 0.322	1.035 ± 1.057
100–104	403 ± 58	0.061 ± 0.022	0.021 ± 0.007	0.080 ± 0.033	0.202 ± 0.038	0.840 ± 0.569	2.070 ± 1.918	0.325 ± 1.985	1.255 ± 1.185
Mean	455 ± 94	0.046 ± 0.012	0.019 ± 0.006	0.066 ± 0.015	0.182 ± 0.037	0.688 ± 0.446	1.919 ± 1.507	0.240 ± 1.288	1.395 ± 1.091
Females									
1–4	506 ± 126	0.038 ± 0.007	0.015 ± 0.011	0.057 ± 0.010	0.167 ± 0.025	0.505 ± 0.197	1.810 ± 1.257		1.010 ± 0.978
5–8	502 ± 133	0.039 ± 0.006	0.017 ± 0.010	0.064 ± 0.017	0.186 ± 0.030	0.560 ± 0.463	1.590 ± 1.220		1.260 ± 1.144
9–12	530 ± 102	0.033 ± 0.007	0.018 ± 0.010	0.063 ± 0.018	0.184 ± 0.045	1.240 ± 1.187	1.815 ± 2.153	0.455 ± 2.121	2.270 ± 2.503
13–16	478 ± 89	0.044 ± 0.010	0.019 ± 0.006	0.062 ± 0.009	0.175 ± 0.021	0.800 ± 0.479	2.450 ± 1.700		1.770 ± 1.104
17–20	448 ± 140	0.040 ± 0.038	0.019 ± 0.006	0.060 ± 0.012	0.165 ± 0.032	1.147 ± 0.832	3.168 ± 1.918		2.611 ± 1.467
21–24	502 ± 101	0.041 ± 0.007	0.019 ± 0.006	0.060 ± 0.010	0.176 ± 0.030	0.825 ± 0.579	2.900 ± 1.746	0.050 ± 0.467	1.500 ± 0.692
37–40	507 ± 68	0.040 ± 0.004	0.020 ± 0.0	0.065 ± 0.011	0.188 ± 0.026	0.685 ± 0.446	1.705 ± 1.007	0.050 ± 0.467	1.320 ± 1.032
48–52	472 ± 126	0.042 ± 0.009	0.020 ± 0.0	0.066 ± 0.014	0.188 ± 0.036	0.455 ± 0.126	1.245 ± 0.726	0.022 ± 0.216	0.985 ± 0.451
74–78	457 ± 84	0.047 ± 0.012	0.020 ± 0.004	0.071 ± 0.015	0.194 ± 0.033	0.740 ± 0.477	2.030 ± 1.923		1.480 ± 1.695
100–104	401 ± 56	0.054 ± 0.014	0.021 ± 0.006	0.072 ± 0.019	0.196 ± 0.045	0.775 ± 0.902	1.535 ± 2.441	0.390 ± 1.561	1.525 ± 0.876
Mean	450 ± 102	0.042 ± 0.008	0.019 ± 0.012	0.064 ± 0.014	0.182 ± 0.032	0.773 ± 0.569	2.025 ± 1.609	0.193 ± 0.483	1.573 ± 1.194

* A standard of 2 cm/mV was used for recording but for comparison purposes increases corrected to a standard of 1 cm/mV.
† Negative values would be read as zero.
Values given are the means and 95% range for groups of 20 rats.

19

variation between the age groups and it is concluded that there were no obvious or consistent changes in amplitude with increasing age. Although mean values of female heart rates tend to be somewhat higher than males, this difference is not statistically significant.

Rhythm was of sinus origin in all animals examined. Some sinus arrhythmia was seen in the older rats. In ECG's recorded using the aforementioned apparatus, P, R and T waves were commonly seen while Q and S waves were uncommon. When the three standard limb leads were recorded, leads I and II appeared to show the individual waves best, while in the augmented limb leads, aVR generally exhibited the clearer complexes. In the ECG recordings made in this work, there was an obvious lack of an S–T segment—the early part of the T wave appeared to be obliterated due to its partial superimposition upon the termination of the R wave. Repolarization was apparently beginning before depolarization was complete. The resulting high take-off of the T wave accounts for the considerable variation in the amplitude of R and T waves seen in Table 1. Because of the high heart rate, the P wave commonly supervened before the T wave had returned to the isoelectric line, resulting in elevation of this waveform in a similar manner as described for the T wave. Correspondingly, variation in the amplitude of the P wave occurred. However, using the restraining tube in conjunction with more modern and sensitive equipment, much clearer rat ECG's can be obtained, a typical example of which is shown in Fig. 3. In this instance, the ECG waveforms are clearly distinguishable, the improvement in ECG quality being due to the use of a machine with frequency response (100 Hz) and a higher paper speed, both of which were not available to the author in his earlier work. Accordingly, the rat ECG amplitude values in Table 1 can only, if anything, be used as guidelines. With the ECG intervals, such problems were not so apparent since comparison of the author's values with the published values available at the time (Table 2) showed reasonable correlation.

In the records obtained from the 400 rats examined, the incidence of abnormalities was limited to the oldest, i.e. two-year, age group. Increasing age, not surprisingly, produces sinus bradycardia and sinus arrhythmia. Also seen in these older animals were instances of atrial extrasystoles and partial A–V block (generally 2 or 3:1) and Wenckenach phenomenon. Typical examples are shown in Fig. 4. These abnormalities support the findings of Berg[2] who studied the ECG of aging rats.

The foregoing investigations permitted the author to ascertain the effects of sex and age on the rat ECG. Attention was subsequently focussed on the effects of anaesthetic, body position and finally pregnancy upon the ECG of this rodent. It was discovered that use of a typical anaesthetic such as "Avertin"* (which induces third-plane deep anaesthesia within five minutes

* Tribromoethyl alcohol with amylene hydrate, Winthrop Laboratories, Surrey, U.K.

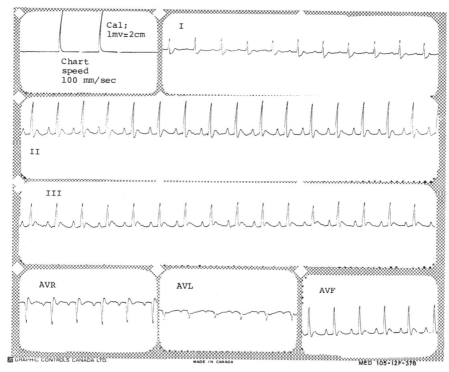

Fig. 3. Typical rat ECG.

in rats) produced the expected reduction in heart rate. The findings are summarized in Table 3 and it can be seen that with the associated slowing of heart rate there was a corresponding lengthening of P–R and Q–T intervals. ECG waveforms and their amplitudes appeared unchanged following administration of this anaesthetic. These findings indicated that use of this anaesthetic produced very few changes on the rat ECG. However, in toxicity studies, the use of anaesthetic agents to aid ECG recording is questionable in view of the potential for synergistic action between the compound being tested and the anaesthetic administered.

One of the contentious areas in interpreting ECG's relates to the position of the animal or its limbs during ECG recording. It has been clearly indicated, for example, in dogs, by Hill[8], that changes in the forelimb position of the animal can produce variations in the ECG waveforms. Such changes would appear to be related in part to heart movement within the thoracic cavity. Determining whether such changes occurred in the ECG of the conscious rat was considered an impractical proposition using the restraining and recording techniques devised by the author. However, investigations were made into ECG changes produced by heart movement

TABLE 2. COMPARISON OF PUBLISHED VALUES OF THE CONSCIOUS AND ANAESTHETIZED RAT ECG WITH FINDINGS IN THE PRESENT STUDY (MEAN VALUES)

Parameter	Hundley et al. (1945)	Hill et al. (1960)	Values derived from Ensor (1946)	Fraser et al. (1967)	Present study
No. of animals	56	50	20	100	400
Age of animals (weeks)	4–19	4–18	4–52	Adult ♂	1–104
Anaesthetic	None	None	None	Ether	None
Recording position	Prone	Supine	Prone	Supine	Prone
Heart rate/min	475–525	380–480	405–540	334	402–502
P–R (sec)	0.035–0.050	0.04–0.06	0.04–0.045	0.065	0.040–0.060
QRS (sec)	0.006–0.013	0.02	0.01–0.015	0.023	0.016–0.021
Q–T (sec)	0.05–0.09	0.08–0.10	—	0.066	0.059–0.075
QTc (sec)	—	—	—	0.153	0.171–0.199
Amplitude					
P	—	—	—	0.072	0.048–0.081
R	—	—	—	0.920	0.175–0.180
S	—	—	—	0.330	0–0.036
T	—	—	—	0.190	0.096–0.141

* No age quoted. Weights quoted as averaging 208 g which is approximately 6 weeks of age.

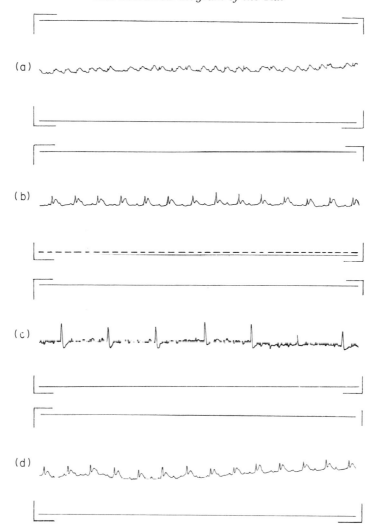

Fig. 4. Examples of abnormalities encountered in normal aging rats: (a) sinus arrhythmia, (b) sinus bradycardia, (c) ectopic beats, (d) partial A-V block.

within the thoracic cavity. This was achieved by placing the rat in the restraining tube and recording its ECG when the tube was placed in positions up to 90° about the normal or reference (horizontal) recording position. When recorded with the rat in a 45° about the reference position, the ECG showed no changes. At 90°, some changes did occur, indicating, not unexpectedly, changes in the heart position within the thoracic cavity. Typical examples are shown in Fig. 5. Such changes appeared to be less

B. E. Osborne

TABLE 3. CHANGES IN THE RAT ECG (LEAD II) FOLLOWING ANESTHETIZATION WITH TRI-BROMOETHYL ALCOHOL FOR APPROXIMATELY 20 MINUTES. MEAN (S.D.) VALUES OF 5 RATS/SEX

Sex	Heart rate/min	P–R	Duration (s) QRS	Q–T	QTc†	Amplitude (mm)* P	R	T
			Conscious					
Male								
Mean	503	0.04	0.02	0.06	0.18	0.7	2.3	1.2
S.D.	37	0.005	—	0.004	0.011	0.210	0.76	0.22
Female								
Mean	526	0.04	0.02	0.06	0.18	0.6	1.8	1.1
S.D.	24	—	—	—	0.004	0.17	0.64	0.23
			Anesthetized					
Male								
Mean	415	0.05	0.02	0.07	0.18	0.7	2.8	1.3
S.D.	33	—	—	0.005	0.012	0.17	0.26	0.28
Female								
Mean	459	0.05	0.02	0.06	0.18	0.5	1.7	0.9
S.D.	20	0.005	—	0.005	0.010	—	0.26	0.08
			Difference following anesthetization					
Male	−88	+0.01	0	0	0	0	+0.5	+0.1
Female	−67	+0.01	0	0	0	−0.1	−0.1	−0.2

* Using a calibration of 1 mV = 20 mm

$$† QT_c = \frac{Q - T(s)}{\sqrt{R - R(s)}} \text{ (Reference 19)}$$

than those seen in similar studies in dogs and primates indicating more restriction of heart movement within the thoracic cavity in the rat.

Finally, changes in the rat ECG which might be induced by the condition of pregnancy were investigated. Recordings were made on groups of 10 rats which were either 7, 14 or 20 days pregnant. In addition, in another study, the ECG of 10 rats was monitored prior to mating and again on day 7, 14 and 20 of pregnancy. Data from such investigations is illustrated in Table 4. Where separate groups of ten animals were examined at different stages during pregnancy, no real changes in heart rate were observed, whereas in a group of ten rats followed through their individual pregnancies, a 17 percent reduction in heart rate was noted. This latter change may be due to the fact that the animals became acclimatized to the recording procedure. Amplitudes of the R wave in particular, in both sets of investigations, decreased as the gestation period increased. This is of course most likely due to the displacement of the heart away from its normal position, by the growing fetuses. Where electrocardiographic monitoring of rats during pregnancy is undertaken, this change should be borne in mind.

As a corollary to determining the effects of pregnancy on the rat ECG, investigations were also made into the epinephrine arrhythmia ED_{50} value in pregnant and non-pregnant rats. The results obtained are illustrated in Table 5. It was found that the epinephrine cardio-arrhythmic ED_{50} tended

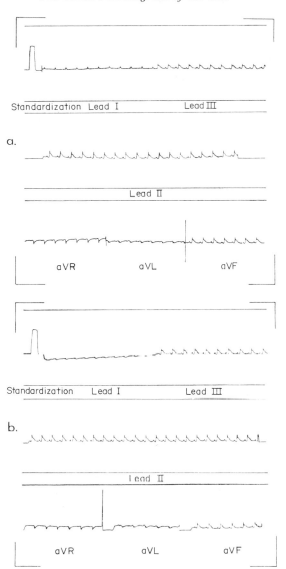

Fig. 5. Changes in the rat ECG induced by changes in body position: (a) reference position, (b) 90° backward.

to increase during the course of pregnancy, while corresponding values for non-pregnant animals showed virtually no changes over a similar period of time. Overall, such ED_{50} values for pregnant rats tended to be higher than those seen in non-pregnant animals. It was inferred that in pregnant animals the increase in ED_{50} was due to a change in the physiological state

TABLE 4. ECG DATA FROM PREGNANT RATS

		Before and during pregnancy							
		(mean values of 10 animals followed through their individual pregnancies)							
	Heart		Duration (sec)				Amplitude (mm*)		
Occasion	rate/min	P–R	QRS	Q–T	QTc	P	R	S	T
Premating	544	0.041	0.021	0.059	0.178	0.45	1.24	0	1.00
Day 7	500	0.042	0.020	0.060	0.174	0.35	1.13	0	0.84
Day 14	503	0.043	0.020	0.061	0.177	0.28	1.18	0	0.79
Day 20	453	0.041	0.020	0.068	0.187	0.17	0.82	0	0.47
		During pregnancy							
		(3 groups of rats each of 20 different animals)							
Day 7	455	0.043	0.021	0.061	0.179	0.63	2.13	0.010	1.09
Day 14	459	0.042	0.020	0.064	0.177	0.58	1.92	0	1.45
Day 20	494	0.042	0.020	0.070	0.202	0.55	1.56	0	1.27

* 1 cm = 1 mV.

and/or the increased body weight of the animal. It has been said that during pregnancy, in man, the heart appears to enlarge, due partly to the change in its position which occurs as the enlarging uterus pushes upwards on the diaphragm. It is not certain whether there is actual pressure on the heart, but cardiac output undoubtedly increases, particularly during the first two-thirds of pregnancy in order to meet the increasing demand for oxygen. It is concluded that during the course of pregnancy in the rat, the cardiac reserve is increased to a level which more than compensates for the increased burden placed upon it by the physiological changes associated with gestation. Such compensation also infers that the threshold effect level of some cardiovascular drugs could be higher in pregnant as compared to non-pregnant animals.

In a similar set of experiments, an investigation was made into the way in which pregnancy influences the cardio-arrhythmic effects of vasopressin. Vasopressin induces typical changes in the rat ECG, i.e. bradycardia and T

TABLE 5. INTRAVENOUS EPINEPHRINE ARRHYTHMIA:* ED_{50} VALUES IN PREGNANT AND NON-PREGNANT RATS

ED_{50} and 95% range	Day 1	Day 7	Day 14	Day 20
Pregnant	7.22	9.21	8.50	9.99
rats	(5.21–10.01)	(6.65–12.76)	(6.15–11.73)	(8.33–11.99)
Non-pregnant	9.21	8.50	9.03	9.03
rats	(6.88–12.34)	(7.88–11.53)	(6.40–12.76)	(5.88–13.88)
Mean ED_{50} and 95% range				
Pregnant rats		9.21 (6.65–12.61)		
Non-pregnant rats		8.50 (6.26–12.77)		

* Arr. = Arrhythmia (as indicated by the presence of ventricular extra-systoles).

TABLE 6. ECG CHANGES IN PREGNANT AND NON-PREGNANT RATS FOLLOWING A SINGLE INTRA-VENOUS DOSE OF VASOPRESSIN (3 U/kg) ON DAY 18 OF PREGNANCY

Rat No.	Weight (g)	Duration of max T wave elev (s)	Heart rate predose	Heart rate-% decrease after injection			
				+1 min	+2 min	+3 min	+5 min
			18 day pregnant rats				
1	400	8.4	532	50	44	44	47
2	340	6.4	532	50	37	33	37
3	390	8.8	556	43	49	41	48
4	340	7.5	357	19	35	31	36
5	380	6.4	500	51	46	46	27
6	400	5.6	556	57	45	36	31
7	395	5.2	578	54	50	45	46
8	380	8.0	441	36	29	33	26
9	391	6.0	429	42	38	27	32
10	410	6.0	500	46	57	47	45
Mean	383	6.8	498	45	43	38	38
			Non-pregnant rats				
1	315	6.8	578	73	73	78	57
2	327	6.4	484	64	66	54	52
3	350	3.4	500	47	50	48	36
4	320	7.6	484	44	46	42	38
5	300	4.4	578	72	73	59	54
6	310	8.8	653	60	58	45	52
8	320	10.0	532	57	40	36	31
9	290	8.4	441	48	55	56	49
10	300	7.6	532	78	68	66	62
Mean	314	7.1	536	59	56	52	41

wave elevation. The values obtained (Table 6) demonstrated that the reduction in heart rate was significantly less ($p < 0.05$) in pregnant rats when compared with non-pregnant animals. While not statistically significant, such reductions were also seen in the duration of the T wave elevation subsequent to administration of vasopressin (3 U/kg). These results together with those obtained in the adrenaline studies indicate that the natural cardiovascular changes associated with pregnancy are more than sufficient to cope with the stresses subsequent to administration of either of these substances.

REFERENCES

1. Beinfield, W. H. and Lehr, D. (1956) Advantages of ventral position in recording the electrocardiogram of the rat. *J. Appl. Physiol.* **9**, 153–156.
2. Berg, B. M. (1955) The electrocardiogram in aging rats. *J. Geront.* **10**, 420–423.
3. Cooper, D. K. C. (1969) Electrocardiographic studies in the rat in physiological and pathological states. *Cardiovasc. Res.* **3**, 419–425.
4. Drury, A. N., Harris, L. J. and Maudsley, C. (1930) Vitamin B deficiency in the rat. *Biochem. J.* **24**, 1632–1649.

5. Ensor, C. R. (1946) The electrocardiogram of rats on vitamin E deficiency. *Am. J. Physiol.* **147**, 477–480.
6. Fraser, R. S., Harley, C. and Wiley, T. (1967) Electrocardiogram in the normal rat. *J. Appl. Physiol.* **23**, 401–402.
7. Heise, E. and Kimbel, K. H. (1955) Das normale Elektrokardiogramm der Ratte. *Z. Kreislaufforsch.* **44**, 212–221.
8. Hill, J. O. (1968) The electrocardiogram in dogs with standardised body and limb positions. *J. Electrocardiol.* **1**, 175–182.
9. Hill, R., Howard, A. N. and Gresham, G. A. (1960) The electrocardiographic appearance of myocardial infarction in the rat. *J. exp. Path.* **41**, 633–637.
10. Hundley, J. M., Ashburn, L. L. and Sebrell, W. H. (1945) The electrocardiogram in chronic thiamine deficiency in rats. *Am. J. Physiol.* **114**, 404–414.
11. Irmak, S. and Aykut, R. (1955) Vergleichende Electrokardiographische Untersuchungen beim Menschen und bei den Laboratoriumstieren. *Münch. med. Wsch.* **97**, 460–461.
12. Jones, D. C., Osborn, G. K. and Kimeldorf, D. J. (1968) Cardiac arrhythmia in the ageing male rat. *Gerontologia*, **13**, 211–218.
13. Kirch, B. (1953) The heart rate and the electrocardiogram of small animals. *Exp. Med. Surg.* **11**, 117–130.
14. Lambard, E. C. (1952) Electrocardiograms of small mammals. *Am. J. Physiol.* **171**, 189–193.
15. Lepeschkin, E. and Wilson, F. N. (1951). *Modern Electrocardiography*, Vol. 1, Bailliere, Tindall and Cox Limited, London.
16. Normann, S. J., Priest, R. F. and Benditt, E. P. (1961) Electrocardiogram in the normal rat and its alteration with experimental coronary occlusion. *Circulation Res.* **9**, 282–287.
17. Osborne, B. E. (1973) A restraining device facilitating electrocardiogram recording in rats. *Lab. Anim.* **7**, 185–188.
18. Sambhi, M. P. and White, F. N. (1960) The electrocardiogram of the normal and hypertensive rat. *Circulation Res.* **8**, 129–134.
19. Taran, L. M. and Szilagyi, N. (1947) The duration of the electrical systole (Q–T) in acute rheumatic carditis in children. *Am. Heart J.* **33**, 14–24.
20. Waller, R. K. and Charipper, H. A. (1945) Electrocardiographic observations in normal thyroidectomized and thiourea-treated rats. *Am. J. med. Sci.* **210**, 443–452.
21. Weiss, S., Haynes, F. W. and Zoll, P. M. (1938) Electrocardiographic manifestations and the cardiac effect of drugs in vitamin B deficiency in rats. *Am. Heart J.* **15**, 206–220.

Relationship between the Scaler Electrocardiogram and Cellular Electrophysiology of the Rat Heart

J. F. SPEAR

ABSTRACT

Experiments were performed on anesthetized, open-chest rats to correlate ventricular depolarization and repolarization with the QRST complex of the scaler electrocardiogram. Bipolar electrograms from the surface of the *in situ* heart were recorded simultaneously with the electrocardiogram. Also, transmembrane potentials were recorded from the ventricular endocardium of excised hearts superfused in a tissue bath. The electrophysiologic properties of the rat heart were contrasted with those of the dog. The atrioventricular node and specialized ventricular conduction system of the rat transmitted the cardiac impulse from atrium to ventricle more rapidly than in the dog heart and the effective refractory period of the atrioventricular node was briefer than in the dog. The epicardial activation sequence of right and left ventricles for both of these species was comparable. However, the total activation time of the ventricle in the rat was about one-third that of the dog. This is accounted for by the smaller heart of the rat and results in a briefer QRS duration. In the adult rat, the T wave follows upon the QRS without an isolectric segment. This is due to the brief duration and lack of a plateau phase of the rat ventricular myocardial action potential. In addition, it was observed that during the initial portion of the T wave there were areas of the ventricles that were simultaneously in depolarization and repolarization phases. Because of the characteristic action potential configuration of the rat heart in which rapid repolarization follows on the depolarization phase, areas of the ventricle that are activated early must be repolarizing during the inscription of the QRS complex. Because of these overlaps there is no clear point on the electrocardiogram that can be used to indicate the end of depolarization and the beginning of repolarization.

The rat electrocardiogram exhibits several unique features which are shared by several other animals such as the kangaroo and bat, but which distinguish it from that of most mammalian species. Two distinguishing characteristics are its brief QT interval and lack of an isoelectric ST segment (Fraser *et al.*, 1967; Beinfield and Lehr, 1968). There is relatively little information available concerning the relationship between the cellular electrophysiology and the scaler electrocardiogram in the rat. Since the rat is a species used in pharmacological and toxicological studies, an understanding of this relationship is important for the electrocardiographic interpretation of the effects of interventions on rat cardiac physiology. In the present paper, I will consider several electrophysiologic features which characterize

29

ventricular depolarization and repolarization in the rat heart and how these determine the peculiar QRST complex of the rat electrocardiogram.

METHODS

The observations were made on Sprague–Dawley laboratory rats weighing approximately 300 grams and anesthetized with sodium pentobarbital (30 mg/kg i.p.). Ventilation was maintained through an endotracheal tube by a positive pressure respirator. The chests were opened by a mid-sternal incision and the hearts exposed by resecting the pericardium. A lead II electrocardiogram was monitored and Teflon-coated stainless steel bipolar electrodes with diameters of 0.2 mm and interelectrode spacing of 1.0 mm were used to record from and stimulate the heart. The frequency response of the amplifiers was from 0.1 to 1000 Hz. All signals were displayed on an oscilloscope and recorded on an instrumentation tape recorder and ink-writing oscillograph with a frequency response from 0 to 2000 Hz. Electrical stimulation was provided by a constant current stimulator delivering a square wave pulse 2 msec in duration with a variable intensity up to 10 mA. The pacing intensity was between 0.4 and 1.0 mA.

In vitro studies were carried out on ventricular tissues superfused with oxygenated Tyrode's solution in a temperature-controlled tissue bath. Transmembrane potentials were recorded using standard 3 M KCl-filled micropipettes. Details of our techniques have been published previously (Horowitz *et al.*, 1976; Moore *et al.*, 1978).

RESULTS

In the following discussions data from the dog heart will also be presented in order to contrast the electrophysiological properties of the rat heart with those of a typical mammal. In the rat, as in other mammalian species, the cardiac impulse reaches the ventricular myocardium after transversing the specialized ventricular conducting system. The impulse upon leaving the atrium engages sequentially the atrioventricular node, the bundle of His, the left and right bundle branches and terminal Purkinje system. The pattern of ventricular muscle activation is determined by the distribution of the terminal Purkinje network.

Atrioventricular Conduction

In Fig. 1 are data which contrast in the dog and rat the characteristics of conduction and refractoriness in the specialized conduction system. These

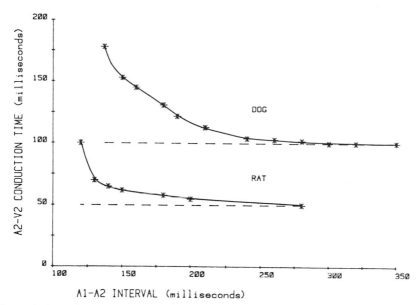

Fig. 1. Atrioventricular refractory curves for dog and rat heart. The abscissa is the coupling interval between the last basic atrial response (A1) and premature atrial responses (A2). The ordinate is the conduction time between atrium and ventricle (A2–V2) for the premature atrial responses. The sinus node was crushed in the rat heart in order to pace the heart at a slower rate.

data were generated in the following way. Recording bipolar electrodes were applied to the right atrium and right ventricular epicardium. A stimulating electrode was also applied to the right atrium. The dog heart was paced at a basic cycle length of 350 msec and the rat at a basic cycle length of 280 msec. The hearts were paced in this manner for 12 basic beats. Following the last basic beat (A1) a premature atrial test pulse was inserted (A2). The conduction time between the atrial recording site and the ventricular recording site (A2–V2) was measured for successive test beats of increasing prematurity. The data were then plotted in Fig. 1 relating the A2–V2 conduction time to the degree of prematurity of the test atrial responses (A1–A2).

In Fig. 1 at the basic cycle length the conduction time between atrium and ventricle for the dog heart was 100 msec. As the atrial beat was introduced more prematurely, the atrioventricular conduction time increased until the effective refractory period was reached at an A1–A2 interval of 137 msec. Beats of shorter A1–A2 interval blocked within the AV node. The atrioventricular conduction time for the rat at the pacing basic cycle length was 50 msec and the effective refractory period 120 msec. The briefer conduction time and shorter refractory period for the rat atrioventricular

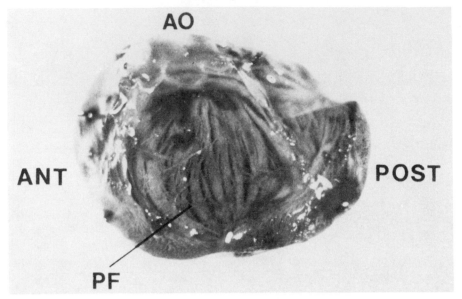

Fig. 2. A view of the left endocardial septal surface of the rat ventricle. The line indicates free-running Purkinje fibers which were stained with 5% iodine solution (PF). The aortic root is indicated by AO.

conduction system accounts for the shorter PR interval and the ability of the rat heart to conduct impulses from atrium to ventricle at the faster heart rate characteristic of this species.

Ventricular Transmembrane Potentials

Differences between the rat heart and most other mammalian species with regard to the QRST complex are primarily due to the characteristics of the ventricular transmembrane potential. To demonstrate these differences, transmembrane potentials were recorded from the endocardia of rat and dog left ventricles. Figure 2 shows a septal endocardial view of the left ventricle of a rat, opened by an incision extending from base to apex through the free wall. The line indicates fine free-running Purkinje fibers originating from the left bundle branch and distributing over the anterior papillary muscle (PF). Recordings were made from both Purkinje fibers and underlying ventricular muscle cells in this area. Table 1 presents transmembrane potential characteristics for both Purkinje fibers and ventricular muscle cells recorded in rat and dog ventricles. The parameters presented in Table 1 are the resting potential, the action potential amplitude and the degree to which the action potential overshoots the zero reference poten-

TABLE 1. TRANSMEMBRANE POTENTIAL CHARACTERISTICS

	Resting potential (mV)	Action potential amplitude (mV)	Overshoot (mV)	Action potential duration at 50% repolarization (msec)
		PURKINJE		
Dog (n = 10)	96.1 ± 3.3	129.5 ± 8.6	33.5 ± 10.1	285.1 ± 46.2
Rat (n = 6)	75.8 ± 2.7	115.2 ± 7.7	39.3 ± 6.1	34.3 ± 4.7
		MUSCLE		
Dog (n = 24)	82.4 ± 5.9	99.3 ± 6.5	16.9 ± 4.9	145.9 ± 48.1
Rat (n = 7)	83.0 ± 8.0	112.0 ± 6.8	29.0 ± 3.9	25.6 ± 2.4

tial. The duration of the action potential measured from the upstroke to the repolarization phase at one-half of the total amplitude of the action potential is also included. Fifty percent repolarization was chosen since this occurs at a time during the rapid repolarization phase (phase 3) of cardiac muscle. It is the asynchronous repolarization of various parts of the ventricles during this rapid phase which generates the major portion of the T wave of the electrocardiogram. It can be seen in Table 1 that the duration of the action potential was greater for Purkinje fibers than ventricular muscle cells. This was true for both the dog and rat ventricle. However, both Purkinje fibers and muscle cell action potentials were considerably shorter in duration for the rat as compared to the dog. Since it is the duration of ventricular muscle action potential which determines the relationship between the QRS complex and T wave, this difference is reflected by the surface electrocardiograms.

Figure 3 presents a schematic demonstrating the relationship between transmembrane potentials in the dog ventricle and the surface electrocardiogram. The two vertical dashed lines align the peak of the T wave and the end of the T wave with the transmembrane potentials recorded from a Purkinje fiber and ventricular muscle. As represented in the schematic the bundle branch-Purkinje system is activated prior to the initiation of the Q wave of the electrocardiogram. Purkinje activation does not contribute to potential changes recorded on the surface of the body using routine electrocardiography. There have been some suggestions, however, that repolarization of the Purkinje system may contribute to the U wave recorded in the electrocardiogram (Hoffman and Cranefield 1960; Watanabe and deAzevedo, 1973). The relationship between ventricular muscle repolarization and the T wave for the dog heart can also be seen in Fig. 3. During the plateau phase of the ventricular action potential transmembrane volt-

J. F. Spear

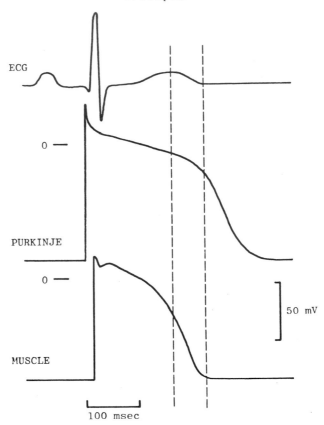

Fig. 3. A schematic demonstrating the relationship between transmembrane potentials recorded from a Purkinje fiber and ventricular muscle cell and the surface electrocardiogram in the dog. The vertical dashed lines indicate the peak and terminations of the T wave. The 0 potential is indicated by the horizontal line for both of the transmembrane potentials.

ages are changing very slowly. Since it takes approximately 40 msec for total ventricular activation, all parts of the ventricle are depolarized during most of the plateau. Therefore extracellular current flow is minimal. Thus there is an isoelectric ST segment in the electrocardiogram. The peak of the T wave of the electrocardiogram corresponds to the phase of rapid repolarization of ventricular muscle and the end of the T wave is coincident with full repolarization.

Figure 4 presents a similar schematic demonstrating the relationship between ventricular transmembrane potentials and the electrocardiogram in the rat. Again the vertical lines indicate the peak of the T wave and the end of the T wave. The Purkinje system in the rat exhibits a plateau phase; however, it is considerably shorter in duration than dog Purkinje fiber

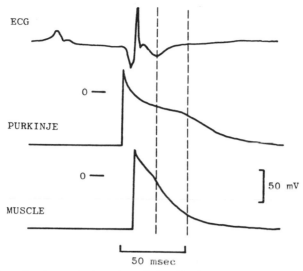

Fig. 4. A schematic demonstrating the relationship between transmembrane potentials recorded from a Purkinje fiber and ventricular muscle cell and the surface electrocardiogram in the rat. The arrangement of this figure is similar to that of Fig. 3.

potentials. The lack of an isoelectric ST segment in the rat is also apparent from this figure. Rat ventricular muscle does not exhibit a prominent plateau phase during repolarization and its total duration is considerably shorter than that of the dog ventricle. Thus, a rapid phase of membrane repolarization follows on depolarization. Therefore, areas activated early must be repolarizing during the QRS complex and the T wave follows immediately on the QRS complex without an isoelectric ST segment.

Ventricular Activation

Epicardial mapping was carried out in the rat heart to determine the sequence and duration of ventricular activation. In Fig. 5 are analog records demonstrating this technique. A surface electrocardiogram is displayed on the top record. Two simultaneously recorded bipolar electrograms are displayed below the electrocardiogram. In the mapping procedure a fixed reference electrode is applied to the surface of the heart. This is necessary since manipulation of the heart during the procedure distorts the electrocardiogram. This electrogram is indicated in the figure as REF. A roving, hand-held bipolar electrode is then applied to the epicardium at multiple sites on both the right and left ventricles. One such electrogram is indicated in the figure by ROV. The dashed vertical lines indicate the activation times for the reference and the selected roving site relative to the

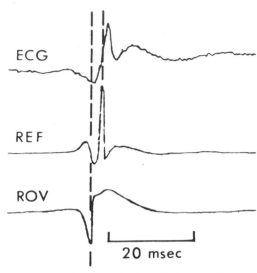

Fig. 5. Analog records demonstrating the scaler lead II electrocardiogram and simultaneously recorded electrograms in the rat. ECG is the lead II electrocardiogram, REF is a reference electrogram recorded from the right ventricle and ROV is an electrogram recorded with a hand-held roving probe. The vertical dashed lines indicate the timing of the intrinsic deflections for the two electrograms. In these studies, activation times were measured from the largest peak of a primarily monophasic complex or the fastest base line crossing of a biphasic complex. The end of local repolarization was measured at the time at which the T wave of the local electrograms had returned to baseline. In these experiments the configuration of the electrocardiogram was somewhat distorted due to it being recorded from an open-chest anesthetized animal.

simultaneously recorded electrocardiogram. The activation times between the roving and reference electrograms are determined for each of the roving epicardial recording sites. After multiple sites have been recorded, the epicardial map is generated by referencing all activation times to the earliest epicardial activation and displaying them relative to the electrocardiogram.

Figure 6 presents a typical epicardial activation map generated from a dog ventricle. The schematic above presents anterior and posterior views of the ventricles of the dog. The numbers indicate the times in msec at which each of the epicardial sites were activated relative to the earliest site of activation indicated by the darkened area. Extrapolated isochronic lines were drawn to connect sites with similar activation times. The lines indicate 5 msec increments. This figure demonstrates for the dog that the earliest sites of epicardial activation occurred simultaneously on the right ventricular anterior free wall and left ventricular apex. Activity proceeded from apex to base. The latest sites activated were on the base of the posterior left ventricle and right ventricular outflow tracts at 29 and 25 msec respectively. This characteristic epicardial activation is due to the

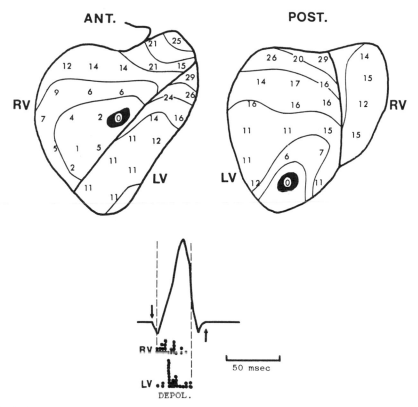

Fig. 6. An epicardial isochronic activation map recorded in the dog ventricle during normal sinus rhythm. The spontaneous basic cycle length was 380 msec. The isochronic lines in the schematic above indicate 5 msec increments. Below, the times of activation for the right ventricular and left ventricular sites are indicated relative to the surface QRS complex. The left arrow indicates the beginning of the Q wave, the right arrow indicates the termination of the S wave.

distribution of right and left bundle branch-Purkinje systems in the dog which terminate at the apical portions of the ventricles. At the bottom of Fig. 6 the relative activation times for the right and left ventricular sites are displayed and time-aligned with the QRS complex of the electrocardiogram. The arrows indicate the beginning of the Q wave and the termination of the S wave in the electrocardiogram. The dashed lines indicate the time of occurrence of earliest epicardial breakthrough and the time of activation of the latest epicardial site. It can be seen that right ventricular and left ventricular epicardial activation encompasses most of the QRS complex except for the initial portion of the Q wave and the terminal portion of the R wave and the S wave. The portions of the QRS complex not accounted for by epicardial activation are due to septal activation. In

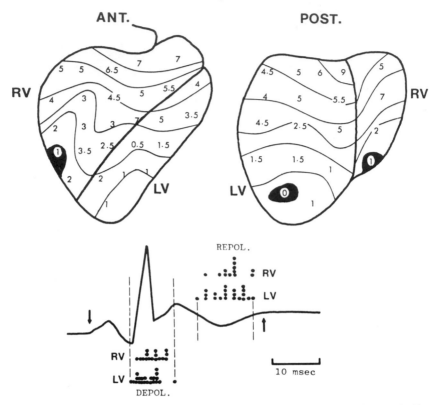

Fig. 7. An epicardial activation map measured in the rat ventricle. The isochronic lines indicate 1 msec increments. Below, the times of right and left ventricular depolarization and end of repolarization are plotted relative to the QRST complex of the rat electrocardiogram. The left arrow indicates the beginning of the Q wave, the right arrow indicates the termination of the T wave. The spontaneous sinus cycle length was 190 msec.

the dog repolarization occurs at approximately 150 msec after the ventricles have been activated and this is not shown in the figure.

The epicardial activation map of a rat ventricle is presented in Fig. 7. The isochronic lines in this map are drawn in 1 msec increments. The earliest epicardial activation sites and the general sequence of depolarization of the rat ventricle was similar to that of the dog. Earliest left ventricular activation occurred at the apex and right ventricular activation occurred on the right ventricular free wall, but more laterally than was seen in the dog (Fig. 6). Total epicardial activation was more rapid in the rat. The base of the left ventricle and the outflow tract of the right ventricle were last to be activated at 9 and 7 msec respectively. This activation sequence suggests that the distribution of the left and right bundle branch system and terminal Purkinje fibers are functionally similar for both rat and dog. The shorter total epicardial activation time in the rat can probably be entirely accounted for by the relative heart size. The size of the rat heart is considerably less than that of the dog, being approximately 1.5 cm from base to apex for the rat and 8 cm from base to apex for the dog. Both rat and dog ventricular muscle conduct with approximately the same velocity of 0.9–1.0 M/sec (Spear and Moore, 1972; Hoffman and Cranefield, 1960).

Below the epicardial maps in Fig. 7 are displayed the rat QRST complex with the times of epicardial depolarization and repolarization aligned to the electrocardiographic waveform. The left arrow indicates the beginning of the Q wave, the right arrow indicates the end of the T wave. The left pair of vertical dashed lines indicate the times of earliest and latest epicardial activations. There are several important observations that can be made from this figure. Right and left ventricular depolarization occurred during the major portion of the R wave. However, the epicardium of the rat was still being activated at a time when the T wave was being inscribed. The end of repolarization for the recording sites are shown above and to the right of the electrocardiographic waveform and indicate that epicardial repolarization was terminating during the latter part of the T wave. The interval between the beginning of the Q wave indicated by the left arrow and initial epicardial breakthrough was presumably associated with ventricular septal activation. If we assume that the duration of activity for septal activation, that is, the interval from depolarization to the end of repolarization, is similar to that of the epicardium, then septal repolarization must have been occurring during the R wave and the initial portion of the T wave. Thus, septal repolarization occurred at a time when the epicardium was being activated. Therefore, the QRST waves of the rat electrocardiogram represent components of both depolarization and repolarization.

DISCUSSION

The cellular electrophysiology of the rat heart determines its characteristic electrocardiographic configuration. The atrioventricular node and specialized ventricular conduction system of the rat transmits the cardiac impulse from atrium to ventricle in approximately 50 msec. In addition, the effective refractory period of the AV node is briefer than in the dog heart. This allows for atrioventricular conduction at the faster spontaneous heart rate of the rat. The functional distribution of the bundle branch-Purkinje system to the ventricles is similar in the rat and dog. Therefore, the overall activation sequence of right and left ventricle for both these species is comparable. However, the total activation time of the ventricle in the rat is about one-third that of the dog. This is accounted for by the smaller heart of the rat and results in a briefer QRS duration. In the rat, the T wave follows upon the QRS without an isoelectric ST segment. This is due to the brief duration and lack of a prominent plateau phase of the rat ventricular myocardial action potential.

Figure 7 demonstrates that during the initial portions of the T wave there are different areas of the rat heart that are simultaneously in depolarization and repolarization phases. In addition, Fig. 4 demonstrates that because of the action potential configuration repolarization of ventricular areas activated early must be occurring during the inscription of the QRS complex. These findings have implications for the use of the rat scaler electrocardiogram to evaluate electrophysiologic characteristics of the heart in response to interventions. Because of this overlap there is no clear point on the electrocardiogram that can be used to indicate the end of depolarization or the beginning of repolarization. This means that it is difficult to distinguish from the electrocardiogram whether changes in the configuration of the QRST waves are due to an effect on the activation process or recovery process of ventricular muscle.

REFERENCES

Beinfield, W. H. and Lehr, D. (1968) QRS–T variations in the rat electrocardiogram. *Am. J. Physiol.* **214,** 197–204.

Fraser, R. S., Harley, C. and Wiley, T. (1967) Electrocardiogram in the normal rat. *J. Appl. Physiol.* **23,** 401–402.

Hoffman, B. F. and Cranefield, P. F. (1960) *Electrophysiology of the Heart.* Futura Publishing Company, Inc., Mt. Kisco, NY.

Horowitz, L. N., Spear, J. F. and Moore, E. N. (1976) Subendocardial origin of ventricular arrhythmias in 24-hour-old experimental myocardial infarction. *Circulation* **53,** 56–63.

Moore, E. N., Spear, J. F., Horowitz, L. N., Feldman, H. S. and Moller, R. A. (1978) Electrophysiologic properties of a new antiarrhythmic drug—Tocainide. *Am. J. Cardiol.* **41,** 703–709.

Spear, J. F. and Moore, E. N. (1972) Stretch-induced excitation and conduction disturbances in the isolated rat myocardium. *J. Electrocardiol.* **5,** 15–24.

Watanabe, Y. and deAzevedo. (1973) Electrocardiographic correlation of bundle branch block and the U wave. *J. Electrocardiol.* **6**(3), 215–220.

The Rat ECG in Acute Pharmacology and Toxicology

R. BUDDEN, G. BUSCHMANN and U. G. KÜHL

ABSTRACT

The effects of selected drugs on ECG and blood pressure in anesthetized rats (1.25 g urethane/kg i.p.) were tested using identical experimental conditions. The drugs were infused continuously into the femoral vein of male Wistar rats prepared for ECG (lead heart axis) and blood pressure (carotid artery) recordings. The ECG and blood pressure signals were evaluated by on-line biosignal processing (Schumacher et al., 1980). The drug infusion was increased logarithmically at 10, 20, and 30 min after the start of the lowest infusion rate. As a rule, toxic signs were seen at the highest infusion rate. According to their mode of action the drugs tested were divided into three groups: Drugs affecting the central nervous system (narcotics, diazepam, chlorpromazine, imipramine, metoclopramide), drugs affecting the autonomic nervous system (carbachol, atropine, adrenaline, noradrenaline, dopamine, dobutamine, propranolol, metoprolol, talinolol), cardiovascular drugs (N-propyl-ajmaline bitartrate, lidocaine, propafenon, sparteine, verapamil, aconitine, clonidine, hydralazine, adenosine, hydrochlorothiazide).

From the presented results the following conclusions were drawn:

1. The rat ECG is a suitable tool in the characterization of pharmacodynamic or toxic cardiac actions of drugs.
2. Computer evaluation is a rapid means for the correct measurement of rat ECG parameters in routine experiments.
3. There is a sufficient correlation of electrocardiographic drug effects between rat and man.
4. The incorporation of the ECG in acute rat experiments may augment the usability of this species.

1. INTRODUCTION

The electrocardiogram (ECG) has proved to be an indispensable tool toward the characterization of the cardiac actions of compounds. In practice it cannot be replaced by other methods, although the ECG is not sufficient to give a complete picture of cardiac function.

Until now the dog has been the preferred species in the pharmacological or toxicological investigation of cardiovascular drug actions. As far as the ECG is concerned, there are obvious similarities between dog and man. The rat ECG, however, differs considerably from the two other species,

41

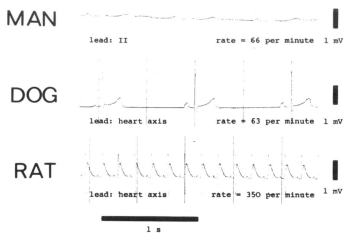

Fig. 1. Species differences in ECG configuration.

particularly in heart rate and configuration (Fig. 1). On the other hand, the use of rats in pharmacological and toxicological experiments undoubtedly has advantages over the dog: rats are well standardized, easily handled, and available in large numbers. But the shortage of published data on drug effects on the rat ECG warrants further investigation in order to establish background data for the transferability of rat ECG results to man.

Owing to the time and technical facilities required and to the "anomalous" configuration of the rat ECG, which differs from that of other laboratory animals and man, especially as the repolarization phase is concerned (Heise and Kimbel, 1955; Grauwiler and Spörri, 1960; Sambhi and White, 1960; Lepeschkin, 1965; Beinfield and Lehr, 1968b) a continuous evaluation of electrocardiograms in rats is rarely performed. Moreover, it is difficult to draw an interlaboratory comparison of rat ECG data, because of the differences in the experimental procedure. So the comments of Beinfield and Lehr (1968a) are still true: "Many of the differences appear to be due to the type of recording technique employed which includes such variables as: the presence or absence of anesthesia, the type of anesthetic agent, the recording position of the animal, the use of mechanical restraining devices, the gain and frequency response of the amplifier, the frequency response and paper speed of the recorder, and the manner in which time duration measurements are made and the leads selected for this purpose. The age, weight, sex, and strain of each animal are also factors contributing to variations which should be considered in the evaluation of any given rat electrocardiogram."

As the subject of this paper, "the rat ECG in acute pharmacology and toxicology", is very extensive, we will restrict ourselves to the discussion of selected methodological problems, results from our laboratory and some published data. In this context the term "acute" defines the single administration of an agent; it does not delimit the duration of the observation period. In a few cases, we will include published results of experiments with repeated administrations for comparison with those from acute tests.

2. OWN METHODS

In our experiments we tested drugs of different clinical indications under identical conditions. Male Wistar rats (Han:Wistar) weighing 300–360 g and aged about 15–20 weeks were anesthetized with 1.25 g urethane/kg intraperitoneally, fixed in the supine position and prepared for ECG and blood pressure recordings as described by Buschmann *et al.* (1980). The ECG was taken by a bipolar lead in the direction of the heart axis (lead A) as advised by Spörri (1944) with the P wave recorded as a positive deflection. The experimental protocol is shown on the following scheme:

Experimental Protocol

	Time [min]		
	−40	← urethane 1.25 g/kg i.p.	(∼15 min)
	−25	← preparation	(∼10 min)
	−15	← equilibration period	(∼10 min)
	−5	← predrug period	(5 min)
no effects	0	← start of drug infusion	(10 min)
	+10	← x-fold initial infusion rate	(10 min)
	+20	← x²-fold initial infusion rate	(10 min)
	+30	← x³-fold initial infusion rate	(max. 20 min)
toxic effects	+50	← end of experiment	

After an equilibration period of at least 10 min, predrug values were taken during a 5-min period immediately before the start of the drug infusion. The drugs were administered by continuous intravenous infusion into the femoral vein. The infusion rate was increased x-fold every 10 min, as a rule starting with no effect and ending with toxic rates, without changing the infusion volume (0.1 ml/min). All data were evaluated by continuous on-line biosignal processing. Details on the technical and biometrical procedure are given by Schumacher *et al.* (see p. 171). Figure 2 shows the ECG parameters measured in our experiments: PR interval, QRS interval, RαT interval (beginning at the onset of QRS, ending at the apex of T), SαT segment (beginning at the minimum of S, ending at the apex of T), and αTP segment. The heart rate was calculated from the RR interval. An isoelectric ST segment is not present in the adult rat.

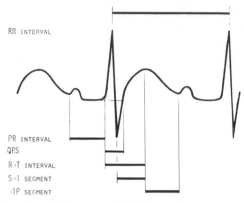

Fig. 2. Routinely-evaluated ECG intervals and segments.

In order to distinguish between drug-induced modifications of the ECG intervals or segments and those depending upon heart rate changes, the relation of these parameters to heart rate was studied in experiments with hypothermia-induced heart rate variations. In these experiments the lowest heart rate was 197 and the highest 441 beats/min, corresponding to RR intervals of 305 to 136 ms.

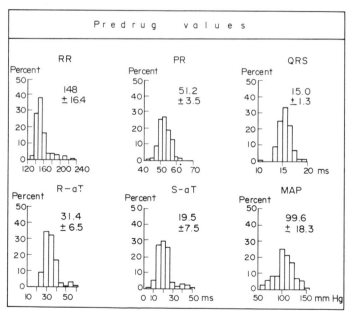

Fig. 3. Predrug values of the measured ECG intervals and segments and of mean arterial blood pressure (MAP), and their frequency distribution (percent) in 132 male Wistar rats anesthetized with 1/25 urethane/kg. Numbers are arithmetic means ± standard deviation.

TABLE 1. EFFECTS OF AN INTRAVENOUS INFUSION OF 0.9% SALINE ON HEART RATE, ECG PARAMETERS AND ON MEAN ARTERIAL BLOOD PRESSURE (MAP) IN ANESTHETIZED MALE WISTAR RATS (1.25 URETHANE/kg INTRAPERITONEALLY)

Experimental time (min)	Cumulated dose (ml)	n	Heart rate (min^{-1})	PR interval (ms)	PR_c interval (ms)	QRS (ms)	RαT interval (ms)	MAP* (mm Hg)
0	0	6	429 ± 28	50 ± 2.5	50 ± 2.9	13 ± 2.6	28 ± 2.4	92 ± 23
8.5	0.85	6	444 ± 20	49 ± 2.5	50 ± 2.7	13 ± 1.2	31 ± 4.1	101 ± 26
17	1.7	6	439 ± 29	50 ± 3.3	50 ± 2.3	13 ± 2.1	28 ± 4.7	96 ± 28
25	2.5	6	437 ± 30	49 ± 3.3	49 ± 3.0	13 ± 1.6	28 ± 2.5	90 ± 25
35	3.5	6	446 ± 36	48 ± 3.6	49 ± 1.9	13 ± 1.2	28 ± 2.1	88 ± 17
50	5.0	5	448 ± 45	48 ± 3.8	48 ± 1.7	13 ± 0.8	28 ± 1.8	83 ± 18

Infusion rate was 0.1 ml min^{-1} throughout the experiment; ECG lead: heart axis (Spörri, 1944).
Means ± SD.
* MAP: Mean arterial pressure: (mm Hg) × 0.1333 = (kPa).

As a close correlation was found between RR and PR intervals, and particularly between RR intervals and αTP segments (Buschmann et al., 1980), PR intervals corrected for intraindividual heart rate changes (PR$_c$) were also considered in the assessment of a drug action (PR$_c$ = PR$_i$ + (RR$_o$ − RR$_i$) × 0.2; cf. Schumacher et al., p. 177). No correction was applied to the αTP segment, since it corresponds to a large extent to the electrical diastole.

Since the prolongation of PR observed in these experiments probably is not only related to the hypothermia-induced bradycardia, but also caused by a direct effect of cooling on the AV conduction, the regression coefficient of 0.2 in the formula may be too high. Therefore—as will be shown later on the basis of some of our own results—this formula tends to an "overcorrection" of the PR interval towards too short PR$_c$ values.

Figure 3 presents the frequency distribution and the mean values of the measured ECG parameters from the predrug periods of our experiments. The longest QRS duration, taken from 132 animals anesthetized by urethane, was 19 ms. So, QRS durations above 20 ms are considered to be abnormal values under our experimental conditions. The parameters did not change considerably during the experimental period, when *isotonic saline* was infused in a control experiment at the rate used for drug infusion in our experiments (0.1 ml/min) (Table 1).

3. DRUGS AFFECTING THE CENTRAL NERVOUS SYSTEM

3.1. Narcotics

Until now, conflicting views exist about the usefulness of anesthesia and the most suitable one in the measurement of ECG parameters in rats. Commonly, barbiturates, urethane, and ether are employed.

Some authors have collected data from rats anesthetized with their preferred anesthesia.

Barbiturates. Mean values of ECG parameters in *thiobarbiturate* anesthetized rats, as measured by Heise and Kimbel (1955) are given in Table 2.

TABLE 2. HEART RATE AND ECG PARAMETERS IN RATS ANESTHETIZED WITH 75 mg/kg NA-METHYL-THIOETHYL-2'-PENTYL-THIOBARBITURIC ACID (THIOGENAL®) AS REPORTED BY HEISE AND KIMBEL (1955). NO DATA ABOUT STRAIN, SEX, WEIGHT, AGE OR THE EXACT ECG LEAD ARE AVAILABLE

	Heart rate (min^{-1})	PQ segment (ms)	QRS (ms)	QT (ms)	P (ms)	R (ms)	S (ms)	T (ms)
Mean	346	33	26	84	17	12	6.3	58
SD	29	3.7	2.2	10.2	2.5	1.4	1.2	10.8
n	122	122	114	122	122	122	122	122

The authors found a rather high mean QRS duration of 26 ms, and a mean heart rate of 346 beats/min. As no information about strain, sex, weight, age, or the exact lead is available, the difference between these values and ours cannot be interpreted as an effect of the different anesthesias.

Ether anesthesia, especially the "light ether anesthesia" is a frequently-used technique in ECG recording. Gessler and Kuner (1959) found a wide correspondence between values obtained from rats in light ether anesthesia and the values obtained by Heise and Kimbel (1955) in thiobarbiturate anesthesia. But if ether anesthesia is badly operated, especially with increasing depth of anesthesia, a marked bradycardia or rhythm disorders have not infrequently been observed, as well as a widening of the T wave and an increase of the T amplitude (Gessler and Kuner, 1959; Werth and Dadgar, 1965; Werth and Wink, 1967). With light ether anesthesia, alterations in amplitude, shape, polarity and duration of the P wave commonly due to shifting of the location of the pacemaker were observed by Beinfield and Lehr (1968b) and attributed to oscillations in the autonomic tone of the heart. Because of the instabilities in the ECG, and as it is very difficult with ether to produce the same degree of anesthesia in different animals as well as to maintain a constant level in one animal, we do not recommend ether anesthesia in the measurement of ECG parameters in acute, non-recovery experiments in rats.

Pentobarbital. In our experiment with *pentobarbital* anesthesia, the ECG parameters remained unchanged during the first 50 to 60 min (Table 3). After 140 min, Driscoll (1979) found a significant increase in PR and a slight, insignificant increase in heart rate (Table 4). In females receiving 40 mg/kg pentobarbital intraperitoneally the same effect was found as in males receiving the double amount, reflecting the well-known sex differences in barbiturate sensitivity (Holk *et al.*, 1937).

Urethane. Comparing the electrocardiograms of conscious with those of anesthetized rats, Heering (1970a) found that *urethane* anesthesia produced

TABLE 3. EFFECTS OF ANESTHESIA WITH PENTOBARBITAL SODIUM (50 mg/kg INTRAPERITONEALLY) ON HEART RATE AND ECG PARAMETERS IN MALE WISTAR RATS

Experimental time (min)	n	Heart rate (min^{-1})	PR interval (ms)	PR_c interval (ms)	QRS (ms)	RαT interval (ms)
0	4	397 ± 42	49 ± 2.0	49 ± 2.0	15 ± 1.4	25 ± 6.4
11	4	403 ± 38	48 ± 1.7	50 ± 3.6	15 ± 1.4	25 ± 6.1
20	4	413 ± 37	48 ± 1.8	50 ± 4.0	14 ± 1.7	24 ± 3.8
30	4	418 ± 29	48 ± 2.7	50 ± 4.1	14 ± 0.9	25 ± 6.0
41	4	421 ± 33	47 ± 1.8	50 ± 3.7	16 ± 2.1	26 ± 6.3
50	4	423 ± 37	47 ± 2.1	49 ± 4.0	14 ± 0.5	26 ± 6.2

ECG lead: heart axis (Spörri, 1944).
Means ± SD.

TABLE 4. HEART RATE AND PR INTERVAL IN MALE AND FEMALE RATS OF THE ROMAN HIGH-AVOIDANCE (RHA) STRAIN. MALES (380 ± 15 g) WERE ANESTHETIZED WITH 80 mg PENTOBARBITAL/kg INTRAPERITONEALLY, FEMALES (229 ± 10 g) WITH 40 mg PENTOBARBITAL INTRAPERITONEALLY (DRISCOLL, 1979)

	Dose (mg/kg i.p.)	Time after injection (min)	Heart rate (1/min)	PR interval (ms)
RHA males	80	20	279 ± 22	53.6
		40	250 ± 16	54.0
		60	258 ± 14	54.3
		100	278 ± 24	56.0
		140	309 ± 15	59.0*
RHA females	40	20	341 ± 26	48.4
		40	326 ± 25	51.2
		60	336 ± 21	54.0
		100	343 ± 15	54.4
		140	357 ± 12	54.7*

* Significantly different to 20 min value.

a fall in heart rate and an increase in PR, QT, and PT intervals (Table 5). The QRS duration remained nearly unchanged. In our experiments, an intraperitoneal dose of 1.25 g urethane/kg was sufficient to produce a stable anesthesia for more than 50 minutes (cf. Table 1). As urethane is long acting and devoid of prominent reflex inhibiting effects (Barnes and Eltherington, 1973), we prefer urethane instead of barbiturates in acute non-recovery experiments.

Ethanol, a drug known to intensify a preexisting anesthesia, did not significantly affect the ECG time measurements and heart rate in our experiments up to the cumulated dose of 2.1 g/kg i.v. (Table 6). After acute peroral administration of ethanol to conscious rats, Hillbom and von Boguslawsky (1978) found an increase in heart rate without changes in PR, QRS and QT (Table 7).

3.2. Tranquilizers

Diazepam, which is the most widely used minor tranquilizer, is a nearly water insoluble compound. In our experiments we tested the commercially

TABLE 5. EFFECTS OF ANESTHESIA (1,4 g URETHANE/kg) ON HEART RATE AND ECG INTERVALS IN FEMALE ALBINO RATS (160–250 g); LEAD II (HEERING, 1970)

Group	n	Heart rate (min^{-1})	PR interval (ms)	QRS (ms)	QT interval (ms)
Untreated, awake	50	472 ± 13.3	41 ± 4.1	21 ± 3.6	58 ± 9.1
Urethane 1.4 g/kg i.p.	25	314 ± 17.5	50 ± 7.0	18 ± 2.7	78 ± 20.0

TABLE 6. EFFECTS OF AN INTRAVENOUS INFUSION OF ETHANOL ON HEART RATE, ECG PARAMETERS AND ON MEAN ARTERIAL BLOOD PRESSURE (MAP) IN ANESTHETIZED MALE WISTAR RATS (1.25 URETHANE/kg INTRAPERITONEALLY)

Experimental time (min)	Cumulated dose (mg kg^{-1})	n	Heart rate (min^{-1})	PR interval (ms)	PR$_c$ interval (ms)	QRS (ms)	RαT interval (ms)	MAP* (mm Hg)
0	0	4	387 ± 16	51 ± 5.1	51 ± 5.1	14 ± 1.2	29 ± 3.5	104 ± 4
10	1	4	387 ± 17	51 ± 5.1	50 ± 4.9	14 ± 1.2	31 ± 7.1	108 ± 7
20	11	4	387 ± 23	51 ± 4.3	49 ± 4.2	14 ± 1.2	31 ± 4.3	113 ± 8
30	111	4	387 ± 23	53 ± 5.1	51 ± 4.9	14 ± 0.9	29 ± 3.3	107 ± 4
40	1111	4	389 ± 25	53 ± 4.5	51 ± 4.5	14 ± 1.5	27 ± 0.9	111 ± 4
50	2111	4	388 ± 29	53 ± 5.0	52 ± 5.4	14 ± 1.1	28 ± 3.1	112 ± 8

Infusion rates were 0.1; 1.0; 10.0; 100.0 mg kg^{-1} min^{-1}; they were increased at 10, 20, and 30 min after the start of the lowest infusion rate. ECG lead: heart axis (Spörri, 1944). Cumul. lethal dose: >2.1 g kg^{-1}.

Means ± SD.

* MAP: Mean arterial pressure: (mm Hg) × 0.1333 = (kPa).

TABLE 7. EFFECTS OF ETHANOL (2.7 g/kg PERORALLY) ON HEART
RATE AND ECG INTERVALS IN CONSCIOUS, ALCOHOL-AVOIDING
MALE RATS; LEAD II (HILLBOM AND VAN BOGUSLAWSKY, 1978)

Time (min)	Heart rate (min^{-1})	PR interval (ms)	QRS (ms)	QT (ms)
0	360 ± 29	56 ± 4	16 ± 2	95 ± 11
10	442 ± 44	53 ± 4	15 ± 2	79 ± 13
20	428 ± 50	54 ± 5	15 ± 2	83 ± 14
40	403 ± 38	56 ± 4	16 ± 2	88 ± 15
70	359 ± 48	58 ± 6	16 ± 3	96 ± 13

Mean ± S.D.

available ampoules (Valium® Amp.); in parallel the diazepam solvent was taken in order to differentiate between drug and solvent effects (Table 8a,b).

Whereas diazepam induced a dose-dependent increase in blood pressure with the three lower infusion rates, no pressure changes were seen with the solvent except for a small and transient hypotension after about 10 min infusion. Comparing the bradycardiac action of both diazepam and the solvent, the former seems to be slightly more potent, whereas there is obviously no appreciable effect of diazepam itself on the PR interval. On the other hand, high doses of diazepam caused a significant prolongation of the RαT interval as well as a slight increase in the QRS duration, suggesting some delay in ventricular de- and repolarization.

As a whole, our findings are consistent with the low incidence of cardiac side effects reported for therapeutic use of diazepam in man (Greenblatt and Koch-Weser, 1973; Greenblatt and Shader, 1974; Pateisky and Wessely, 1975; Stimmel, 1975, 1979). The increase in mean blood pressure observed in our experiments, however, is somewhat surprising, since the pressure effect associated with parenteral diazepam is reported to be a hypo- rather than a hypertension in man (Greenblatt and Koch-Weser, 1973; Greenblatt and Shader, 1974; Stimmel, 1975, 1979) and in both normo- and hypertensive rats (Bolme and Fuxe, 1977; van Zwieten, 1977).

Chlorpromazine, the prototype of the major tranquilizers of the phenothiazine group, had a prominent hypotensive and a weaker negative chronotropic action in our experiments with adult rats (Table 9). Staib (1967) demonstrated a distinct age dependence of the chronotropic chlorpromazine effects: an increase in heart rate in young rats which is also seen in humans (Moccetti et al., 1971), and a fall in heart rate in adult rats. In our experiments the PR interval increased at high doses, but after correcting the values for heart rate changes no slowing of AV conduction was left because of the marked bradycardia present at these dosages. At toxic dosages the QRS complex was slightly prolonged.

With continuous chlorpromazine infusion in pentobarbital-anesthetized rats, Langslet (1970a) found a similar decrease in heart rate and a some-

TABLE 8a. EFFECTS OF AN INTRAVENOUS INFUSION OF DIAZEPAM (VALIUM® AMP.) (mol. wt. 285) ON HEART RATE, ECG PARAMETERS AND ON MEAN ARTERIAL BLOOD PRESSURE (MAP) IN ANESTHETIZED MALE WISTAR RATS (1.25 URETHANE/kg INTRAPERITONEALLY)

Experimental time (min)	Cumulated dose (μmol kg^{-1})	n	Heart rate (min^{-1})	PR interval (ms)	PR$_c$ interval (ms)	QRS (ms)	RαT interval (ms)	MAP* (mm Hg)
0	0	4	414 ± 20	53 ± 4.9	53 ± 4.9	15 ± 1.0	29 ± 1.5	108 ± 17
10	0.1	4	412 ± 26	53 ± 4.9	53 ± 4.9	15 ± 0.8	35 ± 11.2	118 ± 20**
20	1.1	4	410 ± 26	53 ± 5.4	53 ± 5.3	15 ± 0.5	31 ± 4.5	134 ± 8**
30	11.1	4	389 ± 32**	58 ± 6.3	55 ± 6.6	15 ± 0.5	34 ± 4.0	141 ± 8
40	111	4	344 ± 51**	55 ± 6.8	49 ± 9.8	16 ± 0.5	40 ± 2.8†	104 ± 10
50	211	4	328 ± 45**	57 ± 6.0**	49 ± 7.3	17 ± 0.8	48 ± 4.7†	109 ± 14

Infusion rates were 0.01; 0.1; 1.0; 10.0 μmol kg^{-1} min^{-1}; they were increased at 10, 20, and 30 min after the start of the lowest infusion rate. ECG lead: heart axis (Spörri, 1944). Cumul. lethal dose: >211 μmol kg^{-1}.

Means ± SD.

* MAP: Mean arterial pressure: (mm Hg) × 0.1333 = (kPa)

**, † p < 0.05 and p < 0.01 to predrug value (Student's paired t-test).

TABLE 8b. EFFECTS OF AN INTRAVENOUS INFUSION OF SOLVENT FOR DIAZEPAM (VALIUM® AMP.) ON HEART RATE, ECG PARAMETERS AND ON MEAN ARTERIAL BLOOD PRESSURE (MAP) IN ANESTHETIZED MALE WISTAR RATS (1.25 URETHANE/kg INTRAPERITONEALLY)

Experimental time (min)	Diazepam‡ (µmol/kg)	n	Heart rate (min⁻¹)	PR interval (ms)	PR$_c$ interval (ms)	QRS (ms)	RαT interval (ms)	MAP* (mm Hg)
0	0	4	427 ± 8	55 ± 3.1	55 ± 3.1	14 ± 0.5	26 ± 0.9	119 ± 2
10	0,1	4	415 ± 8	55 ± 3.4	55 ± 3.9	13 ± 0.5	26 ± 1.1	106 ± 9**
20	1.1	4	421 ± 16	56 ± 4.3	56 ± 3.8	14 ± 0.8	25 ± 0.5	119 ± 13
30	11.1	4	414 ± 16	57 ± 4.0	57 ± 3.6	14 ± 0.0	26 ± 1.0	124 ± 9
40	111	4	394 ± 27**	58 ± 5.0	56 ± 4.4	13 ± 0.5	26 ± 0.9	114 ± 12
50	211	4	382 ± 29**	59 ± 5.0**	56 ± 4.2	13 ± 0.5	27 ± 0.8	118 ± 12

Infusion rate was 0.1 µmol/min throughout the experiment; they were increased at 10, 20, and 30 min after the start of the lowest infusion rate. ECG lead: heart axis (Spörri, 1944). Cumul. lethal dose: > 5 ml/kg.
Means.
* MAP: Mean arterial pressure (mm Hg) × 0.1333 = (kPa).
**, † $p < 0.05$ and $p < 0.01$ to predrug value (Student's t-test for paired observations).
‡ Corresponding cumulated dose of diazepam (Table 8a).

TABLE 9. EFFECTS OF AN INTRAVENOUS INFUSION OF CHLORPROMAZINE (mol. wt. 355) ON HEART RATE, ECG PARAMETERS AND ON MEAN ARTERIAL BLOOD PRESSURE (MAP) IN ANESTHETIZED MALE WISTAR RATS (1.25 URETHANE/kg INTRAPERITONEALLY)

Experimental time (min)	Cumulated dose (μmol kg^{-1})	n	Heart rate (min^{-1})	PR interval (ms)	PR$_c$ interval (ms)	QRS (ms)	RαT interval (ms)	MAP* (mm Hg)
0	0	4	409 ± 34	52 ± 5.5	52 ± 5.5	15 ± 1.5	31 ± 6.3	104 ± 10
9	0.09	4	407 ± 35	52 ± 6.4	52 ± 6.4	14 ± 1.5	26 ± 6.6	85 ± 9**
13	0.4	4	403 ± 34	52 ± 5.4	52 ± 5.5	15 ± 1.5	30 ± 1.2	68 ± 11***
23.5	4.6	4	359 ± 39	52 ± 3.7	48 ± 9.1	15 ± 1.8	34 ± 8.0	53 ± 18†
35	61.1	4	205 ± 40†	57 ± 2.9	29 ± 2.5**[a]	17 ± 2.9	34 ± 7.5	49 ± 11**
42	131	4	224 ± 15†	71 ± 21.2	45 ± 19.1	22 ± 8.0	44 ± 7.8	46 ± 31†

Infusion rates were 0.01; 0.1; 1.0; 10.0 μmol kg^{-1} min^{-1}; they were increased at 10, 20, and 30 min after the start of the lowest infusion rate. ECG lead: heart axis (Spörri, 1944). Cumul. lethal dose: 190 ± 19 μmol kg^{-1}.

Means ± SD.

* MAP: Mean arterial pressure: (mm Hg) × 0.1333 = (kPa).

[a] n = 3.

,†,* $p < 0.05$, $p < 0.01$ and $p < 0.001$ to predrug value (Student's paired t-test).

TABLE 10. EFFECTS OF A CONTINUOUS INTRA-
VENOUS INFUSION (CONSTANT RATE) OF CHLOR-
PROMAZINE ON HEART RATE AND PR INTERVAL
IN MALE WISTAR RATS (500 g) ANESTHETIZED
WITH PENTOBARBITAL (20 mg/kg INTRAPERI-
TONEALLY) (AFTER LANGSLET, 1970a)

Dose (μmol/kg)	Heart rate (%)	PR interval (%)
1	100	100
10	100	106
25	90	123
40	63	133
60	33	157
80	24	168

Mean values.

what greater increase in the PR interval with varying degrees of AV block at high doses (Table 10). The delay in AV conduction and the negative chronotropism, which is obviously characteristic of the adult rat after acute chlorpromazine administration, has also been demonstrated on isolated rat hearts *in vitro* (Langslet, 1970b; Langslet and Ryg, 1971; Aronson and Serlick, 1977), (Table 11).

In contrast to the results of acute rat experiments, Zbinden *et al.* (1977a) observed an increase in heart rate in relation to the controls and a con-comitant diminution of the PR interval after repeated oral administration of chlorpromazine. A slight widening of the QRS complex of borderline significance became evident in the 17th week. From these results it cannot be decided whether the prolongation of QRS in the acute and chronic experiments is based on the same pathomechanism or not.

Electrocardiographic changes, at times quite impressive, are also known to occur in man on phenothiazines, the degree of abnormality being dose-related. The most frequent alterations are repolarization abnormalities re-sembling those produced by quinidine, including flattening of T waves and prolongation of QT intervals (Moccetti *et al.*, 1971; Stimmel, 1975, 1979). An increase of QT in rats, too has been documented after chlorpromazine administration *in vivo* (Langslet, 1970a) and *in vitro* (Langslet, 1970b; Aronson and Serlick, 1977). Flattened T waves and prolonged RαT inter-vals were also observed in our experiments, the latter results confirming *in vitro* findings (QαT) of Aronson and Serlick (1977) (Table 11).

3.3. Antidepressants

In clinical use, tricyclic antidepressants often produce tachycardia and alterations in blood pressure, the degree varying among others with the

TABLE 11. EFFECTS OF A PERFUSION WITH 5 mg/l CHLORPROMAZINE ON HEART RATE AND ECG INTERVALS IN ISOLATED PERFUSED RAT HEARTS (KREBS-RINGER BICARBONATE SOLUTION, 2.54 mmol CALCIUM, 37°C) (Aronson and Serlick, 1977)

Group	n	Perfusion time* (min)	Heart rate (1/min)	PR interval (ms)	QTa interval (ms)	QT interval (ms)
Control	7	0	291 ± 8.6	42 ± 1.2	19 ± 1.6	73 ± 3.3
		15	279 ± 10.8	41 ± 0.9	20 ± 1.3	72 ± 2.0
		30	274 ± 4.3	42 ± 1.1	20 ± 1.1	73 ± 2.1
		45	261 ± 13.8	43 ± 1.4	19 ± 1.2	74 ± 2.6
		60	261 ± 13.8	41 ± 0.8	19 ± 1.0	74 ± 2.2
Chlorpromazine (5 mg/l)	9	0	280 ± 14.1	40 ± 0.8	16 ± 0.6	70 ± 1.3
		15	257 ± 13.1	53 ± 3.7**	21 ± 1.6	106 ± 5.3**
		30	240 ± 17.3**	65 ± 6.1**	25 ± 3.6	127 ± 5.8**
		45	223 ± 21.9**	78 ± 5.3**	30 ± 6.5**	150 ± 6.5**
		60	190 ± 21.2**	87 ± 5.3**	51 ± 12.8**	165 ± 12.6**

Drug concentrations of 0.05 and 0.5 mg/l had no effect on the ECG mean ± S.E.M.
* Duration of perfusion after initial 15 min equilibration period.
**$p < 0.05$ (paired variate t-test).

TABLE 12. EFFECTS OF AN INTRAVENOUS INFUSION OF IMIPRAMINE (mol. wt. 317) ON HEART RATE, ECG PARAMETERS AND ON MEAN ARTERIAL BLOOD PRESSURE (MAP) IN ANESTHETIZED MALE WISTAR RATS (1.25 URETHANE/kg INTRAPERITONEALLY)

Experimental time (min)	Cumulated dose (μmol kg^{-1})	n	Heart rate (min^{-1})	PR interval (ms)	PR$_c$ interval (ms)	QRS (ms)	RαT interval (ms)	MAP* (mm Hg)
0	0	4	410 ± 52	50 ± 1.7	50 ± 1.7	14 ± 1.2	31 ± 4.0	97 ± 11
9	0.9	4	435 ± 36	51 ± 2.1	53 ± 3.7	15 ± 0.5	38 ± 10.1	98 ± 12
13	2.4	4	441 ± 33	50 ± 2.0	53 ± 3.6	16 ± 1.3	31 ± 8.8	88 ± 6
23.5	13.2	3	418 ± 20	55 ± 4.0	58 ± 5.8	17 ± 0.5	41 ± 12.7	64 ± 4**
30	27.1	3	381 ± 14	57 ± 3.0**	57 ± 5.8	19 ± 1.5**	48 ± 14.7	63 ± 2†
31.5	42.1	4	363 ± 6	59 ± 2.4***	55 ± 6.1	22 ± 3.8	50 ± 9.5	60 ± 4**

Infusion rates were 0.1; 0.464; 2.15; 10.0 μmol kg^{-1} min^{-1}; they were increased at 10, 20, and 30 min after the start of the lowest infusion rate. ECG lead: heart axis (Spörri, 1944). Cumul. lethal dose: 116 ± 20 μmol kg^{-1}.
Means ± SD.
* MAP: Mean arterial pressure (mm Hg) × 0.1333 = (kPa).
,†,* p < 0.05 and p < 0.01 to predrug value (Student's paired t-test).

specific tricyclic and the presence of preexisting cardiac disease. Signs of cardiotoxicity are not uncommon, and sudden deaths have been reported. According to Stimmel (1979) "asymptomatic electrocardiographic changes consisting of prolongation of the QT interval, widening of QRS complexes, and ST- and T-wave changes, are similar to those seen with the phenothiazines and have been noted in up to 20% of persons". T wave changes at therapeutic serum levels, and prolonged PR, QRS, and QT intervals may occur (Moccetti *et al.*, 1971; Moccetti, 1973; Stimmel, 1975, 1979). Even in patients without known cardiac disease, these changes may be followed by conduction disturbances or arrhythmias of clinical importance.

Imipramine. In our rat experiments the tricyclic antidepressant drug *imipramine* induced a slight increase in heart rate at low dosages and a decrease in blood pressure at higher dosages (Table 12). The first toxic sign was a significant decrease in blood pressure at a cumulated dose of 13.2 μmol/kg. At higher doses PR, PR_c, QRS, and RαT were prolonged with the heart rate only slightly decreased. These findings are in good agreement with the results of Lisciani *et al.* (1978), who found a dose-dependent prolongation of PR and a fall in mean blood pressure during continuous imipramine infusion (5 mg/kg/min) in male and female rats. Prolonged PR and QRS intervals have also been observed in rats after repeated (3 days) and particularly after chronic (8–15 weeks) oral imipramine administration with the heart rates unaffected in both experiments (Zbinden *et al.*, 1977a, 1977b).

Amitriptyline, another tricyclic antidepressant with cardiotoxic potency in man, has similar effects on blood pressure and ECG parameters in the rat as imipramine. With acute intravenous administration to pentobarbital-anesthetized rats, Thorstrand (1975) and Thorstrand *et al.* (1976) found a significant prolongation of PR and QRS, and a decrease in heart rate and blood pressure (Table 13). Nemec (1973) was able to demonstrate these cardiac changes only with intravenous amitriptyline infusions in rats anesthetized with pentobarbital. After a single i.v. injection to urethane-anes-

TABLE 13. EFFECTS OF INTRAVENOUS AMITRIPTYLINE ON HEART RATE, PR INTERVAL, QRS DURATION AND MEAN ARTERIAL BLOOD PRESSURE (MAP) IN FEMALE SPRAGUE–DAWLEY RATS (200 g) ANESTHETIZED WITH SODIUM PENTOBARBITAL (n = 10, MAP = 8 ANIMALS) (THORSTRAND *et al.*, 1976)

	Dose (mg/kg i.v.)	Heart rate (min^{-1})	PR-interval (ms)	QRS (ms)	MAP (mm Hg)
Basal values	—	333 ± 26	50 ± 4.3	18 ± 1.8	111 ± 13
Amitriptyline	0.5	310 ± 43	54 ± 4.6	20 ± 1.5	90 ± 16
Amitriptyline	+0.5 =1.0	259 ± 34	56 ± 5.5	22 ± 1.6	74 ± 16

Mean values ± SD.

TABLE 14. EFFECTS OF AN INTRAVENOUS INFUSION OF METOCLOPRAMIDE (mol. wt. 336) ON HEART RATE, ECG PARAMETERS AND ON MEAN ARTERIAL BLOOD PRESSURE (MAP) IN ANESTHETIZED MALE WISTAR RATS (1.25 URETHANE/kg INTRAPERITONEALLY)

Experimental time (min)	Cumulated dose (μmol kg⁻¹)	n	Heart rate (min⁻¹)	PR interval (ms)	PRc interval (ms)	QRS (ms)	RαT interval (ms)	MAP* (mm Hg)
0	0	4	409 ± 22	53 ± 1.4	53 ± 1.4	15 ± 0.5	39 ± 4.7	97 ± 10
4.5	1.42	4	408 ± 16	55 ± 1.2	55 ± 1.4	16 ± 3.1	37 ± 6.5	104 ± 17
9.0	2.84	3	407 ± 19	55 ± 3.5	55 ± 2.7	15 ± 0.5	34 ± 12.5	93 ± 10
19.5	12.7	4	373 ± 30†	58 ± 3.9	55 ± 4.9	16 ± 0.5	42 ± 4.4	87 ± 16
23.5	24.2	4	353 ± 37†	63 ± 4.5**	58 ± 5.9	18 ± 0.9**	40 ± 7.0	81 ± 16
32.0	64.8	4	319 ± 53**	66 ± 6.2	57 ± 9.7	22 ± 5.0	52 ± 9.6	68 ± 19**
49.0	235	3	248 ± 29†	82 ± 1.5**	63 ± 2.8**	31 ± 2.0†	52 ± 7.2	51 ± 17**

Infusion rates were 0.316; 1.0; 3.16; 10.0 μmol kg⁻¹ min⁻¹; they were increased at 10, 20, and 30 min after the start of the lowest infusion rate. ECG lead: heart axis (Spörri, 1944). Cumul. lethal dose: >245 μmol kg⁻¹.
Means.
* MAP: Mean arterial pressure (mm Hg) × 0.1333 = (kPa).
**,† $p < 0.05$ and $p < 0.01$ to predrug value (Student's t-test for paired observations).

thetized rats, amitriptyline prolonged AV conduction as well as the QRS duration, but also increased the heart rate, suggesting some influence of the anesthetic and/or the speed of injection. In chronic experiments Zbinden *et al.* (1977a) observed a prolongation of PR and QRS, too.

3.4. Metoclopramide

Metoclopramide is a drug which not only stimulates the gastrointestinal motility by a direct peripheral action, but which also has strong antiemetic properties. Moreover, metoclopramide has proved to be a central dopamine antagonist (Neeb and Grabner, 1978; Ålander *et al.*, 1980). With the lowest infusion rate of 0.316 μmol/kg/min, the drug was without appreciable effects on ECG and blood pressure. Beginning at a cumulated dose of 12.7 μmol/kg, metoclopramide induced dose-dependent reductions in heart rate and blood pressure and likewise dose-related prolongations of PR, PR_c, QRS, and RαT (Table 14). These results confirm the findings of Marmo and coworkers (1969a, 1969b, 1970) in anesthetized rats, guinea-pigs and cats.

The findings in our rat experiments are in agreement with the absence of blood pressure and heart rate changes with therapeutic dosages in man after single intravenous injections (10–20 mg $\approx$ 0.43–0.85 μmol/kg) (Agabiti–Rosci *et al.*, 1977) as well as after long-term treatment with doses up to 20 mg/day (Neeb and Grabner, 1978).

The rather quinidine-like ECG effect of metoclopramide at higher doses is indeed accompanied by a definite antiarrhythmic activity of the agent, as demonstrated by Ramos *et al.* (1967) and Marmo *et al.* (1970).

4. DRUGS AFFECTING THE AUTONOMIC NERVOUS SYSTEM

4.1. Parasympathetic Nervous System

Carbachol. In agreement with theoretical expectations, the directly-acting parasympathomimetic drug *carbachol* produced a marked decrease in heart rate and blood pressure, whereas PR, QRS, and RαT remained unaffected (Table 15). As the pronounced bradycardia is not accompanied by a prolongation of PR, the correction of PR for heart rate changes gave erroneously shortened PR_c values. After a cumulated dose of 0.28 μmol/kg, AV block of varying degree was found in all animals.

Atropine, the best-known antimuscarinic agent, did not change ECG and blood pressure parameters at therapeutic dosages (0.5–1 mg/kg = 0.7–1.4 μmol/kg) in the anesthetized rat (Table 16). In particular we did not find tachycardia. This result fits the findings reported by Valora *et al.* (1963), but it does not agree with the observation of Heering (1970b), who found

TABLE 15. EFFECTS OF AN INTRAVENOUS INFUSION OF CARBACHOL (mol. wt. 182.7) ON HEART RATE, ECG PARAMETERS AND ON MEAN ARTERIAL BLOOD PRESSURE (MAP) IN ANESTHETIZED MALE WISTAR RATS (1.25 URETHANE/kg INTRAPERITONEALLY)

Experimental time (min)	Cumulated dose (μmol kg^{-1})	n	Heart rate (min^{-1})	PR interval (ms)	PR$_c$ interval (ms)	QRS (ms)	RαT interval (ms)	MAP* (mm Hg)
0	0	4	388 ± 25	54 ± 3.1	54 ± 3.1	15 ± 1.2	27 ± 2.4	83 ± 17
9.5	0.0095	4	398 ± 28	53 ± 2.2	54 ± 3.5	15 ± 1.7	28 ± 2.5	95 ± 10
14.5	0.055	4	315 ± 42**	56 ± 3.3	49 ± 6.8	15 ± 0.9	26 ± 1.6	63 ± 6**
19.5	0.105	4	298 ± 46**	56 ± 4.4	46 ± 2.4**	15 ± 0.9	26 ± 0.9	72 ± 14
21	0.21	4	270 ± 46**	57 ± 3.5	42 ± 8.8**	15 ± 1.2	25 ± 2.2	61 ± 12†
31	2.1	3	144 ± 20†	48 ± 10.5	—	19 ± 5.8	39 ± 6.0	60 ± 9

Infusion rates were 0.001; 0.01; 0.1; 1.0 μmol kg^{-1} min^{-1}; they were increased at 10, 20, and 30 min after the start of the lowest infusion rate. ECG lead: heart axis (Spörri, 1944). Cumul. lethal dose: 7.4 ± 0.5 μmol kg^{-1}. Means.

* MAP: Mean arterial pressure (mm Hg) × 0.133 = (kPa).

**,† $p < 0.05$ and $p < 0.01$ to predrug value (Student's t-test for paired observations).

TABLE 16. EFFECTS OF AN INTRAVENOUS INFUSION OF ATROPINE SULFATE (mol. wt. 695) ON HEART RATE, ECG PARAMETERS AND ON MEAN ARTERIAL BLOOD PRESSURE (MAP) IN ANESTHETIZED MALE WISTAR RATS (1.25 URETHANE/kg INTRAPERITONEALLY)

Experimental time (min)	Cumulated dose (μmol kg^{-1})	n	Heart rate (min^{-1})	PR interval (ms)	PR$_c$ interval (ms)	QRS (ms)	RαT interval (ms)	MAP* (mm Hg)
0	0	4	425 ± 14	55 ± 2.1	53 ± 2.1	15 ± 0.9	28 ± 6.6	103 ± 23
9.5	0.0204	4	438 ± 4	51 ± 0.0	52 ± 1.1	15 ± 1.0	29 ± 5.1	108 ± 16
19.5	0.462	4	429 ± 11	51 ± 1.7	52 ± 2.0	15 ± 1.2	27 ± 5.0	93 ± 20
29.5	10.0	4	406 ± 13	55 ± 1.2**	54 ± 2.3†	16 ± 1.7	27 ± 5.1	64 ± 10**
34	96.5	4	330 ± 22†	75 ± 3.3†	67 ± 0.9†	25 ± 2.2†	42 ± 2.4**	64 ± 13**
37.5	172	4	260 ± 16†	91 ± 4.9†	73 ± 4.8†	30 ± 1.0†	48 ± 3.8†	66 ± 16**

Infusion rates were 0.00215; 0.0464; 1.0; 21.5 μmol kg^{-1} min^{-1}; they were increased at 10, 20, and 30 min after the start of the lowest infusion rate. ECG lead: heart axis (Spörri, 1944). Cumul. lethal dose: 412 ± 74 μmol kg^{-1}.

Means.

* MAP: Mean arterial pressure (mm Hg) × 0.1333 = (kPa).

**,† p < 0.05 and p < 0.01 to predrug value (Student's t-test for paired observations).

TABLE 17. EFFECTS OF AN INTRAVENOUS INFUSION OF ADRENALINE (mol. wt. 219.7) ON HEART RATE, ECG PARAMETERS AND ON MEAN ARTERIAL BLOOD PRESSURE (MAP) IN ANESTHETIZED MALE WISTAR RATS (1.25 URETHANE/kg INTRAPERITONEALLY)

Experimental time (min)	Cumulated dose (μmol kg⁻¹)	n	Heart rate (min⁻¹)	PR interval (ms)	PRc interval (ms)	QRS (ms)	RzT interval (ms)	MAP* (mm Hg)
0	0	5	401 ± 39	52 ± 3.0	52 ± 3.0	14 ± 1.1	29 ± 2.5	92 ± 12
1	0.001	5	413 ± 53	50 ± 2.1	52 ± 3.2	14 ± 1.5	30 ± 3.8	82 ± 22
9.5	0.0095	5	433 ± 44**	50 ± 1.3	53 ± 1.7	14 ± 1.5	30 ± 1.8	90 ± 23
19.5	0.105	5	469 ± 35**	49 ± 2.4	55 ± 2.6	14 ± 2.0	29 ± 4.3	132 ± 7†
28.0	0.91	5	470 ± 53**	49 ± 2.4	54 ± 4.1	18 ± 5.6	33 ± 6.5	184 ± 17†
35.5	6.6	5	425 ± 67	56 ± 33.9	58 ± 36.8	19 ± 8.1	55 ± 30.7	171 ± 39**
40.0	11	4	264 ± 117	92 ± 40.1	69 ± 26.4	34 ± 12.5**	59 ± 14.5†	80 ± 64

Infusion rates were 0.001; 0.01; 0.1; 1.0 μmol kg⁻¹ min⁻¹ they were increased at 10, 20, and 30 min after the start of the lowest infusion rate. ECG lead: heart axis (Spörri, 1944). Cumul. lethal dose: $14.2 \pm 1.7\ \mu mol\ kg^{-1}\ min^{-1}$ (n = 5).

Means.

* MAP: Mean arterial pressure (mm Hg) × 0.1333 = (kPa).

**, † $p < 0.05$ and $p < 0.01$ to predrug value (Student's t-test for paired observations).

the bradycardia caused by 1.4 g urethane/kg restored by an intraperitoneal injection of 25 mg atropine/kg. Only in extremely high dosages, far above the therapeutic range, did we observe toxic signs like bradycardia, hypotension and prolongation of PR, PR_c, QRS, and $R\alpha T$. According to suggestions of Valora *et al.* (1963), the absence of an appreciable indirect sympathetic action of atropine may be attributed to a high sympathetic tone as indicated by the high initial heart rates present under our experimental conditions. Valle *et al.* (1975) did not find significant ECG and heart rate changes after bilateral vagotomy in rats either.

4.2. Sympathetic Agonists

Although directly acting adrenergic drugs have gained wide clinical application, there are few systematic investigations comparing their effects on the ECG in animals, particularly in the rat. As our experiments on four catecholamines have already been published in detail (Buschmann *et al.*, 1980), these results will be discussed here more briefly.

Adrenaline led to a short-lasting fall in mean blood pressure at the beginning of the lowest infusion rate, whereas a pronounced increase in pressure and in heart rate was observed at higher infusion rates (Table 17). A few minutes after the onset of the highest infusion rate, however, both parameters decreased until the death of the animals occurred. As PR remained almost unchanged, a prolongation of PR_c was calculated because of the marked increase in heart rate. A clear widening of QRS was present at the highest infusion rate.

Noradrenaline. During the infusion of *noradrenaline*, the ECG parameters measured were altered essentially in the same way as with adrenaline (Table 18).

Isoproterenol. The beta-receptor stimulating agent *isoproterenol* lowered the mean blood pressure in a dose-related manner (Table 19). As the heart rate showed a moderate increase and the PR interval a concomitant slight shortening throughout the experiment, the calculated PR_c interval remained unchanged. Beginning at 0.01 μmol kg^{-1} min^{-1}, a prominent widening of QRS became apparent in two out of four animals; so the level of statistical significance was not reached. The $R\alpha T$ interval showed a slight prolongation.

After repeated subcutaneous noradrenaline or isoproterenol injections, Noda *et al.* (1970) did not observe ECG changes with noradrenaline, whereas isoproterenol produced a prolongation of QT and a concomitant inversion of the T wave, which we did not find (Table 20).

Dopamine. As far as heart rate and blood pressure are concerned, the actions of *dopamine* resembled those of adrenaline and noradrenaline

TABLE 18. EFFECTS OF AN INTRAVENOUS INFUSION OF NORADRENALINE (mol. wt. 205.7) ON HEART RATE, ECG PARAMETERS AND ON MEAN ARTERIAL BLOOD PRESSURE (MAP) IN ANESTHETIZED MALE WISTAR RATS (1.25 URETHANE/kg INTRAPERITONEALLY)

Experimental time (min)	Cumulated dose (μmol kg^{-1})	n	Heart rate (min^{-1})	PR interval (ms)	PR$_c$ interval (ms)	QRS (ms)	RαT interval (ms)	MAP* (mm Hg)
0	0	4	409 ± 43	50 ± 2.4	50 ± 2.4	14 ± 1.2	28 ± 2.3	93 ± 18
8	0.008	4	425 ± 37**	49 ± 1.7	50 ± 1.9	14 ± 0.9	29 ± 1.5	105 ± 18
19	0.10	4	446 ± 39†	47 ± 5.1	50 ± 4.5	17 ± 3.3	33 ± 3.0	125 ± 13†
23	0.41	4	425 ± 49	51 ± 5.0	53 ± 3.6	14 ± 0.5	32 ± 2.5	173 ± 20†
31.5	2.6	3	442 ± 17	52 ± 6.0	53 ± 5.8	19 ± 3.0	34 ± 3.5**	215 ± 26**
36	7.1	4	421 ± 32	54 ± 6.6	56 ± 6.1	18 ± 1.2†	31 ± 1.4	181 ± 9†

Infusion rates were 0.001; 0.01; 0.1; 1.0 μmol kg^{-1} min^{-1}; they were increased at 10, 20, and 30 min after the start of the lowest infusion rate. ECG lead: heart axis (Spörri, 1944). Cumul. lethal dose: 14.3/16 μmol kg^{-1} (n = 2).
Means.
* MAP: Mean arterial pressure (mm Hg) × 0.1333 = (kPa).
**,† p < 0.05 and p < 0.01 to predrug value (Student's t-test for paired observations).

TABLE 19. EFFECTS OF AN INTRAVENOUS INFUSION OF ISOPROTERENOL (mol. wt. 278.3) ON HEART RATE, ECG PARAMETERS AND ON MEAN ARTERIAL BLOOD PRESSURE (MAP) IN ANESTHETIZED MALE WISTAR RATS (1.25 URETHANE/kg INTRAPERITONEALLY)

Experimental time (min)	Cumulated dose (μmol kg^{-1})	n	Heart rate (min^{-1})	PR interval (ms)	PR$_c$ interval (ms)	QRS (ms)	RαT interval (ms)	MAP* (mm Hg)
0	0	4	411 ± 20	52 ± 6.2	52 ± 6.2	15 ± 1.0	29 ± 3.5	102 ± 26
9.5	0.0095	4	440 ± 27†	50 ± 4.9	52 ± 4.6	16 ± 3.0	33 ± 3.3†	92 ± 22**
19	0.10	4	444 ± 26†	49 ± 3.3	51 ± 2.9	17 ± 2.9	34 ± 4.1†	67 ± 16**
28	0.91	4	445 ± 23†	47 ± 4.2	49 ± 4.1	19 ± 4.6	34 ± 3.4†	53 ± 5**
40	11	4	446 ± 25†	46 ± 3.9	49 ± 3.9	19 ± 6.4	32 ± 6.1	54 ± 6**
50	21	4	453 ± 27†	46 ± 4.2	49 ± 4.1	17 ± 5.2	33 ± 8.0	52 ± 4**

Infusion rates were 0.001; 0.01; 0.1; 1.0 μmol kg^{-1} min^{-1}; they were increased at 10, 20, and 30 min after the start of the lowest infusion rate. ECG lead: heart axis (Spörri, 1944). Cumul. lethal dose: >21 μmol kg^{-1}.
Means.
* MAP: Mean arterial pressure (mm Hg) × 0.1333 = (kPa).
**,† $p < 0.05$ and $p < 0.01$ to predrug value (Student's t-test for paired observations).

TABLE 20. EFFECTS OF REPEATED (7 DAYS) ADMINISTRATION OF NORADRENALINE AND ISOPROTERENOL ON ECG INTERVALS AND CONFIGURATION IN MALE SPRAGUE-DAWLEY RATS (280-320 g) ANESTHETIZED WITH PENTOBARBITAL, 5 ANIMALS PER GROUP; LEAD I AND II (Noda et al., 1970)

	Daily dose (mg/kg sc.)	PR interval (ms)	QRS (ms)	QT (ms)	Inverted T	Deep Q	ST-T depression
Control		37-47	7-22	52-70	0/5	0/5	0/5
Noradrenaline	0.6	42-43	17-18	60-67	0/5	0/5	0/5
	1.0	40-45	7-20	55-67	0/5	0/5	0/5
Isoproterenol	0.7	42-50	8-20	50-78	5/5	5/5	4/5
	1.2	40-47	17-18	58-92	5/5	4/5	5/5

(Table 21). But in contrast to both other catecholamines, no prolongation of the QRS complex was observed. PR_c, too, remained virtually unchanged indicating that the shortening of PR was a direct consequence of the tachycardia. At higher infusion rates $R\alpha T$ was prolonged significantly by a few milliseconds.

Dobutamine. In contrast to dopamine, the newer beta$_1$-adrenergic drug *dobutamine*, which is used for similar clinical indications, induced only a faint increase in heart rate and PR_c with a significant decrease in blood pressure at low dosages (Table 22). At higher dosages a marked fall in blood pressure and heart rate and a prolongation of PR, PR_c, QRS and $R\alpha T$ were found.

A shortening of the PR interval after administration of catecholamines, as also found by others in different species and in man (Haas and Busch, 1967; Surawicz and Lasseter, 1970; Loeb et al., 1974; Martin-Serrano et al., 1975; Vargas et al., 1975; Wit et al., 1975; Graf and Leuschner, 1978), was eliminated in our experiments with most catecholamines when correcting the intervals for heart rate changes. Dobutamine, on the other hand, produced a prolongation of PR irrespective of the heart rate changes, although mainly at rather high dosages; as the increase in PR was paralleled by a marked prolongation of both QRS and $R\alpha T$ as well as by a prominent fall in heart rate and blood pressure, this is probably a toxic rather than a pharmacodynamic effect. The same can be assumed for the change induced by the highest doses of adrenaline and noradrenaline.

The absence of a widening of QRS even at the highest dose of dopamine is consistent with low cardiotoxicity of this drug as evidenced by a comparative study with 15 sympathomimetic amines by Rosenblum et al. (1965). After several weeks of intravenous dopamine treatment, Graf and Leuschner (1978) did not find histological signs of myocardial lesions in rats and dogs. These alterations have frequently been induced in rats by isoproterenol (Rona et al., 1959, 1963; Rosenblum et al., 1965; Noda et al., 1970; Pavlovitchova et al., 1970; Balazs et al., 1972; Wexler and Greenberg, 1974; Wexler et al., 1974; Godfraind and Sturbois, 1979).

4.3. Sympathetic Antagonists

In another series of experiments we compared the effects of the unspecific beta-blocker propranolol with those of the cardioselective blockers metoprolol and talinolol. As the results are presented and discussed in detail in another paper (Buschmann et al., p. 185), we will restrict ourselves to a short survey.

Propranolol caused a dose-dependent fall in heart rate and a prolongation of the PR interval. Applying our formula, a dose-dependent shortening

TABLE 21. EFFECTS OF AN INTRAVENOUS INFUSION OF DOPAMINE (mol. wt. 189.6) ON HEART RATE, ECG PARAMETERS AND ON MEAN ARTERIAL BLOOD PRESSURE (MAP) IN ANESTHETIZED MALE WISTAR RATS (1.25 URETHANE/kg INTRAPERITONEALLY)

Experimental time (min)	Cumulated dose (μmol kg^{-1})	n	Heart rate (min^{-1})	PR interval (ms)	PR$_c$ interval (ms)	QRS (ms)	RαT interval (ms)	MAP* (mm Hg)
0	0	6	395 ± 38	51 ± 3.5	51 ± 3.5	15 ± 0.8	27 ± 2.2	84 ± 15
7.5	0.075	6	415 ± 29	50 ± 4.1	52 ± 4.7	14 ± 0.8	27 ± 2.0	88 ± 19
19.5	1.05	6	457 ± 16†	50 ± 3.3	55 ± 4.5**	14 ± 1.7	29 ± 1.8	98 ± 17†
22.5	3.6	6	468 ± 23†	48 ± 3.5†	54 ± 4.6	14 ± 1.1	29 ± 1.5	112 ± 10†
32.5	36	6	460 ± 30**	48 ± 4.5**	53 ± 4.3	14 ± 1.0	29 ± 1.6†	158 ± 20†
50	211	6	507 ± 20†	43 ± 2.4†	51 ± 3.5	14 ± 1.2	30 ± 1.8†	103 ± 13†

Infusion rates were 0.01; 0.1; 1.0; 10.0 μmol kg^{-1} min^{-1}; they were increased at 10, 20, and 30 min after the start of the lowest infusion rate. ECG lead: heart axis (Spörri, 1944). Cumul. lethal dose: >211 μmol kg^{-1}. Means.
* MAP: Mean arterial pressure (mm Hg) × 0.1333 = (kPa).
**,† $p < 0.05$ and $p < 0.01$ to predrug value (Student's t-test for paired observations).

TABLE 22. EFFECTS OF AN INTRAVENOUS INFUSION OF DOBUTAMINE (mol. wt. 337.9) ON HEART RATE, ECG PARAMETERS AND ON MEAN ARTERIAL BLOOD PRESSURE (MAP) IN ANESTHETIZED MALE WISTAR RATS (1.25 URETHANE/kg INTRAPERITONEALLY)

Experimental time (min)	Cumulated dose (μmol kg^{-1})	n	Heart rate (min^{-1})	PR interval (ms)	PR$_c$ interval (ms)	QRS (ms)	RαT interval (ms)	MAP* (mm Hg)
0	0	4	413 ± 21	49 ± 2.9	49 ± 2.9	15 ± 1.2	31 ± 3.5	110 ± 12
10	0.1	4	413 ± 16	50 ± 2.5	50 ± 2.5	15 ± 0.9	30 ± 3.1	94 ± 6
20	1.1	4	434 ± 29	49 ± 3.3	51 ± 3.7	17 ± 3.7	33 ± 2.7	72 ± 7†
30	11.1	4	420 ± 34	52 ± 3.0**	53 ± 3.5**	17 ± 4.9	34 ± 3.3**	51 ± 7†
39.5	106	4	320 ± 43**	74 ± 2.9†	65 ± 5.9†	26 ± 3.4†	49 ± 5.6†	42 ± 7†
50	211		279 ± 42†	98 ± 9.4†	82 ± 2.3†	35 ± 10.8†	67 ± 11.1†	35 ± 7†

Infusion rates were 0.01; 0.1; 1.0; 10.0 μmol kg^{-1} min^{-1}; they were increased at 10, 20, and 30 min after the start of the lowest infusion rate. ECG lead: heart axis (Spörri, 1944). Cumul. lethal dose: >211 μmol kg^{-1}.

Means.

* MAP: Mean arterial pressure (mm Hg) × 0.1333 = (kPa).

**,† p < 0.05 and p < 0.01 to predrug value (Student's t-test for paired observations).

of PR_c is calculated for the three lower infusion rates. At low and medium doses, the mean arterial pressure was elevated significantly, mainly by increasing the diastolic values; RαT showed a slight shortening. At high dosages propranolol caused a significant widening of QRS with a concomitant prolongation on the RαT interval in our experiments.

Metoprolol. The negative chronotropic action of the cardioselective blocker *metoprolol* as well as its effect on the PR interval was weaker than that of propranolol. Again, as in the propranolol experiment, the slight prolongation of PR turned to a dose-dependent shortening after correction for the heart rate decrease. High doses of metoprolol induced a slight widening of QRS without affecting the RαT interval.

The cardioselective beta-blocker *talinolol*, too, caused a fall in heart rate, a prolongation of the PR interval, and a rise in mean arterial blood pressure. In contrast to metoprolol, talinolol showed an increase in PR_c at high dosages together with a prolongation of QRS and RαT.

5. DRUGS AFFECTING THE CARDIOVASCULAR SYSTEM

5.1. Antiarrhythmic Drugs

For the group of antiarrhythmic agents, ECG analysis is of special interest in the characterization not only of the side effects, but also for the analysis of the mode of action. The results of these experiments are given in detail in another paper (Kühl *et al.*, p. 197). Summarizing the results of these experiments, we compared the ECG profile of selected compounds with what could be expected according to the electrophysiological profile and to the classification of Vaughan Williams (1970, 1979) and Singh and Hauswirth (1974). N-propyl-ajmaline bitartrate (NPAB) was taken as a typical representative of class 1a action, and lidocaine as a class 1b-type agent. Whereas *NPAB* produced a prolongation of PR, PR_c and QRS at therapeutic dose levels, this was not so with *lidocaine*. As far as their effects on the conduction velocity is concerned, the newer antiarrhythmic agent *propafenon* was similar to the class 1a drug NPAB, and the alkaloid *sparteine* was similar to the class 1b compound lidocaine.

With *verapamil*, a representative of class 4 action, no appreciable changes in the measured ECG parameters were observed except for a marked reduction in heart rate.

5.2. Arrhythmogenic Drugs

Aconitine, an alkaloid of the European monkshood, which in experimental pharmacology is frequently used to produce cardiac arrhythmias, did

TABLE 23. EFFECTS OF AN INTRAVENOUS INFUSION OF ACONITINE (mol. wt. 646) ON HEART RATE, ECG PARAMETERS AND ON MEAN ARTERIAL BLOOD PRESSURE (MAP) IN ANESTHETIZED MALE WISTAR RATS (1.25 URETHANE/kg INTRAPERITONEALLY)

Experimental time (min)	Cumulated dose (nmol kg^{-1})	n	Heart rate (min^{-1})	PR interval (ms)	PR$_c$ interval (ms)	QRS (ms)	RαT interval (ms)	MAP* (mm Hg)
0	0	4	462 ± 26	50 ± 3.5	50 ± 3.5	15 ± 2.1	36 ± 9.8	102 ± 16
9.5	0.095	4	467 ± 19	48 ± 2.5	48 ± 2.8	14 ± 1.7	36 ± 11.8	108 ± 9
20	1.1	4	465 ± 21	48 ± 2.4	48 ± 2.5	14 ± 2.8	37 ± 7.0	106 ± 13
24.5	5.6	4	468 ± 20	49 ± 2.1	49 ± 2.8	14 ± 2.1	37 ± 7.7	113 ± 12
27.5	8.6	4	469 ± 32	48 ± 2.7	48 ± 2.8	14 ± 2.0	39 ± 4.7	112 ± 10
32	31.9	3	482 ± 14	47 ± 2.8	48 ± 3.0	13 ± 3.2	32 ± 4.9	114 ± 8

Infusion rates were 0.01; 0.1; 1.0; 10.0 nmol kg^{-1} min^{-1}; they were increased at 10, 20, and 30 min after the start of the lowest infusion rate. ECG lead: heart axis (Spörri, 1944). Cumul. lethal dose: 118 nmol kg^{-1} (n = 1).

Means ± SD.

* MAP: Mean arterial pressure (mm Hg) × 0.1333 = (kPa).

not change any of the measured ECG parameters at infusion rates of 0.01–1 nmol/kg/min (Table 23). However, 3–5 min after changing to the infusion rate of 10 nmol/kg/min the well-known arrhythmias occurred in the characteristic sequence: ventricular extrasystoles, ventricular tachycardia, ventricular flutter (Marmo *et al.*, 1970; Raschack, 1975, 1976). As at the onset of severe ECG irregularities the computer program interrupts, no computer data are available for two minutes after the start of the highest infusion rate.

5.3. Vasodilators/Antihypertensives

With therapeutic doses of antihypertensive agents adverse ECG changes do not play a significant role in clinical use. To the contrary: during antihypertensive drug treatment ECG changes related to hypertension may improve markedly (Poblete *et al.*, 1973; Guazzi *et al.*, 1974).

Clonidine. At low dosages the centrally-acting, alpha-receptor stimulating drug *clonidine* did not produce any changes in the measured parameters except for a significant reduction in heart rate, and a moderate fall in arterial blood pressure (Table 24). At higher dose levels an increase of mean arterial blood pressure occurred, which was probably caused by an alpha-receptor mediated peripheral vasoconstriction (Hoefke and Kobinger, 1966; Kobinger and Walland, 1967; Boissier *et al.*, 1968; Kobinger *et al.*, 1979). At this dosage the QRS duration was increased in all animals. The significant shortening computed for PR_c is due to the strong bradycardiac action without increase in PR. Only at very high doses did clonidine prolong the PR interval. This effect was also found by Hoefke and Kobinger (1966) after 100 µg/kg i.v. in anesthetized rabbits. The absence of ECG changes at low doses is consistent with the obvious lack of electrocardiographic side effects during clonidine therapy in man, although the drug may be a factor in producing atrioventricular block (Kibler and Gazes, 1977).

Dihydralazine. The most prominent effect of *dihydralazine* was a reduction of the mean arterial blood pressure, whereas the heart rate and the ECG parameters remained unaffected up to very high dosages (Table 25).

Nitroglycerin. The first effect seen with *nitroglycerin* was a lowering of mean arterial blood pressure (Table 26). At high infusion rates it was accompanied by a slow fall in heart rate without any ECG changes. Only towards the end of the experiment was the PR interval moderately increased. Our findings are consistent with the absence of ECG changes reported by Fahmy (1978) in normal people after intravenous drug infusion, but do not agree with the increase in heart rate seen in this study as well as in a study with sublingual administration (Sawayama *et al.*, 1973).

R. Budden, G. Buschmann and U. G. Kühl

TABLE 24. EFFECTS OF AN INTRAVENOUS INFUSION OF CLONIDINE (mol. wt. 230) ON HEART RATE, ECG PARAMETERS AND ON MEAN ARTERIAL BLOOD PRESSURE (MAP) IN ANESTHETIZED MALE WISTAR RATS (1.25 URETHANE/kg INTRAPERITONEALLY)

Experimental time (min)	Cumulated dose (μmol kg^{-1})	n	Heart rate (min^{-1})	PR interval (ms)	PR$_c$ interval (ms)	QRS (ms)	RαT interval (ms)	MAP* (mm Hg)
0	0	3	368 ± 39	51 ± 5.5	51 ± 5.5	15 ± 0.5	28 ± 2.6	88 ± 5
4	0.13	3	296 ± 82	49 ± 10.6	38 ± 16.8	15 ± 0.5	24 ± 1.0	66 ± 3**
9	0.28	3	287 ± 52**	53 ± 6.8	42 ± 8.8	15 ± 1.1	23 ± 1.0	98 ± 14
19.5	3.32	3	243 ± 26**	54 ± 7.3	36 ± 7.9**	15 ± 1.0	26 ± 5.2	145 ± 24
28.5	30.3	3	190 ± 18**	55 ± 10.0	—	17 ± 2.5	27 ± 6.3	146 ± 24
40–41.5	350–398	3	163 ± 19†	63 ± 9.3**	—	23 ± 4.7	36 ± 5.1	111 ± 32

Infusion rates were 0.0316; 0.316; 3.16; 31.6 μmol kg^{-1} min^{-1} i.v.; they were increased at 10, 20, and 30 min after the start of the lowest infusion rate. ECG lead: heart axis (Spörri, 1944). Cumul. lethal dose: >670 μmol kg^{-1}.
Means ± SD.
* MAP: Mean arterial pressure (mm Hg) × 0.1333 = (kPa).
**,† $p < 0.05$ and $p < 0.01$ to predrug value (Student's paired t-test).

TABLE 25. EFFECTS OF AN INTRAVENOUS INFUSION OF DIHYDRALAZINE (mol. wt. 288) ON HEART RATE, ECG PARAMETERS AND ON MEAN ARTERIAL BLOOD PRESSURE (MAP) IN ANESTHETIZED MALE WISTAR RATS (1.25 URETHANE/kg INTRAPERITONEALLY)

Experimental time (min)	Cumulated dose (μmol kg^{-1})	n	Heart rate (min^{-1})	PR interval (ms)	PR$_c$ interval (ms)	QRS (ms)	RαT interval (ms)	MAP* (mm Hg)
0	0	4	422 ± 21	52 ± 3.0	52 ± 3.0	15 ± 1.4	31 ± 7.5	106 ± 8
5.5	1.1	4	429 ± 17	50 ± 2.7	50 ± 2.3	15 ± 0.9	32 ± 11.9	82 ± 10**
9	1.8	4	430 ± 17	49 ± 2.2	50 ± 2.2	15 ± 1.5	35 ± 12.7	73 ± 7**
12	6.0	4	426 ± 12	50 ± 1.8	50 ± 2.2	14 ± 1.7	26 ± 6.4	66 ± 6†
27.5	172	4	330 ± 24**	54 ± 1.2	46 ± 2.5†	14 ± 1.2	35 ± 7.7	48 ± 3†
32	622	3	252 ± 32†	59 ± 2.0	39 ± 4.4†	15 ± 1.5	29 ± 3.0	52 ± 6**

Infusion rates were 0.2; 2.0; 20.0; 200.0 μmol kg^{-1} min^{-1}; they were increased at 10, 20, and 30 min after the start of the lowest infusion rate. ECG lead: heart axis (Spörri, 1944). Cumul. lethal dose: 3622 = 569 μmol kg^{-1}.

Means ± SD.

* MAP: Mean arterial pressure (mm Hg) × 0.1333 = (kPa).

**,† p < 0.05 and p < 0.01 to predrug value (Student's paired t-test).

TABLE 26. EFFECTS OF AN INTRAVENOUS INFUSION OF NITROGLYCERIN (mol. wt. 227) ON HEART RATE, ECG PARAMETERS AND ON MEAN ARTERIAL BLOOD PRESSURE (MAP) IN ANESTHETIZED MALE WISTAR RATS (1.25 URETHANE/kg INTRAPERITONEALLY)

Experimental time (min)	Cumulated dose (μmol kg^{-1})	n	Heart rate (min^{-1})	PR interval (ms)	PR$_c$ interval (ms)	QRS (ms)	RαT interval (ms)	MAP* (mm Hg)
0	0	4	419 ± 21	50 ± 2.2	50 ± 2.2	15 ± 1.4	33 ± 14.9	112 ± 7
10	0.15	4	413 ± 21	51 ± 2.9	49 ± 1.7	15 ± 1.4	40 ± 11.3	105 ± 2
20	1.65	4	405 ± 18	51 ± 3.3	49 ± 3.2	14 ± 1.5	38 ± 10.8	96 ± 11**
30	16.7	4	399 ± 21**	52 ± 2.9	49 ± 1.8	14 ± 1.5	35 ± 7.1	65 ± 13†
38	137	4	314 ± 59**	56 ± 4.3	40 ± 6.0	15 ± 1.6	32 ± 4.5	68 ± 13†
45	242	4	300 ± 23†	59 ± 4.1†	46 ± 3.5**	18 ± 3.3	36 ± 3.4	67 ± 8†

Infusion rates were 0.015; 0.15; 1.5; 15.0 μmol kg^{-1} min^{-1}; they were increased at 10, 20, and 30 min after the start of the lowest infusion rate. ECG lead: heart axis (Spörri, 1944). Cumul. lethal dose: 366 ± 36 μmol kg^{-1}.
Means ± SD.
* MAP: Mean arterial pressure (mm Hg) × 0.1333 = (kPa).
**,† $p < 0.05$ and $p < 0.01$ to predrug value (Student's paired t-test).

TABLE 27. EFFECTS OF AN INTRAVENOUS INFUSION OF ADENOSINE (mol. wt. 267) ON HEART RATE, ECG PARAMETERS AND ON MEAN ARTERIAL BLOOD PRESSURE (MAP) IN ANESTHETIZED MALE WISTAR RATS (1.25 URETHANE/kg INTRAPERITONEALLY)

Experimental time (min)	Cumulated dose (μmol kg^{-1})	n	Heart rate (min^{-1})	PR interval (ms)	PRc interval (ms)	QRS (ms)	RαT interval (ms)	MAP* (mm Hg)
0	0	4	381 ± 16	52 ± 3.6	52 ± 3.6	15 ± 1.2	42 ± 9.9	84 ± 16
10	1.0	4	387 ± 17	52 ± 3.2	53 ± 3.4	15 ± 1.0	36 ± 3.4	96 ± 10
20	5.64	4	404 ± 41	53 ± 3.2	55 ± 2.5	16 ± 2.2	39 ± 2.9	47 ± 7†
30	27.1	4	389 ± 37	53 ± 3.9	54 ± 2.0	14 ± 1.7	41 ± 17.3	53 ± 7†
43	157	4	201 ± 87**	65 ± 16.4‡	20 ± 42.9	15 ± 1.2	37 ± 2.5	42 ± 15†
49	217	4	201 ± 93**	63 ± 14.5‡	18 ± 26.1	15 ± 1.2	36 ± 1.5	42 ± 15†

Infusion rates were 0.1; 0.464; 2.15; 10.0 μmol kg^{-1} min^{-1}; they were increased at 10, 20, and 30 min after the start of the lowest infusion rate. ECG lead: heart axis (Spörri, 1944). Cumul. lethal dose: $>230\,\mu$mol kg^{-1}.

Means ± SD.

* MAP: Mean arterial pressure (mm Hg) × 0.1333 = (kPa).

**,† $p < 0.05$ and $p < 0.01$ to predrug value (Student's paired t-test).

‡ n = 3.

Adenosine. The most prominent action of *adenosine* was a marked hypotension, whereas a fall in heart rate and a prolongation of the PR interval were apparent only at rather high doses (Table 27). After correcting the PR values for heart rate dependence no prolongation was left. Essentially, our results agree with the data of Bass *et al.* (1972), who also reported bradycardia and prolongation of PR after intravenous injection of the agent in the rat, though the doses needed were considerably lower (Table 28).

TABLE 28. EFFECTS OF INTRAVENOUS ADMINISTRATION OF ADENOSINE ON HEART RATE, PR INTERVAL AND MEAN ARTERIAL BLOOD PRESSURE (MAP) IN MALE RATS (MENDEL–OSBORNE STRAIN, 250–350 g) ANESTHETIZED WITH DIALLYL-BARBITURIC ACID/URETHANE; LEAD VII (AFTER BASS *et al.*, 1972)

Dose $(mg\ kg^{-1}\ i.v.)$	n	Heart rate (min^{-1})		PR interval (ms)		MAP (mm Hg)	
		pre	post	pre	post	pre	post
0.05	5	432	320	56	59	110	69
0.1	5	420	298	56	60	102	78
0.4	5	416	187	58	67	99	59
0.8	5	388	105	58	70	99	36

Mean values.

Hydrochlorothiazide. The benzothiadiazide diuretic *hydrochlorothiazide* caused only a moderate fall in blood pressure and, at high doses, a small prolongation of both PR and PR_c (Table 29).

6. CONCLUSIONS

From the background of the data presented, the following conclusions may be drawn:

1. The rat ECG is a suitable tool in the characterization of pharmacodynamic or toxic cardiac actions of drugs.

2. Computer evaluation is a rapid means for the correct measurement of rat ECG parameters in routine experiments.

3. There is a sufficient correlation of electrocardiographic drug effects between rat and man.

4. The incorporation of the ECG in acute rat experiments may augment the usability of this species.

TABLE 29. EFFECTS OF AN INTRAVENOUS INFUSION OF HYDROCHLOROTHIAZIDE ON HEART RATE, ECG PARAMETERS AND ON MEAN ARTERIAL BLOOD PRESSURE (MAP) IN ANESTHETIZED MALE WISTAR RATS (1.25 URETHANE/kg INTRAPERITONEALLY)

Experimental time (min)	Cumulated dose (μmol kg^{-1})	n	Heart rate (min^{-1})	PR interval (ms)	PR$_c$ interval (ms)	QRS (ms)	RαT interval (ms)	MAP* (mm Hg)
0	0	4	426 ± 12	50 ± 2.5	50 ± 2.5	14 ± 0.5	40 ± 11.6	100 ± 13
10	10	4	434 ± 13	50 ± 3.5	52 ± 3.4	15 ± 0.0	35 ± 3.5	110 ± 15
20	31.5	4	421 ± 33	51 ± 3.1	51 ± 1.9	14 ± 0.5	32 ± 2.0	88 ± 24
30	77.9	4	420 ± 35	52 ± 3.1	51 ± 2.0	15 ± 0.5	31 ± 2.3	78 ± 16
40	178	4	430 ± 27	53 ± 3.5	54 ± 1.5	15 ± 0.9	34 ± 4.3	81 ± 12
50	278	4	442 ± 23	54 ± 2.9	56 ± 1.9	15 ± 0.5	38 ± 9.1	86 ± 10

Infusion rates were 0; 1.0; 2.15; 4.64; 10.0 μmcl kg^{-1} min^{-}; they were increased at 10, 20, and 30 min after the start of the lowest infusion rate. ECG lead: heart axis (Spörri, 1944). Cural lethal dose: >278 μmol kg^{-1}.
Means ± SD.
* MAP: Mean arterial pressure: (mm Hg) × 0.1333 = (kPa.

78 *R. Budden, G. Buschmann and U. G. Kühl*

REFERENCES

Agabiti–Rosei, E., Alicandri, C. L. and Corea, L. (1977) Hypertensive crisis in patients with phaeochromocytoma given metoclopramide. *Lancet* **I** 8011.

Ålander, T., Andén, N.–E. and Grabowska–Andén, M. (1980) Metoclopramide and sulpiride as selective blocking agents of pre- and postsynaptic dopamine receptors. *Naunyn-Schmiedebergs Arch. Pharmacol.* **312,** 145–150.

Aronson, C. E. and Serlick, E. R. (1977) Effects of chlorpromazine on the isolated perfused rat heart. *Toxicol. Appl. Pharmacol.* **39,** 157–176.

Balazs, T., Ohtake, S. and Noble, J. F. (1972) The development of resistance to the ischemic cardiopathic effect of isoproterenol. *Toxicol. Appl. Pharmacol.* **21,** 200–213.

Barnes, C. D. and Eltherington, L. G. (1973) *Drug Dosage in Laboratory Animals,* 2nd edition, p. 22. University of California Press, Berkeley, Los Angeles, London.

Bass, S. W., Ramirez, M. A. and Aviado, D. M. (1972) Cardiopulmonary effects of antimalarial drugs. VI. Adenosine, Quina-crine and Primaquine. *Toxicol. Appl. Pharmacol.* **21,** 464–481.

Beinfield, W. H. and Lehr, D. (1968a) QRS–T variations in the rat electrocardiogram. *Am. J. Physiol.* **214,** 197–204.

Beinfield, W. H. and Lehr, D. (1968b) P–R interval of the rat electrocardiogram. *Am. J. Physiol.* **214,** 205–211 .

Boissier, J. R., Giudicelli, J. F., Fichelle, J., Schmitt, H. and Schmitt, H. (1968) Cardiovascular effects of 2-(2,6-dichlorophenylamino)-2-imidazoline hydrochloride (ST 155). *Eur. J. Pharmacol.* **2,** 333–339.

Bolme, P. and Fuxe, K. (1977) Possible involvement of gaba mechanisms in central cardiovascular and respiratory control. Studies on the interaction between diazepam, picrotoxin and clonidine. *Med. Biol.* **55,** 301–309.

Buschmann, G., Budden, R. and Kühl, U. G. (1980) Development of ECG changes during the infusion of beta blockers in anesthetized rats. *International Workshop on the Rat Electrocardiogram in Acute and Chronic Pharmacology and Toxicology,* July 14–15, 1980, Hannover.

Buschmann, G., Schumacher, W., Budden, R. and Kühl, U. G. Evaluation of the effect of dopamine and other catecholamines on ECG and blood pressure in rats using on-line biosignal processing (accepted for publication in *J. Cardiovasc. Pharmacol.*)

Driscoll, P. (1979) The electrocardiogram of Roman high- and low-avoidance rats under pentobarbital sodium anesthesia. *Arzneim.-Forsch.* **29,** 897–900.

Fahmy, N. R. (1978) Nitroglycerin as a hypotensive drug during general anesthesia. *Anesthesiology* **49,** 17–20.

Gessler, U. and Kuner, E. (1959) Experimenteller Beitrag zum Einfluß von Äther und Sauerstoffmangel auf das EKG der weißen Ratte. *Z. Kreislaufforsch.* **48,** 870–877.

Godfraind, T. and Sturbois, X. (1979) An analysis of the reduction by creatinol O-phosphate of the myocardial lesions evoked by isoprenaline in the rat. *Arzneim.-Forsch.* **29,** 1457–1464.

Graf, E. and Leuschner, F. (1978) Zur Toxizität von Dopamin. *Arzneim.-Forsch.* **28,** 2208–2218.

Grauwiler, J. and Spörri, H. (1960) Fehlen der ST-strecke im Elektrokardiogramm von verschiedenen Säugetierarten. *Helv. Physiol. Pharmacol. Acta* **18,** C 77–C 78.

Greenblatt, D. J. and Koch–Weser, J. (1973) Adverse reactions to intravenous diazepam: A report from the Boston Collaborative Drug Surveillance Program. *Am. J. Med. Sci.* **226,** 261–266.

Greenblatt, D. J. and Shader, R. I. (1974) Benzodiazepines. *N. Eng. J. Med.* **291,** 1011–1015.

Guazzi, M., Polese, A., Magrini, F. and Fiorentini, C. (1974) Correlation of electrocardiographic changes and hemodynamic functions in the treatment of primary arterial hypertension. *Am. J. Med. Sci.* **267,** 299–309.

Haas, H. and Busch, E. (1967) Vergleichende Untersuchungen der Wirkung von α-Isopropyl-α-[(N-methyl-N-homoveratryl)-γ-amino-propyl]-3,4-dimethoxyphenyl-aceto-nitril, seiner Derivate sowie einiger anderer Coronardilatatoren und β-receptor-affiner Substanzen. *Arzneim.-Forsch.* **17,** 257–272.

Heering, H. (1970a) Das Elektrokardiogramm der wachen und narkotisierten Ratte. *Arch. Int. Pharmacodyn. Ther.* **185**, 308–328.

Heering, H. (1970b) Das EKG der Ratte bei Paraoxon-intoxikation unter Einwirkung von Atropin und Pralidoxim (2-PAM). *Arch. Int. Pharmacodyn. Ther.* **186**, 321–338.

Heise, E. and Kimbel, K. H. (1955) Das normale Elektrokardiogramm der Ratte. *Z. Kreislauf-forsch.* **44**, 212–221.

Hillbom, M. E. and von Boguslawsky, K. (1978) Effect of ethanol on cardiac function in rats genetically selected for their ethanol preference. *Pharmacol. Biochem. Behav.* **8**, 609–614.

Hoefke, W. and Kobinger, W. (1966) Pharmakologische Wirkungen des 2-(2,6-Dichlorphenyl-amino)-2-imidazolin-hydrochlorids, einer neuen, antihypertensiven Substanz. *Arzneim.-Forsch.* **16**, 1038–1050.

Holk, H. G. O., Kanan, M. A., Mills, L. M. and Smith, E. L. (1937) Studies upon the sex-difference in rats in tolerance to certain barbiturates and to nicotine. *J. Pharmacol. Exp. Ther.* **60**, 323–346.

Kibler, L. E. and Gazes, P. C. (1977) Effect of clonidine on atrioventricular conduction. *JAMA* **238**, 1930–1932.

Kobinger, W. and Walland, A. (1967) Kreislaufuntersuchungen mit 2-(2,6-Dichlorphenyl-amino)-2-imidazolin-hydrochlorid. *Arzneim.-Forsch.* **17**, 292–300.

Kobinger, W., Lillie, C. and Pichler, L. (1979) N-allyl-derivative of clonidine, a substance with specific bradycardiac action at a cardiac site. *Naunyn-Schmiedebergs Arch. Pharmacol.* **306**, 255–262.

Kühl, U. G., Buschmann, G. and Budden, R. (1980) Development of ECG and blood pressure changes in anesthetized rats during the infusion of antiarrhythmic compounds. *International Workshop on the Rat Electrocardiogram in Acute and Chronic Pharmacology and Toxicology*, July 14–15, 1980, Hannover.

Langslet, A. (1970a) ECG-changes induced by phenothiazine drugs in the anesthetized rat. *Acta Pharmacol. Toxicol.* **28**, 258–264.

Langslet, A. (1970b) Cardiac effects of antiparkinson drugs, local anesthetics, and tranquil-izers. *Eur. J. Pharmacol.* **9**, 269–275.

Langslet, A. and Ryg, M. (1971) Effects of chlorpromazine and propranolol on left ventricular systolic pressure, ECG, and K$^+$ efflux in the isolated perfused rat heart. *Acta Pharmacol. Toxicol.* **29**, 533–541.

Lepeschkin, E. (1965) The configuration of the T wave and the ventricular action potential in different species of mammals. *Ann. N.Y. Acad. Sci.* **127**, 170–178.

Lisciani, R., Baldine, A., Benedetti, D., Campana, A. and Scorza Barcellona, P. (1978) Acute cardiovascular toxicity of trazodone, etoperidone and imipramine in rats. *Toxicology* **10**, 151–158.

Loeb, H. S., Sinno, M. Z., Saudye, A., Towne, W. D. and Gunnar, R. M. (1974) Electrophysio-logic properties of dobutamine. *Circ. Shock* **1**, 217–220.

Marmo, E., Di Giacomo, S. and Imperatore, A. (1969a) Verhalten des Elektrokardiogramms normaler oder mit verschiedenen Pharmaka vorbehandelter und daraufhin mit Metoch-lopramid perfundierter Ratten. *Jpn. J. Pharmacol.* **19**, 551–562.

Marmo, E., Imperatore, A. and Di Giacomo, S. (1969b) Effetti della metoclopramide sull'ap-parato cardiovascolare e sul relativo SNV. *Clin. Ter.* **51**, 509–539.

Marmo, E., Di Giacomo, S. and Imperatore, A. (1970) Metoclopramid und elektrokardiogra-phische Veränderungen durch KCl, BaCl$_2$, CaCl$_2$, MgCl$_2$, Aconitin, k-Strophanthosid, Vasopressin und durch Asphyxie. *Arzneim.-Forsch.* **20**, 12–18.

Martin-Serrano, G., Cuesta, C. and Lucas Gallego, J. (1975) Diferencias electrocardiográficas y de ATP en ratas tratadas con isoproterenol e inyectadas previamente con propranolol. *Arch. Farmacol. Toxicol.* **1**, 259–268.

Moccetti, T. (1973) Kardiotoxische Medikamente. *Schweiz. Med. Wochenschr.* **103**, 621–630.

Moccetti, T., Lichtlen, P., Albert, H., Meier, E. and Imbach, P. (1971) Kardiotoxizität der trizyklischen Antidepressiva. *Schweiz. Med. Wochenschr.* **101**, 1–10.

Neeb, S. and Grabner, W. (1978) Metoclopramid. *Dtsch. Med. Wochenschr.* **103**, 1572–1575.

Nemec, J. (1973) Cardiotoxic effects of tricyclic antipsychotics. Comparison of some newer derivatives from the 10,11-dihydrodibenzo/b,f/thiepin group with perphenazine and ami-triptyline. *Eur. J. Toxicol.* **6**, 224–231.

Noda, M., Kawano, O., Uchida, O., Sawabe, T., Saito, G. and Fukawa, K. (1970) Myocarditis induced by sympathomimetic amines. *Jpn. Circ. J.* **34**, 7–12.

Pateisky, K. and Wessely, P. (1975) Unterschiedliche Reaktion auf Diazepam bei verschiedener intravenöser Applikationsgeschwindigkeit (polygraphische Studie). *Schweiz. Rundschau Med.* **64**, 962–965.

Pavlovitchova, H., Ancla, M., Laborit, H. and De Brux, J. (1970) Action du dichlorhydrate de l'amino-2 (méthylène isothioureyl)-4 thiazol (Agr 307) sur des altérations biochimiques, électrocardiographiques et histologiques du myocarde du rat provoquées par l'isoprotérénol. *Agressologie* **11**, 333–341.

Poblete, P. F., Kyle, M. C., Pipberger, H. V. and Freis, E. D. (1973) Effect of treatment on morbidity in hypertension. Veterans administration cooperative study on antihypertensive agents: Effect on the electrocardiogram. *Circulation* **48**, 481–490.

Ramos, A. O., Bastos, W. P. and Sakate, M. (1967) Influence of metoclopramide in experimental arrhythmias induced by barium or by chloroform and adrenaline. *Med. Pharmacol. Exp.* **17**, 385–390.

Raschack, M. (1975) Wirkung von Ajmalin und seinen therapeutisch verwendeten Derivaten n-Propylajmalin und Dimonochloracetylajmalin auf funktionelle Refraktärzeit und Kontraktionskraft am Meerschweinchenvorhof sowie Aconitin-arrhythmien an der Ratte. *Arzneim.-Forsch.* **25**, 639–641.

Raschack, M. (1976) Relationship of antiarrhythmic to inotropic activity and antiarrhythmic qualities of the optical isomers of verapamil. *Naunyn-Schmiedebergs Arch. Pharmacol.* **294**, 285–291.

Rona, G., Chappel, C. I., Balazs, T. and Gaudry, R. (1959) An infarct-like myocardial lesion and other toxic manifestations produced by isoproterenol in the rat. *A.M.A. Arch. Pathol.* **67**, 443–455.

Rona, G., Chappel, C. I. and Kahn, D. S. (1963) The significance of factors modifying the development of isoproterenol-induced myocardial necrosis. *Am. Heart J.* **66**, 389–395.

Rosenblum, I., Wohl, A. and Stein, A. A. (1965) Studies in cardiac necrosis. I. Production of cardiac lesions with sympathomimetic amines. *Toxicol. Appl. Pharmacol.* **7**, 1–8.

Sambhi, M. P. and White, F. N. (1960) The electrocardiogram of the normal and hypertensive rat. *Circul. Res.* **8**, 129–134.

Sawayama, T., Tohara, M., Katsume, H. and Nezuo, S. (1973) Polygraphic studies of the effect of nitroglycerin in patients with ischaemic heart disease. *Br. Heart J.* **35**, 1234–1239.

Schumacher, W., Budden, R., Buschmann, G. and Kühl, U. G. (1980) A new method for the evaluation of ECG and blood pressure parameters in anesthetized rats by on-line biosignal processing. *International Workshop on the Rat Electrocardiogram in Acute and Chronic Pharmacology and Toxicology*, July 14–15, 1980, Hannover.

Singh, B. N. and Hauswirth, O. (1974) Comparative mechanism of action of antiarrhythmic drugs. *Am. Heart J.* **87**, 367–382.

Spörri, H. (1944) Der Einfluß der Tuberkulose auf das Elektrokardiogramm–Untersuchungen an Meerschweinchen und Rindern. *Arch. Wiss. Prakt. Tierheilk.* **79**, 1–57.

Staib, A. H. (1967) EKG-Veränderungen bei der Ratte nach Chlorpromazin im Verlauf der postnatalen Entwicklung. *Arch. Int. Pharmacodyn. Ther.* **166**, 11–19.

Stimmel, B. (1975) The effects of mood-altering drugs on the heart. In: *Current Cardiovascular Topics* (E. Donoso, ed.), Vol. I: *Drugs in Cardiology*, part 1, pp. 203–228. Georg Thieme Publishers, Stuttgart.

Stimmel, B. (1979) *Cardiovascular Effects of Mood-altering Drugs.* Raven Press, New York.

Surawicz, B. and Lasseter, K. C. (1970) Effect of drugs on the electrocardiogram. *Prog. Cardiovasc. Dis.* **13**, 26–55.

Thorstrand, C. (1975) Cardiovascular effects of poisoning by hypnotic and tricyclic antidepressant drugs. *Acta Med. Scand. (Suppl.),* **583**, 1–34.

Thorstrand, C., Bergström, J. and Castenfors, J. (1976) Cardiac effects of amitriptyline in rats. *Scand. J. Clin. Lab. Invest.* **36**, 7–15.

Valle, L. B. S., Oliveira-Filho, R. M., Armonia, P. L., Nassif, M. and Saraceni, G., Jr. (1975) Sensibilisation de la bradycardie pendant l'hypotension finale déclenchée par la sérotonine chez le rat: Effet de la lidocaine. *Arch. Int. Physiol. Biochim.* **83**, 647–657.

Valora, N., Salvo, E. and Mei, V. (1963) Azione di alcuni farmaci sull'elettrocardiogramma del ratto. II) L'atropina. *Boll. Soc. Ital. Biol. Sper.* **39**, 152–1555.

Vargas, G., Akhtar, M. and Damato, A. N. (1975) Electrophysiologic effects of isoproterenol on cardiac conduction system in man. *Am. Heart J.* **90**, 25–34.

Vaughan Williams, E. M. (1970) Classification of anti-arrhythmic drugs. *Symposium on Cardiac Arrhythmias* (E. Sandoe, E. Flenstedt-Jensen and K. H. Olesen, eds.). A.B. Astra, Södertalje, Sweden.

Vaughan Williams, E. M. (1979) Characterisation of new antiarrhythmic drugs. In: *Newer Antiarrhythmic Agents* (P. A. van Zwieten and E. Schönbaum, eds.), pp. 13–23. Gustav Fischer Verlag, Stuttgart, New York.

Werth, G. and Dadgar, P. (1965) Zum Elektrokardiogramm der Ratte mit und ohne Narkose, bei Beatmung mit Sauerstoffmangelgemischen sowie bei Intoxikation mit Malachitgrün, unter gleichzeitiger Bestimmung des effektiven Sauerstoffverbrauches. *Arch. Kreislaufforsch.* **48**, 118–131.

Werth, G. and Wink, S. (1967) Das Elektrokardiogramm der normalen Ratte. *Arch. Kreislaufforsch.* **54**, 272–308.

Wexler, B. C. and Greenberg, B. P. (1974) Effect of exercise on myocardial infarction in young vs. old male rats: electrocardiograph changes. *Am. Heart J.* **88**, 343–350.

Wexler, B. C., Willen, D. and Greenberg, B. P. (1974) Progressive electrocardiographic changes in male and female arteriosclerotic and non-arteriosclerotic rats during the course of isoproterenol-induced myocardial infarction. *Cardiovasc. Res.* **8**, 460–468.

Wit, A. L., Hoffman, B. F. and Rosen, M. R. (1975) Electrophysiology and pharmacology of cardiac arrhythmias IX. Cardiac electrophysiologic effects of beta adrenergic receptor stimulation and blockade. Part A. *Am. Heart J.* **90**, 521–533.

Zbinden, G., Bachmann, E., Holderegger, Ch. and Elsner, J. (1977a) Cardiotoxicity of tricyclic antidepressants and neuroleptic drugs. Paper given at the 1st Int. Congress on Toxicology, Toronto, Canada, March 30–April 2.

Zbinden, G., Elsner, J. and Bolliger, H. (1977b) Toxicological evaluation of imipramine in combination with adriamycin and strophanthin. *Agents Actions* **7**, 341–346.

van Zwieten, P. A. (1977) The interaction between clonidine and various neuroleptic agents and some benzodiazepine tranquillizers. *J. Pharm. Pharmacol.* **29**, 229–234.

The Use of Electrocardiography in Toxicological Studies with Rats

D. K. DETWEILER

ABSTRACT

The electrocardiogram was first used in rat studies to monitor for cardiotoxic effects 50 years ago (1930). Since that time, particularly in the past 2 decades, its use has increased in chronic trials of four general categories: (1) nutritional studies; (2) chronic toxicity trials; (3) physiological perturbations; and (4) heart transplantation. A substantial literature on the normal rat electrocardiogram, electrocardiographic effects of various interventions and electrophysiological properties of the rat heart has accumulated during this period.

The adult rat heart, contrasted with that of other common laboratory species (guinea pig, rabbit, dog, monkey), has a variety of anomalous physiological characteristics in: (1) electrophysiological properties (short action potential (AP), short refractory period, absence of plateau in AP and ST segment in ECG, electromechanical dissociation at rapid stimulation rates); (2) ionic exchanges (absence of slow Na current during AP, no K loss with increased frequency of stimulation, hypersensitivity to Mg excitation–contraction uncoupling); (3) negative staircase with increased frequency; (4) resistance to both the positive inotropic and arrhythmogenic effects of digitalis glycosides; (5) heart weight–body weight ratio; and (6) cardiac energetics.

The rat electrocardiogram is characterized by its short QT interval, absence of ST segment, QRS vector orientation like that of carnivores and primates, and fairly stable T wave pattern.

Conventional limb and precordial lead systems have been employed frequently in rats. Precordial leads have the advantage that forelimb position does not alter the electrocardiogram as occurs in the limb leads. The triangular precordial system of Spörri (leads A,D,J) has been the one most widely used for rats.

The P, Ta, QRS, and T waves usually do not share a common isoelectric line, but originate at different levels. P waves may be followed by a measurable discordant Ta wave. The QRS complex often has a single RS, Rs or R configuration. Q waves are rarely present. The modal QRS axes in the frontal plane reported, range from $-37°$ to $130°$. A small r' wave is frequently seen. S waves may be prominent or absent. The ST segment is absent because of the lack of a plateau in the transmembrane AP. The T wave is usually concordant, with an ascending limb steeper than the descending limb. The latter approaches the isoelectric line gradually and is interrupted by the following P wave at rapid heart rates (e.g., $>450/\text{min}$). These characteristics make determination of the end of the QT interval difficult.

The rat ECG electrocardiogram is composed chiefly of frequencies between 50 and 400 Hz. The frequency components that influence the main pattern of the rat ECG are below 200 Hz.

Heart rates can vary from 250 to 750 beats/min, but generally are between 330 and 600 beats/min in electrocardiograms. Whether PR and QT intervals are rate dependent remains controversial. Various spontaneous abnormal arrhythmias and conduction defects occur in a small percentage (say 2–4%) of otherwise normal rats. Despite the small heart size, atrial and ventricular fibrillation occur in rats.

The electrocardiographic effects of drugs and other agents on the rat ECG are comparable to those seen in species without the anomalous features of the rat heart. The rat heart serves as a satisfactory model for cardiotoxicity studies except for agents, such as cardiac glycosides, to which it is insensitive.

83

I. INTRODUCTION

Historically, recording of rodent cardiac electrical potentials probably started with Buchanan (1908, 1910, 1911) who used the capillary electrometer to determine heart rates in a variety of species including the mouse and dormouse. Heart rate values from his mouse data were erroneously quoted by Schinzel (1933) as rat heart rates; these data were later cited by Heise and Kimbel (1955) and included in a table by Werth and Wink (1967). Data from papers on the rat electrocardiogram (ECG) published between 1930 and 1949 were briefly summarized by Lepeschkin (1951). Cooper (1969) cited several papers appearing between 1930 and 1966 in a short introductory review. Much of the remaining literature up to 1970 on the normal rat electrocardiogram (ECG) are referred to in the publications of Grauwiler (1965), Werth and Wink (1967), Beinfield and Lehr (1968a), and Heering (1970).

A survey of representative literature from 1930 to 1979 gives useful information on the types of experimental work with rats in which electrocardiography has been applied, characteristics and normal values for the rat electrocardiogram, types of experiments in which the use of the rat electrocardiogram may be inappropriate or misleading, and the increasing utilization of rat electrocardiography in research. In broad terms the rat ECG has been used to monitor cardiotoxic effects in several types of investigations: (1) nutritional (dietary deficiencies and excesses), (2) toxicological (drugs and various chemical agents), (3) physiological interventions (hypoxia, ischemia, hypothermia, endocrine alterations) and (4) heart transplantation.

The pioneers were Agduhr and Stenström (1930) and Drury *et al.* (1930) Drury and coworkers (1930) gave their reasons for employing electrocardiography in a study of vitamin B_1 deficiency as follows:

> "The heart presents the advantage that certain of its functions can be repeatedly and easily investigated. Electrocardiographic records can be obtained without undue disturbance of the animal, and from these the rate of the heart beat, the position at which it originates and the mode of spread of the contraction process through the heart can be accurately determined."

The effects of vitamin B_1 deficiency on the rat ECG were confirmed by later workers in the same decade (Zoll and Weiss, 1936; Weiss *et al.*, 1938). Heart rates were markedly reduced in deficient animals in these various studies, in contrast to the tachycardia common in human vitamin B_1-deficient states such as pellagra, polyneuritis and beriberi (Zoll and Weiss, 1936), suggesting that the rat heart may behave unexpectedly.

Robertson and Doyle (1937) found heart rates too variable in vitamin B_1-deficient rats to obtain a graded response to B_1 therapy. Agduhr and Stenström (1930) reported cardiac lesions and electrocardiographic changes induced by excessive cod liver oil administration in rats. Both of the 1930 papers provided initial information on normal electrocardiographic values for rats. In 1933 Schinzel, unaware of the previous publications of 1930, presented electrocardiographic data obtained from 12 normal rats, data that he thought might establish his priority. It is interesting that Schinzel's thesis was written under the preceptorship of Prof. Johannes Nörr, whose early contributions to veterinary electrocardiography, beginning in 1913, establish him as the founder of veterinary clinical electrocardiography.

The next decade (1940–1949) did not see a dramatic increase in publications on rat electrocardiography. Moses (1946) determined the heart rate in trained, resting rats, restrained in a special holder. Several authors confirmed the electrocardiographic effects of vitamin B_1 deficiency (Heerswynghels and Thomas, 1945; Hundley *et al.*, 1945; King and Sebrell, 1946); Crismon (1944) reported on the effects of hypothermia; Ensor (1946) found minimum electrocardiographic changes in vitamin E deficiency; Waller and Charipper (1945) studied the effects of thyroidectomy and thiourea administration; Leblond and Hoff (1944) observed the effects of thyroidectomy followed by thyroxine derivatives and dinitrophenol administration; and Rappaport and Rappaport (1943) discussed technical problems encountered in amplifying and recording the high frequency components of small mammal ECGs, using the mouse as their experimental subject.

Interest in rat electrocardiography remained meager in the next decade (1950–1959) as well. During this period, however, attention was given to the characteristics of the rat ECG *per se* and to recording technics. Data on normal rat ECGs were reported by Lombard (1952) and Kisch (1953). The important paper of Heise and Kimbel appeared in 1955, providing statistical data on records obtained from 166 anesthetized rats. These authors claimed that it was virtually impossible to record readable ECGs from unanesthetized rats, an assertion that was to influence later workers even though previous investigators had published satisfactory data and records from unanesthetized subjects in the 1930's and 1940's (q.v.). Beinfield and Lehr (1956) initiated their notable studies of the rat ECG with a paper on the advantages of the prone body position for recording. Their method of recording stabilized foreleg position so that tall R waves were recorded consistently in lead I, in contrast to the variable complexes in lead I obtained by Hundley *et al.* (1945) who restrained their subjects by hand in a crouched position. Berg (1955) described the effects of aging on the ECG in anesthetized rats in the supine position; Irmak and Aykut (1955) com-

D. K. Detweiler

pared the rat ECG with that of other species; and Kayser (1956) observed the effects of hypothermia on electrocardiographic time intervals of anesthetized, curarized and atropinized rats. Grünberg and Hundt (1958) studied the effects of body position, discovered the influence of foreleg position on ECG vectors in rats, and identified a short ST segment in records taken at a paper speed exceeding 100 mm/sec. Gessler and Kuner (1959) investigated the ECG effects of ether and hypoxia. Lepeschkin's useful review appeared in 1951 and Zuckermann (1959) included the rat ECG in an atlas of ECGs from many animal species.

As in most scientific fields, the tempo of research on the rat electrocardiogram and its applications increased dramatically during the next decade (1960–1969). In 1965 Grauwiler published an exhaustive compilation of animal electrocardiographic data from the literature and from original observations.

Grauwiler and Spörri (1960) classified animal species electrocardiographically into two groups on the basis of the relative durations of electrical and mechanical systole. Spörri (1956) and his student Siegfried (1956) had previously reported on the marked dissociation of electrical and mechanical systole in kangaroos, a feature found in various insectivores, bats and rodents including the rat (rat, mouse, Schinzel, 1933; hedgehog, Johansson, 1957; mole, Detweiler and Spörri, 1957; bat, Zuckermann, 1959; hamster, Lombard, 1952; field mouse, gerbil, spiny mouse, dormouse, Grauwiler, 1965). Hamlin and Smith (1965) categorized animals electrocardiographically, in accordance with the pattern of ventricular excitation, into two groups, A and B, placing the rat in group A together with man, monkey, dog and cat.

Werth and Wink's (1967) monumental analysis of 1971 electrocardiograms from ether anesthetized rats followed Werth and Dadgar's (1965) study indicating that light ether narcosis had little effect on the electrocardiogram.

Beinfield and Lehr (1968a, 1968b) confirmed their observations, describing in detail the normal characteristics of the PR and QRST complexes in etherized rats, the effects of induction of anesthesia and the effects of hypercalcemia and hyperkalemia. Fraser *et al.* (1967) presented electrocardiographic data from ether anesthetized rats, and Kenedi (1968) claimed to be able to distinguish the ST segment and U wave in unanesthetized rat electrocardiograms taken at a paper speed of 80 to 100 mm/sec and magnified photographically 5 to 10 times. Angelakos and Bernardini (1963), using a cathode ray oscilloscope, determined that rat QRS complexes are composed of frequencies from 50 to 400 Hz, asserting that gross distortion of the electrocardiographic signals would occur if electrocardiographs with a frequency response less than 250 Hz were employed. These authors concluded therefore, that most direct writing electrocardiographs then available would be inadequate to record rat ECGs. This point of view was refuted by Godwin and Fraser (1965) who compared cathode ray oscilloscope records with those recorded by a direct-writing electrocardiograph with a frequency response 3 db down at 175 Hz and a slow fall off such that at 200 Hz a 50% response remained. These authors concluded that the frequencies influencing the chief patterns of the rat ECG would be less than 200 Hz.

Another important but hitherto neglected contribution during this era is that of Valora and Mei (1963) who published an atlas (44 figures) of electrocardiographic alterations produced by procainamide, quinidine, acetylcholine, atropine, noradrenaline, lanatoside and strophanthin.

Hunt and Kimeldorf (1960) recorded heart rate values in sleeping rats and found that the heart rates corresponded with those obtained under anesthesia. Adolph (1967) determined maximal electrical driving rates for rats under pentobarbital anesthesia for the fetus, newborn and adult. Jones *et al.* (1962) found that the incidence of cardiac arrhythmias increased dramatically with aging from 3 to 28 months.

The remainder of the papers published during this decade dealt with a variety of perturbances affecting the rat electrocardiogram including the effects of various drugs and chemicals such as: digitalis glycosides (Valora and Mei, 1963; Arcasoy and Smuckler, 1969; Franke and Joshi, 1967), adrenergic compounds, reserpine, emetine (Marmo, 1969); metrochlorpyramid (Marmo *et al.*, 1969); chlorpromazine (Staib, 1967); ^{60}Co exposure (Klütsch *et al.*, 1968); hydrocortisone/NaPO$_4$ and 1.0% NaCl drinking water (Badarau *et al.*, 1969); aconitine and calcium chloride (Bianchi *et al.*, 1968); manganese (Conrad and Baxter, 1963). Various interferences were also studied: hypoxia (Hundt and Grünberg, 1960; Scheuer and Stezoski, 1968a, 1968b, 1969; Cooper, 1969); hemorrhage and hypervolemia (Cooper, 1969); hypophysectomy, thyroidectomy (Gargouil, 1960, Gargouil *et al.*, 1960); adrenalectomy (Gargouil *et al.*, 1961; Tricoche *et al.*, 1961); calcium deficiency (Conrad and Baxter, 1966); selenium deficiency (Godwin, 1965); adrenalectomy (Monnereau–Soustre, 1966); daunomycin (Herman *et al.*, 1969); isoproterenol and vasopressin (Leszkovszky *et al.*, 1967). Other studies included: evolution of the neonatal ECG from 1–72 hours after birth (Mei *et al.*, 1964); coronary occlusion, infarction (Normann *et al.*, 1961; Hill *et al.*, 1960); strain differences (Godwin and Fraser, 1965); hypertension (Sambhi and White, 1960); and cardiac transplantation (Abbott *et al.*, 1964, 1965).

Arrigo and Dulio (1964a, 1964b, 1964c) published transmembrane action potential (TMAP) records from unperturbed atrial and ventricular cells and following vagotomy, hypothermia, hypoxia and reserpine administration. Tricoche *et al.* (1963) found that the T waves and the TMAP of *Rattus rattus* differed characteristically from those of *Rattus norvegicus*.

At the beginning of the next decade (1970–1979) Heering (1970) published a detailed analysis of the rat ECG from records taken with a direct-writing electrocardiograph supplemented by computer-averaged data from signals recorded continuously over long periods of time on magnetic tape. This important paper stresses the marked spontaneous variations in time intervals, wave forms and amplitudes of limb lead ECGs from restrained, unanesthetized rats. Manoach et al. (1977) reconfirmed the presence of an ST segment in fetal rat ECGs. Recording telemetered ECGs from unrestrained rats Meinrath et al. (1977) noted genetic strain and weight-related variations in heart rates. Blandon et al. (1974) described the electrocardiographic changes caused by spontaneous Chaga's disease (*Trypanosoma cruzi* infection) in wild rats (*Rattus rattus*) trapped in areas where the disease is epidemic. Heethaar et al. (1973a, 1973b) worked out a mathematical model of atrioventricular conduction in the rat. Osborne (1973) designed a restraining device for recording rat ECGs.

The remainder of studies during the period reflect the increasing use of electrocardiography in toxicological studies with rats. Among the agents studied were: anthracycline antibiotics (Nemec, 1973; Cargill et al., 1974; Bachmann et al., 1975a, 1975b; Zbinden and Brändle, 1975; Zbinden, 1975, 1977; Zbinden et al., 1977a, 1977c, 1977d; Zbinden et al., 1978a, 1978b); tricyclic antidepressants (Bianchetti et al., 1977; Zbinden et al., 1977b, 1977d; Davidson, 1977, Lisciani et al., 1978); phenothiazine tranquilizers (Langslet, 1970; Zbinden et al., 1977b); isoproterenol cardiomyopathy (Kowalczykowa et al., 1971; Balazs, 1973; Wexler and Greenberg, 1974; Guideri et al., 1974, 1975; Davidson, 1977); cobalt cardiomyopathy (Grice et al., 1970; Heggtveit et al., 1970; Davidson, 1977); desoxycorticosterone and 1% NaCl drinking water sensitization to isoproterenol arrhythmias (Guideri et al., 1974, 1975); aerosol propellants (Dorato et al., 1974; Doherty and Aviado, 1975; Durakovic, 1976); cadmium (Hawley and Kopp, 1975; Kopp and Hawley, 1978); rapeseed oil (Hunsacker et al., 1972); mercuric oxycyanide (Juskowa, 1972); benzene, toluene and xylene (Morvai et al., 1976); dehydroemetine (Salako and Durotye, 1972); morphine (Stein, 1976); ouabain (Nadeau and Champlain, 1973; Zbinden et al., 1977d); ajmalene, spartein, aconitine (V. Philipsborn, 1973); β-adrenolytic agents (Marmo and Robertaccio, 1970); palladium compounds (Wiester, 1975); alcohol on B_1-deficient hearts (Yamashita, 1971a, 1971b); high fat diet alone (Zbinden and Rageth, 1978); and with adriamycin (Zbinden et al., 1977c); hypoxia (Calprino et al., 1978); pentobarbital (Driscoll, 1979; ethanol (Hillbom and Boguslawsky, 1978); dopamine (Graf and Leuschner, 1978); lidocaine (Valle et al., 1975). Two papers involved computer analysis of rat ECGs (Caprino et al., 1978; Heering, 1970) and two dealt with telemetered ECGs (Dorato et al., 1974; Meinrath et al., 1977).

II. ANOMALOUS PHYSIOLOGY OF THE RAT HEART

Of the species that have short QT intervals relative to mechanical systole (Grauwiler and Spörri, 1960) physiological characteristics of the heart have been studied most extensively in the rat (Langer, 1978).

The Transmembrane Action Potential (TMAP)

The TMAP of rat ventricular cells is substantially shorter than the duration of mechanical contraction. Phase 2 (plateau) of the TMAP is absent and its total duration relatively shorter than the TMAP duration of species in which the plateau is present (Langer *et al.*, 1975; Langer, 1978; Kelly and Hoffman, 1960; Mainwood and Lee, 1969). The form and duration of rat atrial and ventricular cell TMAPs are similar (Arrigo and Dulio, 1964a) unlike other mammalian species that have long ventricular cell TMAPs with a plateau and shorter atrial cell TMAPs lacking a plateau (Hoffman and Cranefield, 1960; Surawicz, 1972). The short TMAP accounts for the short effective electrical refractory period of less than 50 msec (Mainwood and Lee, 1969).

These characteristics are not present prenatally nor during the early neonatal period, but are gradually acquired during the first 3 to 4 weeks of life (Langer *et al.*, 1975; Langer, 1978; Bernard and Gargouil, 1970; Couch *et al.*, 1969). Similarly, in young kangaroos still in the pouch the QRST has an ST segment (which corresponds to phase 2 of the TMAP) and duration similar to mechanical systole in the adult (Spörri, 1956). Langer *et al.* (1975) and Langer (1978) attribute this progressive loss of plateau and TMAP shortening to a gradual closing of the slow inward Na current channel as the animal ages. Langer *et al.* (1975) demonstrated that a major factor contributing to the prolonged plateau in the neonate is this slow inward Na conductance.

Electromechanical Uncoupling

Mainwood and Lee (1969) have shown in rat papillary muscles, that short-paired pacing intervals uncouple the electrical and mechanical response following the second stimulus. The electrical refractory period was from 50 to 80 msec. At these short pacing intervals the second stimulus evoked no mechanical response. As the paired pacing interval was increased beyond 80 msec, the second mechanical response began to recover. Thus, the rat myocardium cannot be summated or tetanized because of a long mechanical refractory period duration exceeding that of the electrical refractory period. This loss of mechanical response is attributed to depletion of the intracellular releasable Ca for excitation–contraction coupling, i.e., the coupling mechanism has its own refractory period determined by the time required for replenishing Ca ions for release at the next contraction.

Ionic Exchange

Increasing the heart rate in most mammalian species results in K loss from cardiac tissue. This fails to occur in the rat heart (Langer, 1978). In the rat heart Mg perfusion depresses K exchange markedly and has an excitation–contraction uncoupling effect: actions that are minimal in rabbit cardiac tissue (Langer, 1978).

Positive (Bowditch) and Negative (Woodworth) Staircase

The usual response to increasing stimulation frequency is an increase in developed tension (positive or Bowditch staircase). During the first week of life, rat cardiac tissue exhibits a marked positive staircase. This diminishes over the next 3 weeks and in the adult rat increasing frequency reduces contractile force (negative or Woodworth staircase) (Langer *et al.*, 1975; Kruta and Braveny, 1960).

Response to Digitalis Glycosides

The adult rat heart is relatively insensitive to the positive inotropic effect of digitalis glycosides (Langer *et al.*, 1975). Although, it has been suggested that the insensitivity of Na–K ATPase to cardiac glycosides accounts for the lack of response of the adult rat heart (Repke *et al.*, 1965; Allen and Schwartz, 1969; Tobin and Brody, 1972), the sensitivity of Na–K ATPase to cardiac glycosides from the neonatal and adult rat hearts was identical, indicating that the lack of response in the adult heart cannot be attributed to this factor (Langer, 1978). The intact rat is likewise highly resistant to the toxic and arrhythmogenic effects of cardiac glycosides (Detweiler, 1967).

Mechanism of Anomalous Contractile Responses

Langer (1978) has suggested that the negative staircase response and resistance to digitalis glycosides have the same cause, related to the decrease in the slow inward Na current during the TMAP and the associated loss of TMAP plateau. In mammalian hearts with a plateau, both increasing rate of stimulation and digitalis glycosides increase intracellular Na significantly and have a positive inotropic effect. These interventions do not increase intracellular Na (as indicated by absence of a net K loss) in the adult rat (Langer, 1978). The increase in intracellular Na is attributed to a greater opportunity for Na influx with an increased number of excitations per minute or to inhibition of the Na pump by digitalis. Part of the mechanism that introduces Ca into the cell for excitation–contraction coupling is movement across the sarcolemma via a carrier system that couples the movement of 1 Ca ion inward in exchange for the passage of 2 Na ions outward. Increase in intracellular Na is the stimulus activating the Na–Ca carrier. In the adult rat heart the slow Na channel influx during the TMAP is lost. This limits inward flow of Na with each excitation and accounts for the lack of increased intracellular Na with increased rate of digitalis action. This, in turn would result in little increase in intracellular Ca which is thought to be the mechanism for positive inotropy in each case.

Cardiac Energetics

Rats have a lower heart weight/body weight (HW/BW) ratio than man or dog: rat, 3.8 g/kg; man, 5.3 g/kg; dog 8 g/kg (Loiselle and Gibbs, 1979). The rat heart weight/body weight ratio increases with aging from 2.9 g/kg at 219 days of age to 4.8 g/kg at 950 days of age in males (Berg, 1955). Actually, however, this increase is not the result of a relative increase in heart weight. The absolute weight of the heart did not increase significantly in males between day 577 (3.2 g/kg HW/BW) and day 950 (4.8 g/kg HW/BW). Thus, a body weight decrease accounted for the increased HW/BW ratio with aging (Berg, 1955). Although the rat heart has a higher oxygen consumption/hundred g/minute (rat, 17.6; dog, 9.3; man, 8.9 ml $O_2/100$ g min^{-1}), the rat has a high total metabolic rate and the relative contribution of the heart to total body metabolism is lower than in dog or man (i.e., ratio of cardiac oxygen usage ($\dot{E}_H$) to total body oxygen usage ($\dot{E}_B$) or $\dot{E}_H/\dot{E}_B$ = rat, 3.6; dog, 10.4; man, 9.6). Even though both cardiac oxygen consumption per gram of tissue and the basal metabolic rate per gram of body weight are about twice as high in rats as in dogs, the relative contribution of the rat heart to total basal metabolism is only about 1/3 that of the dog even though the heart rate/body weight ratio of the rat is about 1/2 that of the dog (Loiselle and Gibbs, 1979).

In summary, the adult rat heart has a variety of physiological characteristics that differ from those of man and the usual experimental animals (guinea pig, rabbit, dog, and monkey). The unique characteristics include: (1) electrophysiological properties (short TMAP duration; absence of plateau in the TMAP; short electrical refractory period; electromechanical uncoupling at rapid stimulation rates (stimulation intervals of 30–80 msec); absence of an ST segment in the QRST complex); (2) ionic exchanges (absence of slow Na current during the TMAP; no K loss with increased frequency of stimulation; hypersensitivity to Mg excitation–contraction uncoupling); (3) negative staircase with increased frequency; (4) resistance to both the positive inotropic and arrhythmogenic effects of digitalis glycosides; (5) heart weight/body weight ratio; and (6) cardiac energetics.

III. TYPES OF ADULT MAMMALIAN ELECTROCARDIOGRAMS

There are three chief species differences in mammalian electrocardiograms: (1) dissimilarity in the duration of the QT interval relative to the duration of mechanical systole (the short QT intervals are associated with absence of an ST segment); (2) disparity in the direction and sense of the QRS vectors (caused by differences in the pattern of ventricular depolarization); (3) inequality in the degree of T wave lability.

QT Duration and ST Segment

Many rodents, insectivores, bats, and kangaroos have short QT intervals relative to the duration of mechanical systole (Grauwiler and Spörri, 1960). In these species the ST segment is essentially absent so that the QRST complex consists of brief rapid QRS deflections followed immediately by the slower T wave. This is in contrast to the classical QRST complex of the remainder of mammalians that has a distinct ST segment and a QT interval equivalent to mechanical systole.

QRS Vector Direction and Sense

The ventricular activation patterns of various species fall into two general types (Hamlin and Smith, 1965; Roshchevsky, 1978).

Group A. Dog, man, monkey, cat, rat, etc., have QRS vectors that, generally, produce a largely negative deflection in lead V_{10} and positive deflection in the lead aVF.

Group B. Hoofed mammals, dolphins, etc., have QRS vectors that, generally produce largely positive deflections in V_{10} and negative deflections in aVF.

These differences in the pattern of ventricular excitation are associated with the distributive characteristics of the Purkinje network. In group A animals, it is primarily a subendocardial network. In group B animals, the Purkinje network is more elaborate and penetrates deeply into the ventricular myocardium (Robb, 1965).

T Wave lability

In man, primates, and many hoofed mammals, limb lead T wave amplitude and polarity tend to be fairly constant. In dogs and especially in horses T wave vectors are quite labile in polarity and amplitude in limb and some thoracic leads. In dogs T waves in all except two of the conventional leads may vary in polarity in serial records. The two exceptional leads are CV_5RL and V_{10} in which T is normally positive (CV_5RL) or negative (V_{10}) in about 90 percent of individuals (Hill, 1968a, 1968b).

IV. THE NORMAL RAT ELECTROCARDIOGRAM

Leads and Lead Systems

Schinzel (1933) in accordance with concepts of the day, determined the anatomical base–apex axis of the heart and applied bipolar leads on the body surface over the area of the cardiac apex and base. The landmarks were left fourth intercostal space 0.75 mm from the sternum (apex region) and anterior to and 0.5 cm above the dorsal border of the right scapula (base region). This is a so-called axial lead. Since the apical lead is closer to the heart than the base lead, it is essentially a precordial lead with the relatively indifferent electrode at the area of the right dorsal scapula.

The lead system adopted by Spörri (1944) for quadrupeds, reminiscent of the heart triangle of W. Nehb (Lepeschkin, 1951), consists of bipolar leads from the right dorsal scapular region to the sacral area (lead D or dorsal): right dorsal scapular region to cardiac apex region (lead A or axial) and sacral area to the cardiac apex region (lead J or inferior). Employing the conventional limb lead electrodes in this system lead D consists of the RA–LA electrodes (lead I electrodes) lead A the RA–LF electrodes (lead II electrodes), and lead J the LA–LF electrodes (lead III electrodes). Essentially, this system consists of a longitudinal lead (D employing conventional lead I electrodes) equivalent to conventional lead II; and two precordial leads: A and J, in which conventional electrode LF is at the cardiac apex region paired with an indifferent electrode at the scapular region (RA electrode, conventional lead II electrode pair) and at the sacral area (LA electrode, conventional lead III electrode pair). The advantages of this system are that only three electrodes are required, forelimb position has virtually no effect on the records, and ventricular ectopic beats are usually clearly aberrant in at least one of the leads (Fig. 1). Some investigators have routinely employed lead D alone in rat toxicological studies (e.g., Bachmann *et al.*, 1975b; Zbinden and Brändle, 1975; Zbinden *et al.*, 1977a, 1977b, 1977c, 1978a, 1978b).

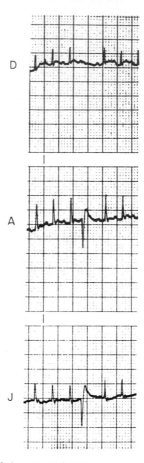

Fig. 1. Leads D, A, and J of the precordial triangular system recorded simultaneously. A premature ventricular ectopic beat (4th complex) is clearly recorded in leads A and J, but a distinct QRST complex cannot be distinguished with certainty in lead D. This illustrates the advantage of recording three leads simultaneously. Were lead D the only record available a certain diagnosis of the arrhythmia would not be possible, in this case. See also Fig. 2, p. 120 in the paper by G. Zbinden.

For the most part, investigators have used the bipolar limb lead system of Einthoven (leads, I, II, III) with or without the augmented unipolar limb leads (aVR, aVL, aVF). The disadvantage of limb leads is that foreleg position changes can alter the scalar ECG wave amplitudes and mimic actual vector changes. The influence of foreleg position on the amplitude and direction of limb lead electrocardiographic waves of the rat was first noted by Grünberg and Hundt (1958) but was largely ignored by subsequent investigators (Fig. 2).

Various thoracic leads paired with the central terminal of Wilson have been applied by several investigators with the exploring electrode attached to the chest in positions somewhat equivalent to the electrode positions used in man (Norman *et al.*, 1961; Fraser *et al.*, 1967; Klütsch *et al.*, 1968; Cooper, 1969; Badarau *et al.*, 1969; Langslet, 1970; Juskowa, 1972; Blandon *et al.*, 1974; Wexler and Greenberg, 1974; Guideri *et al.*, 1975; Abbott, 1975). Some workers used a transthoracic bipolar lead (Stein, 1976) or a right to left shoulder bipolar lead (Jones *et al.*, 1967).

Form and Amplitude

The conventional waves of mammalian electrocardiograms, P, QRS, and T are all identifiable in the rat electrocardiogram (Werth and Wink, 1967; Heering, 1970) although there is controversy about the presence or absence of the ST segment (Grauwiler and Spörri, 1960; Grünberg and Hundt, 1958; Kenedi, 1968). At rapid heart rates (e.g., >450/min) the P wave is often superimposed on the descending limb of the preceding T wave and a distinct Ta (atrial T wave) is frequently present (Beinfield and Lehr, 1968a).

The isoelectric line. Determining amplitudes of the electrocardiographic waves in rat ECGs presents a special problem because the points at which P, Ta, QRS and T waves originate are often at different levels (Beinfield and Lehr, 1968a), i.e., there is no isoelectric line during the electrocardiographic complex. Thus, no common baseline is shared by the deflections. The termination of the P wave often appears lowered by the inscription of a discordant Ta wave. The level of the junction of the termination of QRS and origin of T often appears displaced upwards or downwards from the T–P baseline level. This QRS–T junction is actually being inscribed at the time when ventricular repolarization is rather well advanced in those areas first depolarized but just beginning in the parts of the ventricles activated terminally (Beinfield and Lehr, 1968b; Spear, 1980).

The P and Ta waves. The P wave is normally positive in leads I, II, III and aVF, negative in aVR and flat or negative in aVL. Negative P waves in lead III are common (Werth and Wink, 1967; Heise and Kimbel, 1955). The Ta wave is usually discordant relative to the P wave and appears to terminate prior to the onset of the QRS complex or is of such low amplitude at this point that the remainder of atrial repolarization activity is no longer registered (Beinfield and Lehr, 1968a).

The QRS complex. In leads I, II, III, the Q wave is usually absent (Werth and Wink, 1967; Heering, 1978) but small Q waves are sometimes recorded (Lepeschkin, 1951; Hundley *et al.*, 1945). In bipolar limb leads there is usually a prominent R wave and the S wave may be prominent or absent

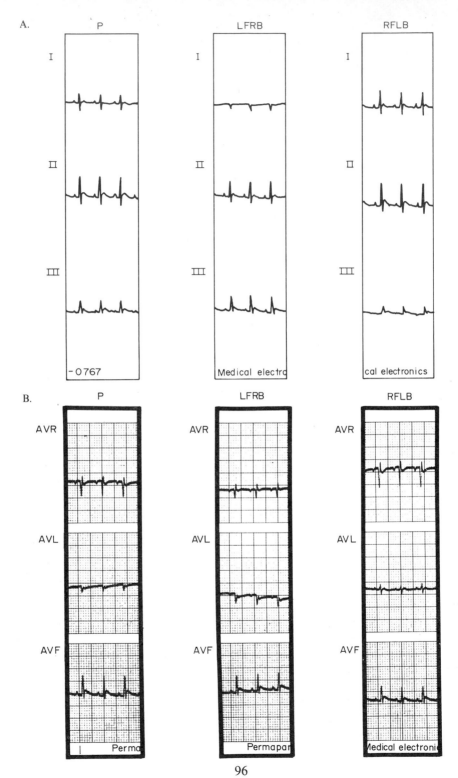

96

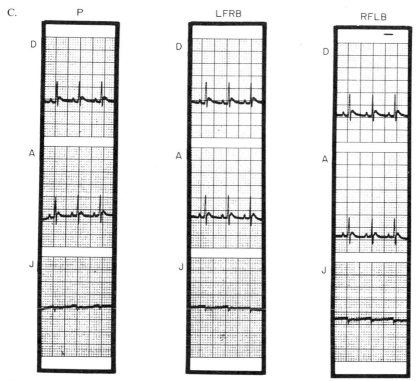

Fig. 2. The effect of foreleg position on the electrocardiograms in limb leads and thoracic leads. The rat was placed in the prone position P, forelegs held parallel; LFRB, left foreleg pulled forward, right foreleg pulled backward; RFLB, right foreleg pulled forward, left foreleg pulled backward. A. Leads I, II, III. B. Leads aVR, aVL, aVF. C. Leads D, A, J. Note especially the changes in QRS pattern produced by these foreleg position shifts in limb leads I, III, aVR and aVL. Configurational changes are minor in leads II and aVF in this subject. As expected, all three thoracic leads D, A, and J were unaffected by forelimb positional changes.

(Heering, 1970; Werth and Wink, 1967). It is often difficult to separate the termination of the S wave and the onset of the T wave.

The QRS axis (frontal plane). The QRS axis determined from limb lead records can be influenced by changes in foreleg position and body position (Grünberg and Hundt, 1958) (Fig. 2). Since body positioning and foreleg positioning has not been standardized, available data on the QRS axis is difficult to evaluate. Lepeschkin (1951) concluded that the QRS axis is about 80° and decreases with growth. This change toward the left with aging corresponds to the finding of Werth and Wink (1967) that the percentage of rats with a left type QRS axis increases in older and post-partum groups of rats. According to Angelakos and Bernardini (1963), in rats at 2 to 3 months (150–200 g) of age the right ventricle has not completely regressed from its neonatal condition. The modal QRS axis shifts progressively toward the left during the next 1 to 2 months and reaches the adult pattern at the fourth or fifth month of life. Since in the dog the evolution to the adult ECG pattern requires only 2 to 3 months (Trautvetter *et al.*, 1980) this long delay is unexpected in the rat. Angelakos and Bernardini (1963) determined the modal QRS axis to be 87° with a range of 57°–130°. Beinfield and Lehr (1968a) gave values of 49.6° $\pm$ 22.6° S.D. (range $-22°$ to 120°) with 86 of 91 rats falling between 1° and 90°. Fraser *et al.* (1967) reported values of 47° $\pm$ 33° S.D. from 100 rats. Juskowa's (1972) values were: 81.4%, 25° to 70°; 11.1%, 2° to $-37°$ and 7.4%, 85° to 125°. The scatter of these data would undoubtedly be reduced were positioning of the subjects standardized as recommended for the dog (Detweiler and Patterson, 1965; Hill, 1968; Detweiler, 1981).

A small r' wave that may appear after the ascending limb of the S wave intersects the isoelectric line can sometimes be detected (e.g., in limb lead electrocardiograms I, II, III) (Heering, 1970). It corresponds to the small wave designated by Heise and Kimbel (1955) as "Nachschwankung". When present it is separated from the T wave by a small negative wave.

ST segment. It is generally agreed that the rat electrocardiogram does not have an isoelectric ST segment with a duration relative to the QT interval comparable to that of species in which the QT interval and mechanical systole are equivalent (Grauwiler and Spörri, 1960; Werth and Wink, 1967; Beinfield and Lehr, 1968b). At rapid paper speeds, however, a short (about 10 to 12 msec), somewhat inconstant isoelectric segment separating the QRS complex and T wave may be recorded (Grünberg and Hundt, 1958; Mei *et al.*, 1964; Kenedi, 1968). This has led to controversy and several authors refer to ST segment deviation following certain interventions such as hypoxia.

Actually, the absence of a distinct ST segment in the rat electrocardiogram can be correlated with the characteristics of the rat ventricular muscle TMAP (Arrigo and Dulio, 1964a, 1964b, 1964c; Spear, 1980) (Fig. 3). As noted previously the TMAP of the rat ventricular cell lacks a distinct plateau normally, although a slowing of the repolarization curve descent may occur.

In rats anesthetized with pentobarbital, Na, Spear (1980) found the following values: heart rate 315/min; PR, 56; QRS, 16; and QT, 50 msec. The duration of the TMAP from onset to 50% repolarization ($TMAP_{50}$) averages 25 msec. The point of 50% repolarization is chosen because in all types of hearts repolarization is rapid at this level. It is this rapid drop in potential, occurring in masses of cells out of phase with the same event in other masses of cells in the ventricles, that generates the T wave in the electrocardiogram. This is true both for species that have and those that do not have an ST segment. Since the entire repolarization curve of the normal rat TMAP descends rapidly, the T wave of the rat electrocardiogram

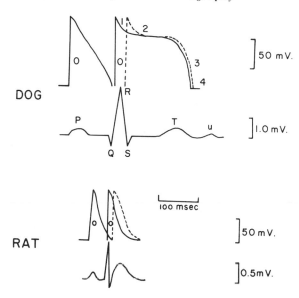

Fig. 3. Schema of atrial and ventricular transmembrane action potentials (TMAP) and the electrocardiogram (ECG) drawn on the same time scale. The five phases of the dog TMAP are labeled: 0, initial rapid depolarization or spike; 1, initial rapid repolarization; 2, slow repolarization or plateau; 3, final rapid repolarization; 4, resting or diastolic transmembrane potential. Note that the rat and dog atrial and the rat ventricular TMAPs have no plateau. The TMAPs drawn with a solid line represent excitation of ventricular cells early during the QRS interval; those drawn with a dashed line represent excitation of ventricular cells later during the QRS interval. Note that in the dog the plateaus of the TMAPs overlap so that there is little difference in charge between groups of cells. This period of overlap coincides with the isopotential ST segment of the ECG. The T wave of the dog ECG is generated during final rapid repolarization, phase 3, when at any given instant in time the charges of different masses of cells are not the same. In the rat, the ventricular TMAPs do not have a plateau and there is no period during repolarization when most cells are isopotential. Thus, no ST segment appears in the ECG.

begins to be generated within a few milliseconds after the onset of ventricular activation, i.e., as soon as a sufficient number of cells have been activated and are repolarizing so that measurable potential differences are generated.

Because the activation time (QRS interval) is short (e.g., 16 msec) relative to the total duration of the rat ventricular muscle TMAP (e.g., TMAP 50–80 msec) almost all of the ventricular muscle cells have been activated before any of the cells have repolarized to 50% of the resting potential (e.g. $TMAP_{50}$ may be 25 msec). Thus, the ventricular repolarization interval extends beyond the QRS interval for about 2.5 or more times the QRS interval duration (e.g., from Werth and Wink (1967) data, the mean QRS is 21 msec, QT, 75 msec and T, 54 msec.). For this reason a large portion of the repolarization phase follows the excitation phase and is reflected as a distinct T wave in the rat ECG. It is important to emphasize, however, that the generation of the T wave begins before excitation (QRS interval) is completed and thus, part of the T wave is buried (or masked) by the larger QRS waves. Thus, potential differences exist all during the QT interval and no ST segment is formed (Fig. 3). Therefore, the apparent beginning of the T wave may be above or below the isoelectric level because the early portion of the R potential generated by repolarizing cells has displaced the baseline. The actual beginning of the T wave occurs during the latter complex and atrial TMAPs have no plateau (Fig. 3). Further, the extracellular record of cardiac action potential (either electrogram or electrocardiogram) approximates the first time derivative of the TMAP, dV/dt (Noble and Cohen, 1978). Thus, a plateau in the TMAP must be present to produce an isoelectric segment in the extracellular record. These considerations support the concept that absence of the TMAP plateau is crucial to the lack of an ST segment.

Another reason for the T wave taking off at a point above or below the isopotential point is that the frequency response of the instrument is too slow to record a rapid potential reaching the isopotential level. If a distinct ST segment appears in the rat electrocardiogram it is abnormal, except when part of the T wave is isopotential in a given load because the lead line is so oriented that part of T wave vector is not recorded. Werth and Wink (1967) have noted that hypoxemia produces ST segment formation with a broad rounded T wave and bradycardia (250–300 beats/min) in normal rats deeply anesthetized with ether. This is probably because TMAP duration is increased and a plateau is produced by hypoxia, as shown by Arrigo and Dulio (1964c). These latter authors showed that a plateau develops in the rat ventricular TMAP when bradycardia is induced by such interventions as hypothermia, hypoxia and reserpine administration (Arrigo and Dulio, 1964a, 1964b, 1964c). Obviously, many agents affecting cardiac cell membrane electrophysiologic properties could have this effect.

Electrocardiographers find it hard to give up the concept of the ST segment, even in records where it cannot be identified. In the classical (textbook) ECGs the ST segment, as an isoelectric period separating the QRS complex and the T wave, shifts from its isoelectric position when injury potentials occur as the result of damage to the myocardium.

Actually, in numerous species (e.g., in the dog) the ST segment is not a flat isoelectric line in many leads. The presence of a stable isoelectric ST segment depends on 2 factors: (1) the occurrence of a distinct plateau and consequent long duration of the TMAP and (2) in large hearts the presence of a rapid conduction system that spreads the excitation quickly. Ventricular ectopic beats, for example, in large hearts result in slowing of depolarization throughout the ventricle such that synchrony of the plateau period in various parts of the heart is reduced and the ST segment, consequently, is abbreviated.

The same perturbations that produce ST segment deviations in species with a distinct ST segment, may produce a similar shift of the slow wave portion of QRST complex in the rat. This has sometimes been referred to as ST segment deviation in damaged rat hearts (Cooper, 1969), although, normally, an ST segment cannot be identified. To avoid confusion in terminology, it is suggested that when an abnormal ST segment appears in a rat electrocardiogram the term should be placed in quotation marks (e.g., "ST" segment elevation or depression) since this term is not entirely equivalent for the two groups of animals distinguished by the presence or absence of a distinct ST segment.

The T wave. The T wave is usually positive and concordant with QRS in leads II and III, not infrequently negative and discordant in lead I (Werth and Wink, 1967) and may be reversed in this lead by such interventions as anesthesia (Beinfield and Lehr, 1968a). The ascending limb of the T wave is characteristically steeper than the descending limb. The latter usually approaches the isoelectric line gradually and its end is the most difficult of all the ECG waves to define (Heering, 1970). Added to this is the complication that the following P wave may interrupt its descent. This led Heering (1970) to define the termination of the T wave as the point at which it becomes horizontal or the point at which the next P wave begins. This latter criterion would clearly misrepresent the true duration of the QT interval. These difficulties have caused some investigators to measure the QTa interval (Lepeschkin, 1965) (i.e., the interval from the beginning of QRS to the apex of T) as an indication of the QT duration. The problem with this is that the form of the T wave may change in serial records so that the T apex shifts within the QT segment while the QT interval remains constant.

The ST–T complex in all species is the most variable part of the ECG and the most subject to drug-induced effects. This is because the recovery phases 2 and 3 (plateau and final rapid repolarization) of the TMAP are markedly affected by drug action or electrolyte changes (Surawicz, 1972) that have little effect on the spread of excitation and therefore, do not alter the form of the QRS complex. Since these changes are not secondary to alterations in the spread of excitation they are called primary T wave changes (Surawicz, 1966). The T wave changes produced by drugs are generally primary.

As pointed out by Beinfield and Lehr (1968b) and Heering (1970) the conformations of the ECG complexes tend to vary somewhat in continuous records, especially the terminal portions of the QRS complex and the T waves.

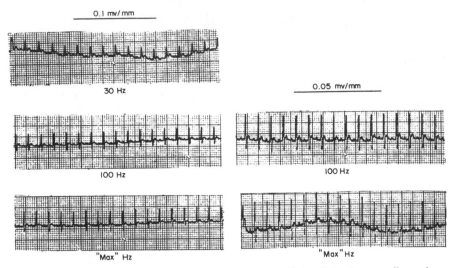

Fig. 4. The effect of changing frequency response and sensitivity of the electrocardiograph on the form of the rat ECG. The two sensitivity settings 0.1 and 0.05 mV/mm are indicated above each set of records. Frequency response was changed by interposing a 2 pole filter. At each frequency setting (30 Hz, 100 Hz and "Max" Hz (about 200 Hz)) there is 70% transmission of the signal. Note that at 30 Hz the S wave of the ECG is not present. There is no great difference between the ECGs recorded at the 2 higher frequency settings. The higher sensitivity recording (0.05 mV/mm) produces an apparent change in the form of the T wave. This is because its amplitude is doubled by greater amplification, but its width is not changed since the paper speed is the same. (Record courtesy of Mr. Paul Struve)

Frequency Components of the Rat ECG

In 1943 Rappaport and Rappaport found that electrocardiographs of that era were incapable of faithfully recording the cardiac action potentials of small mammals such as the mouse, because of an inadequate frequency response. Angelakos and Bernardini (1963) studied the frequency components of the rat electrocardiogram employing a cathode ray oscillograph (frequency response 0 to 40,000 Hz). Fourier analysis of the rat ECG demonstrated that it is composed chiefly of frequencies between 50 and 400 Hz. These authors took as the fundamental frequency the duration of QRS (e.g., 20 msec) or 50 cycles/sec. Gross distortion of the rat electrocardiographic waves was caused by recording with a frequency response less than 250 Hz. They concluded that direct-writing electrocardiographs of that period were incapable of reproduction of rat QRS complexes with sufficient fidelity. This view was refuted by Godwin and Fraser (1965). Their studies compared records taken with a cathode ray oscillograph and a direct writer with a frequency response 3 db down at 175 Hz and 50% response at 200 Hz. These authors concluded that the frequencies influencing the main pattern of the rat ECG are below 200 Hz, a frequency range approached by many current direct-writing electrocardiographs. In Figure 4 ECGs taken at 3 different maximal frequency responses (30 Hz, 100 Hz and 10 to 30% reduction at 200 Hz) are illustrated. In considering the literature on rat ECGs, Werth and Wink (1967) pointed out that the frequency response of the recording apparatus could explain differences in authors' findings about the absence of Q and S waves in limb lead records.

Amplitudes

In general, time interval and configurational changes in PQRST complexes are of greater diagnostic significance than amplitude changes. Other than amplitude changes resulting from major vector alteration, variations in PQRST amplitudes must be substantial to be considered significant. Heering (1970) gave the following amplitude values for lead II in mV. (mean and (range)): P, 0.11 mV (0.02 to 0.20); R, 1.06 (0.22 to 1.50); S, 0.20 (0 to 0.50); T, 0.15 (0.05 to 0.30) mV. These amplitude values for P, S and T compare favorably with the values of Werth and Wink (1967) but the latter found R amplitudes of 0.6–0.8 mV to be more common.

Heart Rate and Time Intervals

Heart rate. The heart rate in rats is relatively slow at birth, increases rapidly during the first few weeks of life, then decreases during continued growth and continues to fall in old age (Everitt, 1958). Heart rates recorded in electrocardiograms taken from restrained adult rats generally range from 330 to 600 beats/min with mean values from different studies ranging from 443 to 492 beats/min (Hundley *et al.*, 1945; Schinzel, 1933; Conrad and Baxter, 1963, 1966; Heering, 1970; Wiester, 1975). Moses (1946) found that emotional stimuli caused greater increases in heart rate than movement, which probably accounts for the fairly high rates found in restrained rats.

Minimal heart rates may be obtained when especial pains are taken to minimize external stimuli. Earlier attempts at determining resting heart rates included auscultation of the heart beat in rats dozing in a cage (281 ± 18 beats/min, Hoskins *et al.*, 1927); auscultation while rats were wrapped in a towel (about 300/min, Fishburne and Cunningham, 1938); palpation of the apex beat with the rats held in the crook of the arm (300–330/min, Meyer and Yost, 1939). Moses (1946) registered ECGs from the feet in rats restrained in a special holder and obtained mean values of 264 ± 18 S.D. after a one-month training period; minimal values were 234 to 246 beats/min. In the sleeping state, Hunt and Kimeldorf (1960) recorded means of 338 ± 24 S.D. to 357 ± 28 S.D. beats/min in young versus older groups of rats, respectively. V. Philipsborn (1973) attached electrocardiographic leads and recorded heart rates of 265 to 315 beats/min, after a period of quiet rest in a cage.

Maximal heart rates probably can exceed the 600 beats/min reported from electrocardiograms. As noted in the foregoing, Mainwood and Lee (1969) in perfused rat papillary muscles at 26°C found that with paired pacing mechanical responses to the second stimulus decreased as the intervals were reduced until at pulse intervals of 80 to 100 msec, the mechanical response to the second action potential became practically undetectable (excitation–contraction uncoupling). If these data can be applied to the intact rat, corresponding heart rates would be 600 to 750 beats/min. Possible electrical responses would be faster, however, from 1200 to 2000/min, corresponding to short intervals between paired stimuli of 30 to 50 msec, that resulted in an electrical response following the second stimulus. Consistent electrical responses to the second stimulus did not occur below 50 msec intervals with paired pacing. Adolph (1965), in intact anesthetized rats, found that maximal electrical drive rates increased with age: mean values; fetus, 350/min; newborn, 430/min; adult, 750/min. These rates were determined by counting the electrocardiographic R waves, not mechanical responses. From the foregoing, the adult rat heart should be capable of a mechanical response at rates up to 750/min. In ether-anesthetized *Rattus rattus* with Chaga's disease, Blandon *et al.* (1974) recorded electrocardiographically heart rates up to 840/min, although, it is not known whether a mechanical response followed each electrical complex. Hoskins *et al.* (1927) claimed to have counted heart rates of up to 792/min (i.e., about 13/sec) by auscultation. The accuracy of these values may be doubted since Meyer and Yost (1939) found it difficult to count rates in excess of 360/min by palpation.

Under anesthesia, reported mean heart rates tend to be lower than in unanesthetized animals in most studies (e.g., mean values ranging from 331 to 400/min) (Werth and Wink, 1967; Heise and Kimbel, 1955; Beinfield and Lehr, 1968a, 1968b; Fraser *et al.*, 1967; Badarau *et al.*, 1969; Zbinden and Rageth, 1978). Higher mean values, however, were reported in anesthetized animals by some investigators (490/min, Agduhr and Stenström, 1930; 506/min, Klütsch *et al.*, 1968).

Heart rate in the rat varies with body temperature. In anesthetized rats over rectal temperature ranges from 30° to 40°C (Drury *et al.*, 1930) and 13° to 35°C (Crismon, 1944) the heart rate fell approximately 15 beats/min per 1°C reduction in temperature.

In summary, the heart rate of rats can vary from about 250 to 750 beats/min and perhaps higher. Heart rates during registration of electrocar-

TABLE 1. REPRESENTATIVE RANGES OF ECG TIME INTERVALS REPORTED IN
RATS (MILLISECONDS)

	Heart rate	Unanesthetized	Anesthetized
P	Mean $\pm$ S.D.	264 ± 18 to 492 ± 36	$331 \pm$ to 507 ± 40
	Ranges	228 to 600	
PR	Ranges	11 to 16	10 to 30
QRS	Mean $\pm$ S.D.	40 ± 4 to 46 ± 8	33 ± 4 to 65 ± 13
	Ranges	33 to 50	25 to 72
QT	Mean $\pm$ S.D.	16 ± 2 to 19 ± 2	16 ± 1 to 26 ± 2
	Ranges	12 to 26	10 to 40
	Mean $\pm$ S.D.	64 ± 7 to 70 ± 6	47 ± 7 to 84 ± 10
	Ranges	38 to 80	60 to 200

Data, rounded to the nearest whole number, for unanesthetized rats
from Drury *et al.*, 1930; Schinzel, 1933; Zoll and Weiss, 1936; Weiss *et
al.*, 1938; Hundley *et al.*, 1945, Moses, 1946; Conrad and Baxter, 1963,
1966; Heering, 1970; Philipsborn, 1973; Wiester, 1975; Zbinden and
Brändle, 1975; Zbinden *et al.*, 1978a. Data for anesthetized rats from
Agduhr and Stenström, 1930; Heise and Kimbel, 1955; Angelakos and
Bernardini, 1963; Fraser *et al.*, 1967; Franke and Joshi, 1967; Werth and
Wink, 1967; Beinfield and Lehr, 1968a, 1968b; Klütsch *et al.*, 1968;
Cooper, 1969; Badarau *et al.*, 1969; Juskowa, 1972; Blandon *et al.*, 1974;
Zbinden and Rageth, 1978. There is disparity between some ranges given
and possible range estimates from corresponding mean $\pm$ S.D. values.
This is because some authors giving mean $\pm$ S.D. values did not state the
range.

diograms are generally between 330 and 600 beats/min. Trained and
quieted animals can have rates in the range of 250 to 350 beats/min. In
anesthetized animals, heart rates usually range from 300 to 400 beats/min.

Time intervals. In Table 1 published values for the various ECG time
intervals from unanesthetized and anesthetized rats are summarized. The
broader ranges and longer duration in the anesthetized rats represent the
influence of varying depth and type of anesthesia. Barbiturates and urethane anesthesia tended to prolong the time intervals more than light-ether
anesthesia. The differing heart rate values for the unanesthetized rats were
related to the degree of excitement induced by the method of restraint,
training, and elimination of environmental stimuli. The criteria used to
determine the measurements are known to be inconsistent among investigators. The frequency response of the electrocardiograph and the lead
selected for measurement (Beinfield and Lehr, 1968b) will also influence the
determination of these time intervals. These several factors account for
varying results among investigators that cannot be resolved by statistical
methods. Reasonable normal ranges for the time intervals in unanesthetized rats would seem to be: P, 10 to 20; PR, 35 to 50; QRS, 12 to 25; and

QT, 38 to 80 msec. Deep anesthesia can be expected to prolong the intervals. Heering (1970) found the average ratio of QT/PR intervals to be 6/5 (range 4/4 to 9/5).

The effect of heart rate on PR and QT intervals. Most investigators have not found a consistent relationship between the duration of the PR and QT intervals and heart rate in rats (Drury *et al.*, 1930; Weiss *et al.*, 1938; Werth and Wink, 1967; Beinfield and Lehr, 1968a, 1968b; Philipsborn, 1973). Others (e.g., Klütsch *et al.*, 1968) report that these intervals are rate-related and some authors calculated QTc values (Beinfield and Lehr, 1956; Fraser *et al.*, 1967; Zbinden and Rageth, 1978). Wildt and Nemec (1976) found that the relationship between PR and QT intervals and heart rate was closest in the guinea pig, less close in rats, and least close in mice. There seem to be three reasons for these conflicting views: (1) At high heart rates (475 to 600/min) and paper speed of 50 mm/sec or less, any changes in PR and QT interval duration with rate are small (i.e. a few msec) and therefore, difficult to measure accurately. (2) Also, at rapid rates (e.g., >450/min) the succeeding P waves are superimposed on the descending limb of the previous T wave and the true QT interval cannot be determined accurately. (3) At lower heart rates (250 to 350/min) that occur most frequently with anesthesia, these interval changes with rate are greater and become easily measurable, but it is uncertain whether this is a rate effect or the result of anesthetic action on the myocardium. The anesthetic might slow both heart rate, and atrioventricular conduction (PR interval), intraventricular conduction and TMAP duration (QT interval) proportionately.

Incidence of Spontaneous Arrhythmias and Conduction Disturbances

Moses (1946) noted occasional ventricular extrasystoles among 113 otherwise normal rats. Werth and Wink (1967) in 1971 rats lightly anesthetized with ether reported the following incidences of arrhythmias and conduction disturbances: respiratory sinus arrhythmia, 1067 (54.13%); isolated supraventricular extrasystoles, 18 (0.91%); sinus arrhythmia, 17 (0.86%); 1st° and 2nd° AV block, 13 (0.66%); 3rd° AV block, 13 (0.66%); isolated ventricular extrasystoles, 10 (0.50%); wandering pacemaker, 7 (0.36%); atrial fibrillation, 3 (0.15%); frequent ventricular extrasystoles, 2 (0.10%); frequent supraventricular extrasystoles, 1 (0.05%). Davidson (1977) reported that about 7% of adult male rats in his colony had electrocardiographic abnormalities such as elevated "ST" segment, conduction defects, and arrhythmias. The incidence of spontaneous arrhythmias and conduction disturbances in control rats appears to be of about the same order of magnitude as observed in Beagles (Detweiler, 1981), swine (Grauwiler, 1965; Detweiler, 1979) and monkeys (Malinow, 1966).

Comparing data on the incidence of arrhythmias from literature sources such as the foregoing or in dose groups of a toxicological study is fraught with uncertainty. The unreliability of detecting an event that occurs at irregularly varying time intervals by sampling over a brief period of time is clear. This has' been documented by a study in human patients with ventricular tachyarrhythmias (Rydén *et al.*, 1975). Intermittent ECG sampling of fairly brief duration (e.g., 1, 2 or 5 minute recordings) when compared with continuous recording for 3 hours had a low detection rate for infrequent arrhythmias and can result in exaggerating or underrating the estimate of true arrhythmia occurrence. The use of groups of animals, however, improves the suitability of intermittent ECG sampling to some extent. Obviously, the period of recording should be the same for each animal and the period of recording should be as long as feasible to obtain comparable results (see also Detweiler, 1981).

Because of their small size one might expect the rat atria and ventricles to be too small to sustain fibrillation (Detweiler and Spörri, 1957). Apparently, this is not the case, probably because of the short QT interval and refractory period. Several authors have published records meeting the electrocardiographic criteria for atrial fibrillation: Hundley *et al.* (1945); King and Sebrell (1946); Werth and Wink (1967); Cargill *et al.* (1974); Blandon *et al.* (1974); Stein (1976); Morvai *et al.* (1976). Ventricular fibrillation has also been reported by several authors: Juskowa (1972); Wiester (1975); Guideri *et al.* (1975); Morvai *et al.* (1976).

V. ELECTROCARDIOGRAPHIC CHANGES IN TOXICITY STUDIES

In general, the electrocardiographic changes induced by drugs, chemicals, hypothermia, nutritional deficiencies, etc. in rats are qualitatively similar to those induced in species with a distinct ST segment. Even the digitalis glycosides, to which the adult rat is highly resistant, can apparently induce many of its typical electrocardiographic effects when given in sufficient dosage (Valora and Mei, 1963; Arcasoy and Smuckler, 1969).

Because of the short refractory period of the rat TMAP, the rat heart may be more susceptible to arrhythmogenic drugs than species with a relatively longer refractory period. This possibility, however, has not been investigated systematically, and may not be true.

Accordingly, despite certain anomalous physiologic characteristics of the rat heart, there is no indication from the literature reviewed here that it has not served as a suitable model for cardiotoxicity studies.

The exception is the specific resistance to the toxic effects of cardiac glycosides that has been known for a long time (Detweiler, 1967). The possibility that such a specific difference in sensitivity to other agents might be found in the future must be kept in mind.

REFERENCES

Abbott, C. P., Creech, O., Jr. and DeWitt, C. W. (1964) Histologic and electrocardiographic changes of the transplanted rat heart. *Surg. Forum* **15**, 253–255.

Abbott, C. P., DeWitt, C. W. and Creech, O., Jr. (1965) The transplanted rat heart: Histologic and electrocardiographic changes. *Transplantation* **3**, 432–445.

Adolph, E. F. (1967) Ranges of heart rates and their regulations at various ages (rat). *Am. J. Physiol.* **212**, 595–602.

Agduhr, E. and Stenström, N. (1930) The appearance of the electrocardiogram in the heart lesions produced by cod liver oil treatment. *Acta Paediat. (Uppsala)* **9**, 280–306.

Allen, J. C. and Schwartz, A. (1969) A possible biochemical explanation for the insensitivity of the rat to cardiac glycosides. *J. Pharmacol. Exp. Ther.* **168**, 42–46.

Angelakos, E. T. and Bernardini, P. (1963) Frequency components and changes in electrocardiogram of the adult rat. *J. Appl. Physiol.* **18**, 261–263.

Arcasoy, M. M. and Smuckler, E. A. (1969) Acute effects of digoxin intoxication on rat hepatic and cardiac cells. *Lab. Invest.* **20**, 190–201.

Arrigo, L. and Dulio, C. (1964a) Sulla morfologia dell'elettrogramma intracellulare derivatos dal curve di ratto *in situ. Boll. Soc. Ital. Biol. Sper.* **40**, (11).

Arrigo, L. and Dulio, C. (1964b) Sull'elettrocardiogramme intracellulare in varie condizioni di vagotomia nel ratto. *Boll. Soc. Ital. Biol. Sper.* **40**, (11).

Arrigo, L. and Dulio, C. (1964c) Modificazioni indotte dalla frequenza sulla morfologia dell'elettrogramma intracellulare del coure di ratto *in situ. Boll. Soc. Ital. Biol. Sper.* (11).

Bachmann, E., Zbinden, G. and Weber, E. (1975a) Anthracycline antibiotics: Correlations between cardiotoxicity, mitochondrial metabolism and drug levels in serum and heart of rats. In: *The Prediction of Chronic Toxicity from Short-term Studies. Proc. Europ. Soc. Study Drug Tox.* **17**, 309–314.

Bachmann, E., Weber, E. and Zbinden, G. (1975b) Effects of seven anthracycline antibiotics on electrocardiogram and mitochondrial function of rat hearts. *Agents and Actions* **5**(4), 383–393.

Badarau, G., Wasserman, L. and Dolinesco, S. (1969) Recherches sur les relations entre les modifications electrocardiographiques et les processus morphopathologiques au cours de l'évolution des myocardodystrophies expérimentales chez le rat. *Rev. Roum. Med. Int.* **2**, 121–130.

Balazs, T. (1973) Cardiotoxicity of sympathomimetic bronchodilator and vasodilating antihypertensive drugs in experimental animals. In: *Experimental Model Systems in Toxicology and their Significance in Man. Proc. Europ. Soc. Study Drug Tox.* **15**, 71–79.

Beinfield, W. H. and Lehr, D. (1956) Advantages of ventral position in recording electrocardiogram of the rat. *J. Appl. Physiol.* **9**, 153–156.

Beinfield, W. H. and Lehr, D. (1968a) P–R interval of the rat electrocardiogram. *Am. J. Physiol.* **214**, 205–211.

Beinfield, W. H. and Lehr, D. (1968b) QRS–T variations in the rat electrocardiogram. *Amer. J. Physiol.* **214**, 197–204.

Berg, B. N. (1955) The electrocardiogram in aging rats. *J. Gerontol.* **10**, 420–423.

Bernard, G. and Gargouil, Y. M. (1970) Électrophysiologie. Acquisitions successives, chez l'embryon de rat, des perméabilites specifiques de la membrane myocardique. *C.R. Acad. Sci.* **270**, 1495–1498.

Bianchetti, G., Bonaccorsi, A., Chiodaroli, A., Franco, R., Garattini, S., Gomeni, R. and Morselli, P. L. (1977) Plasma concentrations and cardiotoxic effects of desipramine and protriptyline in the rat. *Br. J. Pharmac.* **60**, 11–19.

Bianchi, C., Sanna, G. P. and Turba, C. (1968) Anti-arrhythmic properties of 1,5-dimorpholino-3-(1-naphthyl)-pentane(DA 1686). *Arzneim. Forsch.* **18**(7), 845–850.

Blandon, R., Edgcomb, J. H., Guevara, J. F. and Johnson, C. M. (1974) Electrocardiographic changes in Panamanian *Rattus rattus* naturally infected by *Trypanosoma cruzi. Am. Heart J.* **88**, 758–764.

Buchanan, F. (1908) The frequency of the heart-beat in the mouse. *J. Physiol.* **37**, lxxix–lxxx.

Buchanan, F. (1910) The frequency of the heart-beat in the sleeping and waking dormouse. *J. Physiol.* **40**, xlii–xliv.

Buchanan, F. (1911) Dissociation of auricles and ventricles in hibernating dormice. *J. Physiol.* **42**, xix–xx.

Caprino, L., Borrelli, F., Falchetti, R., Biader, U. and Franchina, V. (1978) A new computerized system for automatic ECG analysis: An application to hypoxic rat ECG's. *Comput. Biomed. Res.* **11**, 195–207.

Cargill, C., Bachmann, E. and Zbinden, G. (1974) Effects of daunomycin and anthramycin on electrocardiogram and mitochondrial metabolism of the rat heart. *J. Natl. Cancer Inst.* **53**, 481–486.

Chau, T. T., Dewey, W. L. and Harris, L. S. (1973) Mechanism of the synergistic lethality between pentazocine and vasopressin in the rat. *J. Pharmacol. Exp. Ther.* **186**, 288–296.

Conrad, L. L. and Baxter, D. J. (1963) Effects of manganese on Q–T interval and distribution of calcium in rat heart. *Am. J. Physiol.* **205**, 1209–1212.

Conrad, L. L. and Baxter, D. J. (1966) Effect of calcium deficiency on Q–T interval and distribution of Ca^{45} in rat heart. *Am. J. Physiol.* **210**, 831–832.

Cooper, D. K. C. (1969) Electrocardiographic studies in the rat in physiological and pathological states. *Cardiovasc. Res.* **3**, 419–425.

Couch, J. R., West, T. C. and Hoff, H. E. (1969) Development of the action potential of the prenatal heart. *Circul. Res.* **24**, 19–31.

Crismon, J. M. (1944) Effect of hypothermia on the heart rate, the arterial pressure and the electrocardiogram of the rat. *Archiv. Intern. Med.* **74**, 235–243.

Davidson, W. J. (1977) Psychotropic drugs, stress, and cardiomyopathies. In: *Stress and the Heart* (D. Wheatley, ed.). Raven Press, New York, 63–85.

Degkwitz, R., Heushgem, C., Hollister, L. E., Jacob, J., Julou, L., Lambert, P. A., Marsboom, R., Meier-Ruge, W., Schaper, W. K. A. and Tuchmann-Duplessis, H. C. (1970) Toxicity and side effects in man and in the laboratory animal. In: *Neuroleptics* (D. P. Bobon, P. A. J. Janssen and J. Bobon, ed.) *Mod. Probl. Pharmacopsychiat.* **5**, 71–84.

Detweiler, D. K. (1967) Comparative pharmacology of cardiac glycosides. *Fed. Proc.* **26**, 1119–1124.

Detweiler, D. K. (1979) Spontaneous arrhythmias in normal miniature swine. Unpublished.

Detweiler, D. K. (Due 1981) The use of electrocardiography in toxicological studies with Beagle dogs. In: *Cardiac Toxicology* (T. Balazs ed.). Boca Raton, Fla., CRC Press.

Detweiler, D. K. and Patterson, D. F. (1965) The prevalence and types of cardiovascular disease in dogs. *Ann. N.Y. Acad. Sci.* **127**, 481–516.

Detweiler, D. K. and Spörri, H. (1957) Absence of "physiological" auricular fibrillation in the mole. *Cardiologia* **30**, 372–375.

Doherty, R. E. and Aviado, D. M. (1975) Toxicity of aerosol propellants in the respiratory and circulatory systems. VI. Influence of cardiac and pulmonary vascular lesions in the rat. *Toxicology* **3**, 213–224.

Dorato, M. A., Ward, C. O. and Sciarra, J. J. (1974) Evaluation of telemetry in determining toxicity of aerosol preparations. *J. Pharmaceutical Sci.* **63**(12), 1892–1896.

Driscoll, P. (1979) The electrocardiogram of Roman high- and low-avoidance rats under pentobarbital sodium anesthesia. *Arzneim. Forsch.* **29**(6), 887–900.

Drury, A. N., Harris, L. J. and Maudsley, C. (1930) Vitamin B deficiency in the rat. Bradycardia as a distinctive feature. *Biochem. J.* **24**, 1632–1649.

Durakovic, Z., Stilinovic, L. and Bakran, I. (1976) Electrocardiographic changes in rats after inhalation of dichlorotetrafluoroethane, arcton 114, $C_2 Cl_2 F_4$. *Jap. Heart J.* **17**, 753–759.

Ensor, C. R. (1946) The electrocardiogram of rats on vitamin E deficiency. *Am. J. Physiol.* **147**, 477–480.

Everitt, A. V. (1958) The electrocardiogram of the ageing male rat. *Gerontologia* **2**, 204–212.

Fishburne, M. and Cunningham, B. (1938) Replacement therapy in thyroidectomized rats. *Endocrinol.* **22**, 122.

Franke, F. R. and Joshi, M. J. (1967) Digitoxin resistance of the rat as demonstrated by electrocardiograms. *Exp. Med. Surg.* **25**, 80–85.

Fraser, R. S., Harley, C. and Wiley, T. (1967) Electrocardiogram in the normal rat. *J. Appl. Physiol.* **23**, 401–402.

Gargouil, Y. M. (1960) La sécrétion endocrinienne et l'activité cardiaque ventriculaire chez les mammiferes (activité électrique et mecanique) *J. Physiol.* **52**, 104–106.

Gargouil, Y. M., Tricoche, R. and Laplaud, J. (1960) Électrogramme intracellulaire, électrocardiogramme et mecanogramme du coeur de rat hypophysectomisé. *Compt. rend. Seances Acad. Sci.* **250**, 761–763.

Gargouil, Y. N., Tricoche, R. and Monnereau, H. (1961) Modification chez le rat, de l'electrocardiogramme et de l'electrogramme intracellulaire ventriculaire, par la surrenalectomie. *J. Physiol.* **53**, 346–347.

Gessler, U. and Kuner, E. (1959) Experimental contribution to the influence of ether and oxygen deficiency on the EKG of the white rat. *Z. Kreislaufforsch.* **48**, 870–877.

Godwin, K. O. (1965) Abnormal electrocardiograms in rats fed a low selenium diet. *Quart. J. Exp. Physiol.* **50**, 282–288.

Godwin, K. O. and Fraser, F. J. (1965) Simultaneous recording of ECG's from disease free rats, using a cathode ray oscilloscope and a direct writing instrument. *J. Exper. Physiol.* **50**, 277–283.

Graf, E. and Leuschner, F. (1978) On the toxicity of dopamine. Toxicity acute and subacute and teratology (authors transl.) *Arzneim. Forsch.* **28**, 2208–2218.

Grauwiler, J. (1965) *Herz und Kreislauf der Säugetiere*. Birkhauser, Basel.

Grauwiler, J. and Spörri, H. (1960) Fehlen der ST-Strecke im Elektrokardiogramm von verschiedenen Säugetierarten. *Helv. Physiol. Acta* **18**, C77–C78.

Grice, H. C., Heggtveit, H. A., Wiberg, G. S., Van Petten, G. and Willes, R. (1970) Experimental cobalt cardiomyopathy: correlation between electrocardiography and pathology. *Cardiovasc. Res.* **4**, 452–456.

Grünberg, H. and Hundt, H. J. (1958) Über Typenwechsel im Elektrokardiogramm der Ratte bedingt durch die Körperhaltung. *Z. Kreislaufforsch.* **47**, 874–877.

Guideri, G., Barletta, M. A. and Lehr, D. (1974) Extraordinary potentiation of isoproterenol cardiotoxicity by corticoid pretreatment. *Cardiovasc. Res.* **8**, 775–786.

Guideri, G., Barletta, M., Chau, R., Green, M. and Lehr, D. (1975) Method for the production of severe ventricular dysrhythmias in small laboratory animals. In: *Recent Adv. Cardio. Structure and Metab.* (P. E. Roy and G. Rona, ed.). University Park Press, Baltimore, **10**, 661–679.

Hamlin, R. L. and Smith, C. R. (1965) Categorization of common domestic mammals based upon their ventricular activation process. *Ann. N.Y. Acad. Sci.* **127**, 195–203.

Hawley, P. L. and Kopp, S. J. (1975) Extension of PR interval in isolated rat heart by cadmium (39102). *Proc. Soc. Exp. Biol. Med.* **150**, 669–671.

Heering, H. (1970) Das Elektrokardiogramm der wachen und narkotisierten Ratte. *Arch. int. Pharmacodyn.* **185**, 308–328.

Heerswynghels, J. V. and Thomas, J. (1945) Variations du glycogène et de l'acide pyruvique du coeur lors des modifications électrocardiographiques obsereés dans l'avitaminose B_1 chez le rat. Rôle de l'acide pyruvique. *Cardiologia* **9**, 211–230.

Heethaar, R. M., Denier van der Gon, J. J. and Meijler, F. L. (1973a) A mathematical model of A–V conduction in the rat heart. *Cardiovasc. Res.* **7**, 106–115.

Heethaar, R. M., Burchart, R. M., Denier van der Gon, J. J. and Meijler, F. L. (1973b) A mathematical model of A–V conduction in the rat heart. II. Quantification of concealed conduction. *Cardiovasc. Res.* **7**, 542–556.

Heggtveit, H. A., Grice, H. C. and Wiberg, G. S. (1970) Cobalt cardiomyopathy. *Path. Microbiol.* **35**, 110–113.

Heise, E. and Kimbel, K. H. (1955) Das normale Elektrokardiogramm der Ratte. *Z. Kreislaufforsch.* **44**, 212–221.

Herman, E. H., Schein, P. and Farmar, R. M. (1969) Comparative cardiac toxicity of daunomycin in three rodent species. *Proc. Soc. Exp. Biol. Med.* **130**, 1098–1102.

Hill, J. D. (1968a) The electrocardiogram in dogs with standardized body and limb positions. *J. Electrocardiol.* **1**, 175–182.

Hill, J. D. (1968b) The significance of foreleg position in the interpretation of electrocardiograms and vectorcardiograms from research animals. *Am. Heart J.* **75**, 518–527.

Hill, R., Howard, A. N. and Gresham, G. A. (1960) The electrocardiographic appearance of myocardial infarction in the rat. *J. Exp. Path.* **41**, 633–637.

Hillbom, M. E. and v. Boguslawsky, K. (1978) Effect of ethanol on cardiac function in rats genetically selected for their ethanol preference. *Pharmacol. Biochem. Behav.* **8**, 609–614.

Hoffman, B. F. and Cranefield, R. J. (1960) *Electrophysiology of the Heart*. McGraw-Hill, New York.

Hoskins, R. G., Lee, M. O. and Durrant, E. P. (1927) The pulse rate of the normal rat. *Am. J. Physiol.* **82**, 621–629.

Hundley, J. M., Ashburn, L. L. and Sebrell, W. H. (1945) The electrocardiogram in chronic thiamine deficiency in rats. *Am. J. Physiol.* **144**, 404–414.

Hundt, H.-J. and Grünberg, H. (1960) Vergleichende Untersuchungen über das Ratten-EKG bei Sauerstoffmangelzustanden verschiedener Genese. *Z. Kreislaufforsch.* **49**, 769–780.

Hunsaker, W. G., Hulan, H. W., Kramer, J. K. G. and Corner, A. H. (1972) Electrocardiograms of male rats fed rapeseed oil. *Can. J. Physiol. Pharmacol.* **55**, 1116–1121.

Hunt, E. L. and Kimeldorf, D. J. (1960) Heart, respiration and temperature measurements in the rat during the sleep state. *J. Appl. Physiol.* **15**, 733–735.

Irmak, S. and Aykut, R. (1955) Vergleichende elektro-kardiographische Untersuchungen beim Menschen und bei den Laboratoriumstieren. *Münch. Med. Wschr.* **97**, 460–461.

Johansson, B. (1957) The electrocardiogram and phonocardiogram of the non-hibernating hedgehog. *Cardiologia* **30**, 37–45.

Jones, D. C., Osborn, G. K. and Kimeldorf, D. J. (1967) Cardiac arrhythmia in the aging male rat. *Gerontologia* **13**, 211–218.

Juskowa, J. (1972) The effect of mercuric oxycyanide on the electrocardiographic curve in rat. *Acta Med. Pol.* **13**, 285–308.

Kayser, Ch. (1956) L'incremént thermique de la durée des différents accidents de l'électrocardiogramme chez le rat blanc, le hamster et le spermophile en hypithermie expérimentale. *Comp. rend. des Seances Soc. Biol.* **7**, 1442–1445.

Kelly, J. J., Jr. and Hoffman, B. F. (1960) Mechanical activity of rat papillary muscle. *Am. J. Physiol.* **199**, 157–162.

Kenedi, I. (1968) The correct interpretation of the rat electrocardiogram. *Acta Physiol. Acad. Sci. Hung.* **34**, 29–35.

King, W. D. and Sebrell, W. H. (1946) Alterations in the cardiac conduction mechanism in experimental thiamine deficiency. *Pub. Hlth. Rep.* **61**, 410 414.

Kisch, B. (1953) The heart rate and the electrocardiogram of small animals. *Exptl. Med. Surg.* **11**, 117–130.

Klütsch, K., Wende, W., Braun, H. and Bohndorf, W. (1968) Das Ekg der Ratte unter hochdosierter ^{60}Co-Bestrahlung. *Arch. Kreislaufforsch.* **55**, 185–210.

Kopp, S. J. and Hawley, P. L. (1978) Cadmium feeding: Apparent depression of atrioventricular-His-Purkinje conduction system. *Acta Pharmacol. Toxicol.* **42**, 110–116.

Kowalczykowa, J., Gryglewski, R., Bigaj, M., Jaszcz, W., Kulig, A., Kostka-Trabka, E., Swies, J. and Ocetkiewicz, A. (1971) Dynamics of myocardial damage by isoprenaline in rats and an attempt to correlate the morphologic changes in the myocardium with electrocardiographic, biochemical and hematologic changes. *Acta Med. Pol.* **12**, 1–12.

Kruta, V. and Braveny, P. (1960) Potentiation of contractility in the heart muscle of the rat and some other mammals. *Nature* **187**, 327–328.

Langer, G. A. (1978) Interspecies variation in myocardial physiology: the anomalous rat. *Environ. Hlth. Persp.* **26**, 175–179.

Langer, G. A., Brady, A. J., Tan, S. T. and Serena, S. D. (1975) Correlation of the glycoside response, the force staircase, and the action potential configuration in the neonatal rat heart. *Circul. Res.* **36**, 744–752.

Langslet, A. (1970) ECG-changes induced by phenothiazine drugs in the anaesthetized rat. *Acta Pharmacol. Toxicol.* **28**, 258–264.

Leblond, C. P. and Hoff, H. E. (1944) Comparison of cardiac and metabolic actions of thyroxine, thyroxine derivatives and dinitriphenol in thyroidectomized rats. *Am. J. Physiol.* **141**, 32–37.

Lepeschkin, E. (1951) *Modern Electrocardiography*. Williams and Wilkins, Baltimore.

Lepeschkin, E. (1965) The configuration of the T wave and the ventricular action potential in different species of mammals. *Ann. N.Y. Acad. Sci.* **127**, 170–178.

Leszkovszky, G. P., Gal, G. and Tardos, L. (1967) Correlation between functional and morphological heart changes due to isoproterenol. *Experientia* **23**(2), 112–113.

Lisciani, R., Baldini, A., Benedetti, D., Campana, A. and Barcellona, P. S. (1978) Acute cardiovascular toxicity of trazodone, etoperidone and imipramine in rats. *Toxicology* **10**, 151–158.

Loiselle, D. S. and Gibbs, C. L. (1979) Species differences in cardiac energetics *Am. J. Physiol., Heart Circ. Physiol.* **6**(1), H90–H98.

Lombard, E. C. (1952) Electrocardiograms of small mammals. *Am. J. Physiol.* **171**, 189–193.

Mainwood, G. W. and Lee, S. L. (1969) Rat heart papillary muscles: Action potentials and mechanical response to paired stimuli. *Science* **166**, 396–397.

Malinow, M. R. (1966) An electrocardiographic study of *Macaca mulatta*. *Folia Primat.* **4**, 51–65.

Manoach, M., Aygen, M. M., Netz, H. and Pauker, T. (1977) Q–T interval in young and old mammalian embryos. *Adv. Cardiol.* **19**, 52–54.

Marmo, E. (1969) Verhalten des EKG normaler, reserpinisierter oder emetinisierter Ratten, die mit verschiedenen β-Adrenolytika perfundiert wurden. *Arch. Kreislaufforsch.* **59**, 325–350.

Marmo, E. and Robertaccio, A. (1970) Analisi digli effetti sull'ECG del ratto di vari β-adrenolitici. *Ann. Soc. Ital. Cardiol.* **30**(2), 221–222.

Marmo, E., De Giacomo, S. and Imperatore, A. (1969) Verhalten des Elektrokardiogramms normaler oder mit verschiedenen Pharmaka vorbehandelter und daraufhin mit Metochlopramid perfundierter Ratten. *Jpn J. Pharmacol.* **19**, 551–562.

Mei, V., Fidanza, A. and Valora, N. (1964) Studio comparativo dell'elettrocardiogramma del neonato nel ratto, nel topino e nella cavia. *Boli. Soc. Ital. Sper.* **61**, 319–322.

Meinrath, M., Collins, P. and D'Amato, M. R. (1977) A nonobtrusive heart rate telemetry system for rats. *Behav. Res. Methods Instrument.* **9**(3), 253–246.

Meyer, A. E. and Yost, M. (1939) The stimulating action on metabolism and heart beat of various thyroid preparations, determined in the thyroidectomized rat. *Endocrinol.* **24**, 806–813.

Monnereau-Soustre, H. (1966) Electrocardiogramme du rat surrénalectomisé en hypothermie. *Compt. rend. Seances Soc. Bil.* **160**, 623–629.

Morvai, V., Hudak, A., Ungvary, Gy. and Varga, B. (1976) ECG changes in benzene, toluene and xylene poisoned rats. *Acta Med. Sci. Hung.* **33**(3), 275–286.

Moses, L. E. (1946) Heart rate of the albino rat. *Proc. Soc. Exp. Biol. Med.* **63**, 58–62.

Nadeau, R. and Champlain, J. (1973) Comparative effects of 6-hydroxy-dopamine and of reserpine on ouabain toxicity in the rat. *Life Sci.* **13**, 1753–1761.

Nemec, J. (1973) Cardiotoxic effects of tricyclic antipsychotics. Comparison of some newer derivatives from the 10,11-dihydrodibenzo/b,f/thiepin group with perphenazine and amitriptyline. *J. Europ. Toxicol.* **4–5**, 224–231.

Noble, D. and Cohen, I. (1978) The interpretation of the T wave of the electrocardiogram. *Cardiovasc. Res.* **13**, 13–27.

Normann, S. J., Priest, R. E. and Benditt, E. P. (1961) Electrocardiogram in the normal rat and its alteration with experimental coronary occlusion. *Circul. Res.* **11**, 282–287.

Osborne, B. E. (1973) A restraining device facilitating electrocardiogram recording in rats. *Lab. Anim.* **7**, 185–188.

v. Philipsborn, G. (1973) Zur Wirkung von n-Propyl-ajmalinium-hydrogentartrat (NPAB), sparteinsulfat (Spartein) und NPAB + Spartein auf das Elektrokardiogramm und auf Akonitinarrhythmien von SIV-Ratten. *Arzneim Forsch. Drug Res.* **23**, 1729–1733.

Rappaport, M. B. and Rappaport, I. (1943) Electrocardiographic considerations in small animal investigations. *Am. Heart J.* **26**, 662–680.

Repke, K., Est, M. and Portius, H. J. (1965) Über die Ursache der Specieunterschiede in der Digitalisempfindlichkeit. *Biochem. Pharmacol.* **14**, 1785–1802.

Robb, J. S. (1965) *Comparative Basic Cardiology.* Grune and Stratton, New York.

Robertson, E. C. and Doyle, M. E. (1937) Difficulties in the use of bradycardia method of assaying vitamin B_1. *Proc. Soc. Exp. Biol.* **37**, 139–140.

Roshchevsky, M. P. (1978) *Elektrokardiologia Kopytnych Zivotnych.* Nauka, Leningrad.

Salako, L. A. and Durotye, A. O. (1972) The electrocardiogram in acute dehydroemetine intoxication. *Cardiovasc. Res.* **6**, 150–154.

Sambhi, M. P. and White, F. M. (1960) The electrocardiogram of the normal and hypertensive rat. *Circul. Res.* **8**, 129–134.

Scheuer, J. and Stezoski, S. W. (1968a) Relationship of ATP to the electrocardiogram in the isolated rat heart. *J. Lab. Clin. Med.* **72**, 631–630.

Scheuer, J. and Stezoski, S. W. (1968b) Effects of high-energy phosphate depletion and repletion on the dynamics and electrocardiogram of isolated rat hearts. *Circul. Res.* **23**, 519–530.

Scheuer, J. and Stezoski, S. W. (1969) Discordance between the electrocardiogram and ATP levels in the isolated rat heart. *Am. J. Med. Sci.* **257**, 218–227.

Schinzel, G. (1933) *Das Elektrokardiogramm der kleinen Laboratoriumstiere.* Inaug. Diss. München.

Siegfried, J. P. (1956) *Elektrokardiographische Untersuchungen an Zoo-Tieren.* Inaug. Diss. München.

Spörri, H. (1944) Der Einfluss der Tuberkulose auf das Elektrokardiogramm. Untersuchungen an Meerschweinchen und Rindern. *Arch. Wiss. Prakt. Tierheilk.* **79**, 1–57.

Spörri, H. (1956) Starke Dissoziation zwischen dem Ende der elektrischen und mechanischen Systolendauer bei Känguruhs. *Cardiologia* **28**, 278–284.

Staib, A. H. (1967) EKG-Veränderungen bei der Ratte nach Chlorpromazin im Verlauf der postnatalen entwicklung. *Arch. int. Pharmacodyn.* **166**, 11–19.

Stein, E. A. (1976) Morphine effects on the cardiovascular system of awake, freely behaving rats. *Arch. int. Pharmacodyn.* **223**, 54–63.

Surawicz, B. (1966) Primary and secondary T wave changes. *Heart Bulletin* **15**, 31–35.

Surawicz, B. (1972) The pathogenesis and clinical significance of primary T-wave abnormalities. In: *Advances in Electrocardiography* (R. C. Schlant and I. W. Hurst, eds.). Grune and Stratton, New York, pp. 377–421.

Tobin, T. and Brody, T. M. (1972) Rates of dissociation of enzyme-ouabain complexes and $K_{0.5}$ values in $(Na^+ + K^+)$ adenosine triphosphatase from different species. *Biochem. Pharmacol.* **21**, 1460–1553.

Trautvetter, E., Detweiler, D. K. and Patterson, D. F. (1980) Evolution of the electrocardiogram in young dogs during the first 12 weeks of life. Submitted for publication. *J. Electrocardiol.*

Tricoche, R., Jallageas, M. and Gargouil, Y. M. (1963) Activité électrique comparée chez le rat noir (Rattus rattus) et chez le rat blanc (Rattus norvegicus). *Compt. rend. Seances Soc. Biol.* **157**, 1096–1099.

Tricoche, R., Monnereau, H., Galand, G. and Gargouil, Y. M. (1961) Electrocardiogramme, électrogramme intracellulaire et mécanogramme du rat surrénalectomisé. *Compt. rend. Seances Soc. Biol.* **155**, 1372–1375.

Valle, L. B. S., Oliveira-Filho, R. M., Arnomia, P. L., Nassif, M. and Saraceni, G. (1975) Sensitizing effect of lidocaine on bradycardia in the nadir of the final hypotension determined by serotonin in the rat. *Arch. Int. Physiol. Biochem.* **83**, 647–657.

Valora, N. and Mei, V. (1963) Studio delle modificazioni elettrocardiografiche indotte nel ratto dall' acetilcolina, dalla nor-adrenalina e da alcuni farmace ad azione elettiva sul cuore. *Quad. Nutrizione* **23**, 230–291.

Waller, R. K. and Charipper, H. A. (1945) Electrocardiographic observations in normal thyroidectomized and thiourea treated rats. *Am. J. Med. Sci.* **210**, 443–452.

Weiss, S., Haynes, F. W. and Zoll, P. M. (1938) Electrocardiographic manifestations and the cardiac effect of drugs in vitamin B_1 deficiency in rats. *Am. Heart J.* **15**, 206–220.

Werth, G. and Dadgar, P. (1965) Zum Elektrokardiogramm der Ratte mit und ohne Narkose, bei Beatmung mit Sauerstoffmangelgemischen sowie bei Intoxikation mit Malachitgrün, unter gleichzeitiger Bestimmung des effektiven Sauerstoffverbrauches. *Arch. Kreislaufforsch.* **48**, 118–131.

Werth, G. and Wink, S. (1967) Das Elektrokardiogramm der normalen Ratte. *Arch. Kreis. Forschung* **54**, 272–308.

Wexler, B. C. and Greenberg, B. (1974) Effect of exercise on myocardial infarction in young *vs.* old male rats: electrocardiograph changes. *Am. Heart J.* **88**, 343–350.

Wiester, M. J. (1975) Cardiovascular actions of palladium compounds in the unanesthetized rat. *Environ. Hlth. Persp.* **12**, 41–44.

Wildt, S. and Nemec, J. (1976) Correlation of the duration of the PR and QT interval to the heart rate in small laboratory animals. *Physiol. bohemoslov.* **25**, 285.

Yamashita, S. (1971a) Effect of alcohol on thiamine deficient cardiac lesions. *Jap. Heart J.* **12**(4), 354–367.
Yamashita, S. (1971b) Effect of alcohol on normal rat's heart. *Jap. Heart J.* **12**(3), 242–250.
Zbinden, G. (1975) Inhibition of adriamycin cardiotoxicity by acetyldaunomycin. *Experientia* **31**, 1058–1060.
Zbinden, G. (1977) *Methodes Pharmacologiques en Toxicologie.* Actualites Pharmacologiques 30ᵉ Serie. Masson et Cie, 101–111.
Zbinden, G. and Brändle, E. (1975) Toxicologic screening of daunorubicin (NSC-82151), adriamycin (NSC-123127), and their derivatives in rats. *Cancer Chemother. Rep.* **59**, 707–715.
Zbinden, G. and Rageth, B. (1978) Early changes of cardiac function in rats on a high-fat diet. *Fd. Cosmet. Toxicol.* **16**, 123–127.
Zbinden, G., Bachmann, E. and Bolliger, H. (1977a) Study of coenzyme Q in toxicity of adriamycin. In: *Biomedical and Clinical Aspects of Coenzyme Q* (K. Folkers and Y. Yamamura, ed.). Elsevier, Holland, 219–227.
Zbinden, G., Bachmann, E., Holderegger, Ch. and Elsner, J. (1977b) *Cardiotoxicity of Tricyclic Antidepressants and Neuroleptic Drugs.* Lecture, Smith Kline and French Laboratories.
Zbinden, G., Brändle, E. and Pfister, M. (1977c) Modification of adriamycin toxicity in rats fed a high fat diet. *Agents and Actions* **7**(1), 163–170.
Zbinden, G., Elsner, J. and Bolliger, H. (1977d) Toxicological evaluation of imipramine in combination with adriamycin and strophanthin. *Agents and Actions* **7**(3), 341–346.
Zbinden, G., Bachmann, E. and Holderegger, C. (1978a) Model systems for cardiotoxic effects of anthracyclines. *Antibiotics Chemother.* **23**, 255–270.
Zbinden, G., Pfister, M. and Holderegger, Ch. (1978b) Cardiotoxicity of N, N-dimethyladriamycin (NSC-261 045) in rats. *Toxicol. Letters* **1**, 267–274.
Zoll, P. M. and Weiss, S. (1936) Electrocardiographic changes in rats deficient in vitamin B_1. *Proc. Soc. Exp. Biol.* **35**, 259–262.
Zuckermann, R. (1959) *Grundriss und Atlas der Elektrokardiographie.* Georg Thieme, Leipzig.

ADDENDUM

The first full report on the use of fetal electrocardiography in teratological studies with rats appeared since the present paper was submitted for publication (Grabowski and Payne, 1980). On day $18\frac{1}{2}$ of pregnancy the rats were anesthetized with sodium pentobarbital intraperitoneally, the fetuses removed one at a time and three lead (leads I, II, III with intramuscular electrodes attached to the shoulders and left thigh) electrocardiograms taken. Placental attachment was maintained during recording. In 81 untreated control fetuses the heart rate was 149 ± 4.95 (SEM) beats per minute. One fetus had a transient episode of premature atrial contractions with atrioventricular block. In fetuses from rats treated with the pesticide Mirex, 1st° and 2nd° AV block, atrial flutter and other supraventricular arrhythmias occurred. The ECG abnormalities correlated with the degree of visible fetal edema and their incidence increased with maternal dosage. With this method Grabowski and Tunstall (1977) had previously demonstrated a 12% incidence of fetal electrocardiographic abnormalities in fetuses from rats treated with Trypan blue.

Grabowski *et al.* do not mention taking maternal ECGs at the time the fetal ECGs are registered. This would be an important omission for two reasons: (1) The fetal and maternal hearts have different physiological properties (as discussed in the foregoing; e.g., the lack of response of the adult rat heart to digitalis glycosides in contrast to the positive inotropic action in the neonatal heart) and may respond differently to the same drug. (2) Abnormal fetal ECGs may suggest a morphogenetic change but may actually only represent a cardiotoxic action affecting both mother and fetus.

In any case, the method has merit because functional disorders of the heart can be inferred from the fetal ECG whether caused by specific cardiac abnormalities or by a non-specific general deterioration of the health of the fetus.

BIBLIOGRAPHY

Grabowski, C. T. and Payne, D. B. (1980) An electrocardiographic study of cardiovascular problems in Mirex-fed rat fetuses. *Teratology* **22,** 167–177.

Grabowski, C. T. and Tunstall, A. C. (1977) An electrocardiographic study of rat fetuses treated with Trypan blue (Abstract). *Teratology* **15,** 32A.

Grabowski, C. T. (1978) ECG analysis of effects of Mirex on cardiovascular physiology of rat fetuses (Abstract). *Teratology* **17,** 34A.

Grabowski, C. T. (1979) An analysis of the causes of perinatal deaths induced by prenatal exposure to Mirex (Abstract). *Teratology* **19,** 27A.

Grabowski, C. T. (1973) Fetal cardiac physiology and hypoxia-induced hyperkalemia. *Teratology* **7,** A16.

Spontaneous and Induced Arrhythmias in Rat Toxicity Studies

G. ZBINDEN

GENERAL CONSIDERATIONS

Arrhythmias are changes of the heart function that range from physiological alterations of sinus automaticity coupled to respiration, to ventricular fibrillation, the predominant cause of sudden death in patients with coronary heart disease. Although most arrhythmias do not have such immediate deleterious effects, they often represent undesirable disturbances of cardiac function and frequently necessitate medical treatment. Therefore, all factors promoting the development of rhythm disturbances must be regarded as undesirable. Chemical substances, such as drugs, pesticides, or industrial poisons, may facilitate the occurrence of arrhythmias, particularly in patients with pre-existing cardiac disease. It is, therefore, important to recognize arrythmogenic properties of new chemicals, before they are introduced into commerce.

For a systematic review of cardiac arrhythmias, their pathogenesis and their electrophysiological diagnosis, readers are referred to textbooks, e.g. the popular work of Goldman (1979), and the excellent monograph on cardiac arrhythmias of Watanabe and Dreifus (1977). The present paper deals with arrhythmias observed during acute and chronic toxicity studies in rats. In addition, certain experimental procedures that can be used to facilitate the development of arrhythmias and that can also be included into the toxicological evaluation process will be mentioned.

Table 1 summarizes the most important arrhythmias occurring in man. It is based on the monograph of Watanabe and Dreifus (1977), but uses the nomenclature of the Criteria Committee of the New York Heart Association (1973). From this table it is evident that there are 2 main types of arrhythmias, namely abnormalities of frequency and regularity of impulse formation and conduction blocks. Many of these arrhythmias can also be observed in rats that are exposed to chemical substances.

In the following sections several studies conducted in my laboratory will be presented. The experimental techniques, recording equipment, methods

TABLE 1. THE IMPORTANT CLASSES AND TYPES OF ARRHYTHMIAS

I	Abnormalities of sinus rhythm
	Sinus tachycardia, sinus bradycardia
	Sinus arrhyhthmia and wandering pacemaker
	Sinoatrial exit block, sinus arrest, sick sinus syndrome
II	Atrial arrhythmias
	Atrial tachycardia
	Atrial flutter
	Atrial fibrillation
III	Atrioventricular junctional arrhythmias
	AV junctional escape beats
	AV junctional premature contractions
	AV junctional tachycardia
IV	Atrioventricular and intraventricular block
V	Ventricular arrhythmias
	Ventricular premature contraction
	Ventricular rhythm
	Ventricular tachycardia
	Ventricular fibrillation

of evaluation, strain, sex, and age of animals, housing and nutrition, are described in the literature cited, and in a recent review (Zbinden, 1981).

SPONTANEOUS ARRHYTHMIAS

Spontaneous arrhythmias are defined as arrhythmias occurring in animals that are not subjected to an experimental procedure especially designed to elicit or facilitate the development of a disturbance of cardiac function. Strictly speaking, however, the ECG recording procedure itself represents a potential arrhythmogenic stimulus. In unanesthetized rats the placing of the electrodes and restraining of the animals cause a rapid increase in heart rate from approximately 300 beats per minute (b.p.m.) to about 450 to 600 b.p.m. This is due to sympathetic stimulation that might be expected to precipitate arrhythmic events. However, spontaneous arrhythmias in untreated but restrained rats are rare. They consist almost exclusively of sporadic ventricular premature contractions (VPC). In mature rats of the ZUR:SIV-Z strain used in my laboratory they occur approximately once in 200 routine ECG.

The occurrence of arrhythmias in the course of toxicity experiments must thus be judged against this background. For example, in 338 rats treated with 29 different anthracycline antibiotics at tolerated and subtoxic doses only 3 VPC were observed in a total of 2432 ECG (1 per 811 ECG). From this finding it is concluded that this class of drugs does not possess significant arrhythmogenic properties, although its cardiotoxic characteristics are well recognized. In a group of 10 rats treated for 22 weeks with a

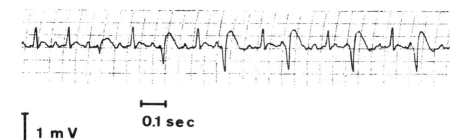

Fig. 1. ECG of a rat 4 days after the 6th i.p. dose of 50 mg/kg of the anthracycline antibiotic NSC 246131 (AD 32). Development of a bigeminy, i.e. a regular alternation of sinus beats and VPC. This may be an instance of ventricular parasystole, but the record was too short to confirm this diagnosis.

tolerated dose of thioridazine 4 VPC were observed in 220 ECG (1 per 55 ECG). There was 1 VPC in 200 ECG obtained from 10 rats treated with the same dose of chlorpromazine, and no arrhythmias occurred in 220 ECG from 10 rats with the same dose of prothipendyl, another phenothiazine neuroleptic. This does, of course, not prove that thioridazine is an arrhythmogenic drug. But the observation should be viewed as a cue to conduct further experiments. Since arrhythmias often occur sporadically, intermittent ECG sampling has a low detection rate especially if the arrhythmias are infrequent in a given individual. This makes comparisons of incidences of arrhythmias in routine ECG from different groups of animals unreliable. For a fuller discussion of this problem see Rydén *et al.*, 1975 and Detweiler, p. 107 in this book.

In rats treated with various cardiotoxic substances other types of arrhythmias may occur. Figure 1 demonstrates the development of ventricular bigeminy in a rat treated with an anthracycline antibiotic. As pointed out above, treatment of rats with this class of cardiotoxic drugs is rarely associated with arrhythmias. The drug used in this case, however, was surprisingly well tolerated by the animals, so that large doses could be administered.

Atrial premature contractions (APC) are rarely observed in drug-treated animals. Another rare disturbance is sinus arrest, a depression of the sinus node, characterized by missing a P wave followed by a pause which is not an exact multiple of a sinus cycle. An example of wandering pacemaker is shown in Fig. 2.

If anesthesia is required for the recording of the ECG, arrhythmias may be caused by the anesthetic used. An example is shown in Fig. 3. It demonstrates episodes of irregular sinus activity occurring during anesthesia with Imobilon®. It should also be noted that anoxia may induce severe disturbances of cardiac function and can manifest itself in the ECG as atrioventri-

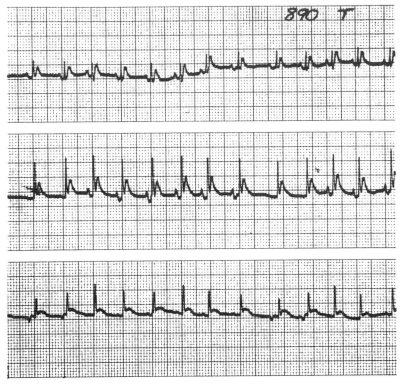

Fig. 2. Wandering pacemaker within the sino-atrial node (SAN). Simultaneously, recorded leads I, II, III (from top to bottom). P waves are consistently present in lead I. In lead III P waves are inverted when they are absent in lead II. Sinus arrhythmia is present and the absent P waves in lead II coincide with the longer RR intervals. When there is no marked shortening of the PR interval this phenomenon is interpreted as shifting of the pacemaker from the head to the tail of the SAN with increased vagal tone during sinus arrhythmia, with resultant alteration in the direction of the P wave vector. It is considered a normal variant that is present from time to time in healthy rats. The absent P waves have only occurred in lead II of the Einthoven limb leads or lead D of the D, A, and J triangular precordial system, in records examined thus far. (Figure courtesy of I.C.I. Americas Inc.).

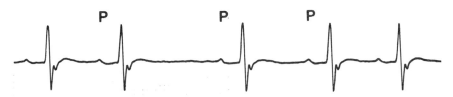

Fig. 3. ECG of a rat in Imobilon® anesthesia (ethorpine 0.037 mg/kg and methotrimeprazine 0.9 mg/kg i.m.). Sinus arrhythmia in which the largest PP interval exceeds 28 msec. Paper speed and voltage calibration as in Fig. 1.

cular (AV) block (Cooper, 1969), or, if severe, as ventricular fibrillation (Erker and Baker, 1980).

ACUTE TOXICITY STUDIES

In single dose experiments in rats, monitoring of the ECG may permit the recognition of potent arrhythmogenic agents. Test compounds are either administered by i.v. bolus injection or by i.v. infusion. A typical example is shown in Figure 4. The rat received an i.v. injection of aconitin, a highly toxic plant alkaloid which activates the development of ectopic automatic centers. The ECG changes recorded after a single dose of $20 \mu/kg$ permit a detailed analysis of the cardiotoxic effects of this compound.

Acute experiments with monitoring of ECG have been used to compare cardiotoxic properties of drugs. For example, various tricyclic anti-depressants were infused i.v. into guinea pigs. The time of appearance of arrhythmias or the cumulative dose required to cause such changes were used as screening parameters (Dumovic *et al.*, 1976). Similar experiments were also performed in rats (Lechat *et al.*, 1972). For the evaluation of potentially toxic gases, the test substances may also be given by inhalation. This procedure was used in mice exposed to various propellants. The occurrence of VPC and AV block was taken as an indicator for the cardio toxic action (Aviado and Belej, 1974).

INDUCED ARRHYTHMIAS

It is a well-established fact that arrhythmias may be provoked by stress-ful events. Lown *et al.* (1973) have shown that dogs required a low threshold current to induce a repetitive ventricular response, if they were brought into a situation that they associated with a previous experience of electric shock. Moreover, VPC and ventricular tachycardia developed in dogs recovering from coronary ligation if they were placed in an environment in which they anticipated administration of electric shock (Corbalan *et al.*, 1974).

It is appropriate to explain these arrhythmias as a consequence of released endogenous catecholamines (CA). These substances increase the rate of firing of automatic cells, induce a shift in pacemaker sites, cause oscillation in membrane potential, increase conduction velocity and de-crease the refractory period of the ventricle muscle. Thus, they create favor-able conditions for re-entry and perpetuated arrhythmias (Leon and Abrams, 1971). Toxicologists can make use of these physiological mechan-isms and can attempt to unmask arrhythmogenic effects of test compounds

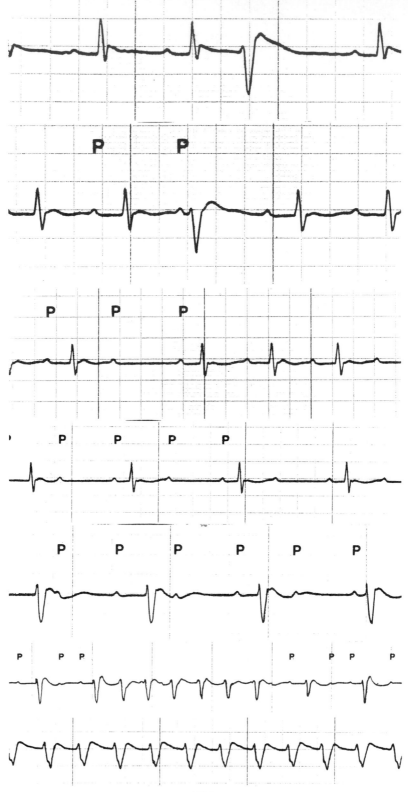

by subjecting the animals to a stressful situation or by treating them with CA.

Placing rats in a warm (50°C) environment for periods of up to 10 minutes represents a mild stress and leads to tachycardia with an increase in heart rate of about 20%. In a damaged heart this can sometimes suffice to provoke an arrhythmia. For example, in a rat chronically treated with the cardiotoxic anthracycline N,N-dimethyl-doxorubicin, thermic stimulation led to the development of an incomplete AV block (Zbinden, 1978). Figure 5 shows another arrhythmia occurring under this experimental condition: multiple VPC developed in a rat chronically treated with chlorpromazine.

Heat stress is only one of many experimental procedures that can be used to elicit arrhythmias in drug-treated animals. With the increasing awareness of the importance of psychologically induced disturbances of heart rhythm it is probable that more sophisticated test methods will soon be developed.

Instead of releasing endogenous CA by stress it is also possible to administer these substances by injection. Experimental procedures to detect a sensitization of experimental animals against the cardiac effects of CA have already been introduced into the toxicological routine. Various chemical substances have been shown to promote the arrhythmogenic effects of epinephrine (E), among them the fire-extinguisher bromochlorodifluoromethane (Beck *et al.*, 1973) and the cholesterol-lowering agent probucol (Marshall and Lewis, 1973). In mice, various propellant gases also sensitized the heart against the arrhythmogenic effect of E (Aviado and Belej, 1974). Norepinephrine (NE) was used to induce arrhythmias in phenobarbital-pretreated rats (Eastwood *et al.*, 1977).

In the procedure developed in my laboratory both NE and E are used. Rats are taken off drug treatment for 1 to 3 days. They are then anesthetized with urethane. For the determination of cardiac output by a thermodilution method a polyethylene catheter is introduced through the left carotid artery with the tip 3 mm distal to the aortic valve (Zbinden and Rageth, 1978). After cardiac function is stabilized 2 μg/kg NE, 0.5 μg/kg E, 10 μg/kg NE, and 1 μg/kg E are injected i.v. with an interval of 10 minutes. ECG, femoral blood pressure, and cardiac output are measured.

Fig. 4. ECG of a rat after 20 μg/kg aconitin i.v. 2nd tracing, 66 sec. PVC following immediately after a normal P wave. 3rd tracing, 72 sec. Second degree (incomplete) Mobitz AV block, Type 1 (Wenckebach). 4th tracing, 77 sec. Second degree AV block with 2:1 AV response: every other atria impulse is blocked. 5th tracing, 120 sec. Third degree (complete) AV block. Impulse transmission from atria to ventricles is completely blocked. Subsidiary pacemaker takes over to control ventricular depolarization. 6th tracing, 140 sec. Third degree AV block with short bursts of paroxysmal ventricular tachycardia, i.e. a series of rapid, repetitive ventricular excitations. 7th tracing, 150 sec. Ventricular tachycardia. Paper speed and voltage calibration as in Fig. 1.

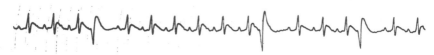

Fig. 5. ECG of a rat treated with 2 × 16 mg/kg chlorpromazine p.o. per day on 5 days per week for 10 weeks. Multiple PVC with constant coupling intervals, after 10 minutes at 50°C. Paper speed and voltage calibration as in Fig. 1.

TABLE 2. UNTREATED CONTROLS (n = 88) ARRHYTHMIAS INDUCED BY NOR-
EPINEPHRINE (NE) AND EPINEPHRINE (E) I.V.

	NE 2 μg/kg	NE 10 μg/kg	E 0.5 μg/kg	E 1 μg/kg
Sporadic APC	3	8	0	0
Multiple APC	0	0	1	0
Sporadic VPC	10	15	3	2
Multiple VPC	1	0	0	0
Total	14 (16%)	23 (26%)	4 (5%)	2 (2%)

APC = Atrial premature contractions. VPC = Ventricular premature contractions.
Multiple = > 5.

In untreated controls the injection of the CA is often followed by the occurrence of sporadic (< 5), rarely multiple VPC and, less frequently, APC (Table 2).

In rats previously treated with certain chemicals VPC and APC may occur more frequently (Figures 6–9). In addition, other arrhythmias can be

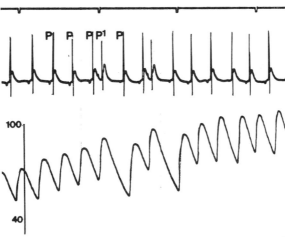

Fig. 6. ECG of a rat treated for 22 weeks with a maximally tolerated dose of an experimental butyrophenone neuroleptic p.o. Taken off drug for 3 days. Urethane anesthesia. Tracing starts 10 sec after 10 μg/kg NE i.v. Two APC. Note the slight drop in femoral blood pressure after each APC. Paper speed 5 cm/sec. Voltage calibration 1 mV = 16 mm.

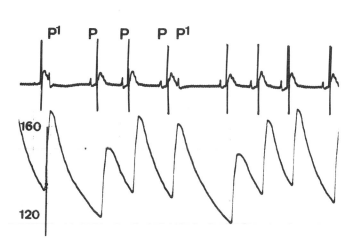

Fig. 7. ECG of a rat treated for 22 weeks with a maximally tolerated dose of an experimental tricyclic antidepressant p.o. Taken off drug for 3 days. Urethane anesthesia. Tracing starts 21 sec after 10 μg/kg NE i.v. Two blocked (non-conducted) APC. Premature atrial excitation hits effective refractory period of AV conducting system. Note marked drop in femoral blood pressure after each APC. Sinus arrhythmia is also present and accounts for the third long RR interval with drop in femoral pressure. Paper speed and voltage calibration as in Fig. 6.

seen. An example is shown in Table 3. It summarizes the results of an experiment with 8 psychotropic drugs. Only the arrhythmias observed after i.v. injection of 10 μg/kg NE are shown. It is evident that arrhythmias were most frequently recorded in rats pretreated with thioridazine. In addition to VPC and APC, 2 rats also exhibited incomplete AV block (type II). This disturbance of conduction was not seen with any of the other drugs. These findings suggest a certain arrhythmogenic quality of thioridazine, a suspicion that is supported by anecdotal clinical reports (Crane, 1970).

Incomplete type II AV block precipitated by CA injections has also been observed in rats treated with emetine (Zbinden *et al.*, 1980) and a high fat diet (Zbinden and Rageth, 1978). The latter observation was of particular interest, since the block that was provoked by NE occurred after 1 week on the high fat diet and was still present in 2 of 7 rats after 2 weeks on the high fat diet followed by 2 weeks on regular food.

Other arrhythmias observed after injection of CA include periods of sinus bradycardia, sinus arrest, sino-atrial exit block, rare occasions of short bursts of ventricular tachycardia (Figure 9), etc.

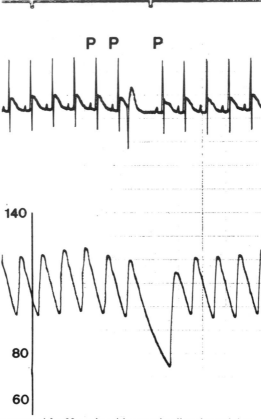

Fig. 8. ECG of a rat treated for 22 weeks with a maximally tolerated dose of bromperidol p.o. 10 μg/kg NE i.v. Taken off drug for 3 days. Urethane anesthesia. Tracing starts 10 sec after 10 μg/kg NE i.v. VPC and marked drop in femoral blood pressure. Paper speed and voltage calibration as in Fig. 6.

CONCLUSIONS

The electrocardiographic technique appears to be a useful tool for the detection of arrhythmogenic properties of chemical compounds. It can easily be applied in rats. Monitoring of the occurrence of spontaneous arrhythmias in rats treated chronically has a low probability of success, since ECG are only recorded for a few seconds. Acute toxicity studies in which high doses of the test compounds are given by i.v. injections, i.v. infusion or inhalation are able to detect potent arrhythmogenic agents. In these studies, due consideration must be given to the total dose adminis- tered, and purely non-specific intoxications must be distinguished from relevant cardiotoxic effects. Provocation of arrhythmias in chronically pre- treated rats by mild stressful procedures or by injection of catecholamines

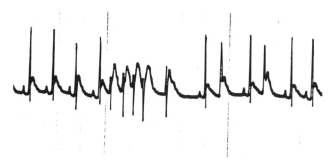

Fig. 9. ECG of a rat treated for 22 weeks with a maximally tolerated dose of an experimental butyrophenone neuroleptic p.o. Taken off drug for 3 days. Urethane anesthesia. Tracing starts 16 sec after 10 μg/kg NE i.v. Short burst (paroxysm) of ventricular tachycardia. Following the paroxysm of ventricular tachycardia two pairs of bigeminal beats occur with slightly different coupling intervals. The second ventricular complex of each pair is slightly aberrant in form and amplitude. These are most probably re-entrant beats arising from a focus in the AV junctional tissues or bundle of His. The small positive deflections at the onset of the T waves in these two ectopic complexes are probably superimposed P waves. Paper speed and voltage calibration as in Fig. 6.

permits the unmasking of potential arrhythmogenic properties. Such experimental procedures appear to be well suited for application in routine toxicology. It should be remembered, however, that other mechanisms than sensitization against CA may also be responsible for arrhythmogenic properties of chemicals. The toxicological evaluation should, therefore, also include other cardiovascular assays. The available methods have recently been reviewed by Brunner and Gross (1979).

TABLE 3. ARRHYTHMIAS INDUCED BY 10 μg/kg NOREPINEPHRINE IN RATS PRETREATED WITH PSYCHOTROPIC DRUGS*

Drug	n	Sp. APC	M APC	Sp. VPC	M VPC	AVB	SAB	Rat without arrh.
Dibenzepine	10	0	0	1	0	0	0	9 (90%)
Imipramine	6	0	0	1	0	0	1	5 (83%)
Maprotiline	8	0	1	1	3	0	0	4 (50%)
Prothipendyl	6	0	0	1	2	0	0	3 (50%)
Thioridazine	8	2	0	2	2	2	0	2 (25%)
Bromperidol	6	0	0	1	1	0	0	4 (67%)
Lenperone	6	3	0	0	1	0	0	3 (50%)
Controls	23	2	1	7	0	0	0	14 (61%)

* 22 weeks, off drug for 3 days, dosing started with 2 × 1 mg/kg per day on 5 days per week and doses were doubled weekly until maximally tolerated doses were reached (Zbinden *et al.*, 1978).
Sp. = sporadic (< 5).
M = multiple (> 5).
SAB = sino-atrial exit block.

ACKNOWLEDGEMENT

Work reported in this paper was supported by a grant from the Swiss National Science Foundation.

REFERENCES

Aviado, D. M. and Belej, M. A. (1974) Toxicity of aerosol propellants on the respiratory and circulatory systems. I. Cardiac arrhythmia in the mouse. *Toxicology* **2**, 31–42.

Beck, P. D., Clark, D. G. and Tinston, D. J. (1973) The pharmacologic action of bromochloro-difluoromethane (BCF). *Toxicol. Appl. Pharmacol.* **24**, 20–29.

Brunner, H. and Gross, F. (1979) Cardiovascular pharmacology: report of the main working party. *Pharmac. Ther.* **5**, 63–97.

Cooper, D. K. C. (1969) Electrocardiographic studies in the rat in physiological and pathological states. *Cardiovasc. Res.* **3**, 419–425.

Corbalan, R., Verrier, R. and Lown, B. (1974) Psychological stress and ventricular arrhythmias during myocardial infarction in the conscious dog. *Am. J. Cardiol.* **34**, 692–696.

Crane, G. E. (1970) Cardiac toxicity and psychotropic drugs. *Dis. Nerv. Syst.* **31**, 534–539.

The Criteria Committee of the New York Heart Association (1973) *Nomenclature and Criteria for Diagnosis of Diseases of the Heart and Great Vessel*, 7th edition. Little, Brown and Co., Boston.

Dumovic, P., Burrows, G. D., Vohra, J., Davies, B. and Scoggins, B. A. (1976) The effect of tricyclic antidepressant drugs on the heart. *Arch. Toxicol.* **35**, 255–262.

Eastwood, I., Forshaw, P. J., Jeyeratnam, J. and Magos, L. (1977) Cardiac sensitization induced by phenobarbitone and prolonged by CS_2. *Arch. Toxicol.* **37**, 237–240.

Erker, E. F. and Baker, T. (1980) Development of a cardiac antiarrhythmic screening test utilizing theophylline in the rat. *Arch. int. Pharmacodyn.* **243**, 86–89.

Goldman, M. J. (1979) *Principles of Clinical Electrocardiography*, 10th edition. Lange Medical Publications, Los Altos, Calif.

Lechat, P., Auclair, M. C. and Adolphe, M. (1972) Comparative effects of chlorpromazine and imipramine on cultured heart cells of the rat. *Proc. Europ. Soc. Study Drug Tox.* **14**, 214–221.

Leon, A. S. and Abrams, W. B. (1971) The role of catecholamines in producing arrhythmias. *Am. J. Med. Sci.* **262**, 9–13.

Lown, B., Verrier, R. and Corbalan, R. (1973) Psychologic stress and threshold for repetitive ventricular response. *Science* **182**, 834–836.

Marshall, F. N. and Lewis, J. E. (1973) Sensitization to epinephrine-induced ventricular fibrillation produced by probucol in dogs. *Toxicol. Appl. Pharmacol.* **24**, 594–602.

Rydén, L., Waldenström, A. and Holmberg, S. (1975) The reliability of intermittent ECG sampling in arrhythmias detection. *Circ.* 52, 540–5s45.

Watanabe, Y. and Dreifus, L. S. (1977) *Cardiac Arrhythmias. Electrophysiologic Basis for Clinical Interpretation.* Grune and Stratton, New York, San Francisco, London.

Zbinden, G. (1978) Méthodes pharmacologiques en toxicologie. *Actualités Pharmacologiques*, 30e Série. Masson et Cie., Paris, pp. 101–111.

Zbinden, G. (1981) Assessment of cardiotoxic effects in chronic rat toxicity studies. In: *Cardiac Toxicity* (T. Balazs, ed.). CRC Press Inc., Boca Raton, FL, in press.

Zbinden, G., Bachmann, E., Holderegger, Ch. and Elsner, J. (1978) Cardiotoxicity of tricyclic antidepressants and neuroleptic drugs. *Proc. 1st Int. Cong. Toxicol.* Academic Press, 285–308.

Zbinden, G. and Rageth, B. (1978) Early changes of cardiac function in rats on a high-fat diet. *Fd. Cosmet. Toxicol.* **16**, 123–127.

Zbinden, G., Kleinert, R. and Rageth, B. (1980) Assessment of emetine cardiotoxicity in a subacute toxicity experiment in rats. *J. Cardiovasc. Pharmacol.* **2**, 155–164.

Cardiac Arrhythmias Accompanying Sialodacryoadenitis in the Rat

D. K. DETWEILER, R. A. SAATMAN AND P. J. DE BAECKE

ABSTRACT

A high incidence of atrial and ventricular arrhythmias associated with an outbreak of sialodacryoadenitis occurred during a chronic drug trial with rats. The cardiac arrhythmias were not more prevalent in treated animals than in controls. They persisted long after physical evidence of the disease subsided. In 5 of 6 rats with high incidences of ectopic arrhythmias myocardial lesions were found histopathologically. It is speculated that the virus of sialodacryoadenitis can produce a lingering myocardosis causing cardiac arrhythmias.

INTRODUCTION

During the course of a routine 6 months chronic toxicity trial with rats, a high prevalence rate of cardiac arrhythmias developed in the animals. The distribution of affected animals in control and dose groups did not indicate this was a drug-related change. Since an intercurrent outbreak of sialodacryoadenitis occurred after the study was under way, it was speculated that the presence of this disease was responsible for the high prevalence of ectopic arrhythmias.

METHODS

Sixty-four Sprague–Dawley rats were divided into four dose groups: Group I, vehicle control; Group II, low dose; Group III, mid-dose; Group IV, high dose. The vehicle was 0.5% aqueous solution of hydroxypropyl-methylcellulose with 0.1% TWEEN 80. Lead I, II, III electrocardiograms were recorded twice pretest, at week 1, week 2, month 1, week 6, month 3, month 6, three times during a 2-week period after withdrawal of the drug, but continuation of the vehicle and at 2 days and 2 weeks after substituting normal saline solution for the vehicle. The animals were unanesthetized and restrained by hand during recording the electrocardiograms with a three-channel direct recording electrocardiograph.

D. K. Detweiler, R. A. Saatman and P. J. De Baecke

TABLE 1. INCIDENCES OF VENTRICULAR AND ATRIAL ECTOPIC BEATS

Date	Gp. I	Gp. II	Gp. III	Gp. IV	Total
4-14-78	0	0	1	0	1
4-21-78	0	0	0	0	0
4-28-78	1	0	1	0	2
5-05-78	0	0	1	0	1
5-26-78	4	1	4	1	10
6-09-78	4	2	3	1	10
7-21-78	1	2	2	1	6
10-12-78	4	3	3	1	11
10-26-78	3	1	2	2	8
11-02-78	4	4	3	2	13
11-09-78	3	1	1	2	7
11-29-78	4	5	1	3	13
12-11-78	5	6	2	4	17
Total	33	25	24	17	99

RESULTS

There were no changes in heart rate or configuration of nomotopic ECG complexes indicating drug action in any of the control or treated groups.

The occurrences of ectopic beats are tabulated in Table 1 by dose groups. In two pretest records one ventricular ectopic beat occurred in 1/64 rats. In the next two sets of records taken at weeks 1 and 2 the prevalences of ectopic beats were 2/64 and 1/64 rats, respectively.

In the month 1 records 5/26/78 ventricular ectopic beats were present in 10/64 rats, a striking increase in overall prevalence rate. Also, at this time there was an increase in the prevalence of 2nd° AV block and sinus arrhythmia. From this date on until the drug was withdrawn, the prevalence varied from 6 to 11/64 rats. A similar prevalence rate continued in three records taken during a 2-week period (10/26/78, 11/2/78, 11/9/78) after the drug had been withdrawn. In two records taken 2 days and 2 weeks (11/29/78 and 12/11/78) after normal saline solution was substituted for the vehicle, the prevalence rates were 13/64 and 17/64 respectively (see Fig. 1).

The incidence of ectopic beats was highest in Group I (vehicle control) and lowest in Group IV (high dose).

The incidences of records containing ectopic beats in each rat are tabulated in Table 2. Note that the highest incidences in individual rats and the highest number of affected rats occurred in Group I (vehicle control) while the reverse was true in Group IV (high dose).

Hearts from 6 rats with high incidences of ectopic arrhythmias were selected for evaluation of myocardial changes histopathologically. Minimal

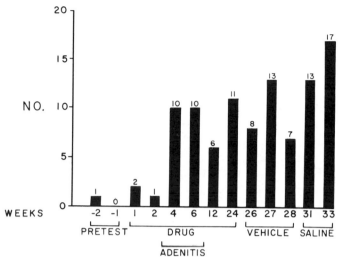

PREVALENCE of ECTOPIC ARRYTHMIAS in 64 RATS
BEFORE, DURING and AFTER SIALODACRYOADENITIS OUTBREAK

Fig. 1.

changes were found in 5 of these 6 hearts consisting of a focus of fibrous tissue in one rat, foci of mononuclear cell infiltration in 4 rats, 1 or 2 necrotic muscle fibers in 2 rats, and medial changes in muscular arteries in 3 rats.

TABLE 2. INCIDENCE OF RECORDS CONTAINING ECTOPIC BEATS (VEN-
TRICULAR OR ATRIAL) IN EACH RAT

Rat No. Gp I	Inc.	Rat No. Gp. II	Inc.	Rat No. Gp. III	Inc.	Rat No. Gp. IV	Inc.
513	7	515	4	511	0	512	2
567	1	573	0	570	2	568	0
601	2	605	0	603	1	598	0
619	1	620	0	621	3	614	0
675	1	672	2	670	0	674	1
726	1	730	0	729	1	727	2
738	7	739	1	734	1	741	3
788	2	784	4	785	3	782	0
516	2	517	1	514	2	510	0
671	2	566	0	572	0	569	0
604	0	599	4	602	1	600	2
617	0	616	3	618	0	615	1
676	3	673	0	677	2	671	2
731	1	732	2	728	2	733	0
736	3	740	1	737	1	735	2
783	0	786	3	787	5	789	2
Total	33		25		24		17

DISCUSSION

It appears that prior to the time of the month 1 electrocardiographic records some event occurred which affected the hearts of many of the animals on test so that a high prevalence of ectopic beats was produced in all animals on test. Prior to recording these month 1 electrocardiograms there was an outbreak of sialodacryoadenitis visibly affecting about 40% of the rats on test. Gland enlargement subsided within a few weeks; the unusually high prevalence of arrhythmias continued, however, throughout the entire study, persisting after withdrawal of the drug in groups II, III, and IV and after withdrawal of the vehicle in all groups.

Therefore, the cardiac effect was chronic and could not be related to either drug or vehicle administration with certainty. It appears possible that a chronic myocardosis resulted from the sialodacryoadenitis and persisted during the course of the study. Neither restraint of the animals during electrocardiographic recording nor passage of the gavage cannula is known to produce ectopic beats in such a high percentage of rats, although Zbinden (personal communication, 1978) has noted that extrasystoles occur when rats are squeezed during restraint for electrocardiographic recording.

Although ventricular ectopic beats are known to occur in control rats, their prevalence is far lower than found during this trial. Davidson[1], on the basis of records from 6000 rats, states that approximately 7% of male rats in their colony have electrocardiographic abnormalities such as elevated ST segment, conduction defects and arrhythmias. He did not indicate the prevalence of ventricular arrhythmias in this material, but it must be far less than 7%. Werth and Wink[3] found 1.56% with ventricular or supraventricular extrasystoles among 1971 electrocardiograms from normal rats lightly anesthetized with ether.

In any case, the increased prevalence of ectopic beats was chronic and leads to the speculation that a chronic process affecting the myocardium may have been present. Immunosuppressant drugs (e.g. aspirin) have been associated with the development of polyarteritis nodosa involving intramural coronary arteries in dogs (personal observation). In this case the resultant myocardial lesions were chronic, although cardiac arrhythmias did not occur. Rather, the electrocardiographic changes resulted from ischemic lesions in the myocardium which apparently accounted for T wave reversal in leads V_{10} and CV_5 RL. Such electrocardiographic evidence of relatively large myocardial lesions in the rat heart did not develop in the present study, i.e. there was no electrocardiographic evidence of intraventricular conduction disturbances.

The pathological changes were minimal and, as such, could be found in routine examination of rat hearts. The incidence, however, in this small series was high and such minimal damage could cause ventricular extrasystoles. Whether they represent the remnants of myocardial lesions caused by the virus of sialodacryoadenitis is uncertain since cardiac lesions have not been reported previously[2].

The high prevalence rates of cardiac arrhythmias were not present in pretest records, but developed in control and all dose groups and persisted after the drug had been withdrawn and after the vehicle had been withdrawn later. Accordingly, it does not appear that any of the treatments can be held responsible.

The possibility that exposure to the virus of sialodacryoadenitis can produce a lingering myocardosis associated with ventricular arrhythmias is, admittedly, speculative. This possibility has not been specifically investigated in the reports available on this disease.

REFERENCES

1. Davidson, Wm. J. (1977) Psychotropic drugs, stress, and cardiomyopathies. *Stress and the Heart*, Raven Press, New York, p. 63.
2. Jacoby, R. O., Bhatt, P. N. and Jonas, A. N. (1975) Pathogenesis of Sialodacryoadenitis in gnotobiotic rats. *Vet. Pathol.* Vol. 12, pp. 196–209.
3. Werth, G. and Wink, S. (1967) Das Elektrokardiogramm der normalen Ratte. *Arch. Kreislaufforsch*, Vol. 54, 272–308.
4. Zbinden, G. (1978) Personal communication.

Measurements of the Electrocardiogram of the Colworth Wistar Rat

G. W. CAMBRIDGE, J. F. PARSONS AND R. SAFFORD

Mean values were derived for the duration and amplitude of the main components of the electrocardiogram (ECG) of the Colworth Wistar rat.

Preliminary studies showed that to avoid movement and muscle artefact anaesthesia was necessary: Pentobarbital anaesthesia was contra-indicated since it produced T wave depression and QRS-notching, but a stable ECG could be obtained under light ether anaesthesia with minimal differences from the ECG of the unanaesthetized animal (Table 1).

Recordings were made from 6 male rats (9 months old) which had been maintained from weaning on a conventional pelleted diet (Spital); the animals were placed in a prone position and conventional limb leads were used with needle electrodes.

The recording equipment was selected to have an adequate frequency response (flat to 3000 Hz), overall sensitivity (2 cm per mV) and paper speed (up to 80 cm per second) which allowed accurate measurement of the parameters.

The equipment used was a D.C. amplifier (Rochar Type A 1338) at a gain of × 500, a galvanometer amplifier (Bell Howell 1-72xx), and a U-V recording oscillograph (Bell Howell S127) with a 7-326 galvanometer.

Mean values were derived from measurements on 10 consecutive beats from each animal (Table 2). A complex from a typical recording (Lead II) is shown in Figure 1.

TABLE 1. EFFECT OF ANAESTHESIA ON THE RECORDING OF THE RAT EGG (LEAD II)

		Conscious	Ether	Nembutal
P Wave	Duration msec	12.5	14.3	12.8
	Amplitude mV	0.145	0.16	0.15
QRS complex	Duration msec	14.5	14.7	14.1
	Amplitude mV	1.09	1.02	0.92
P-R Interval	Duration msec	49.8	49.5	49.3
Q-T Interval	Duration msec	51.0	53.6	52.8
Heart rate	(from R–R interval)	458	379	357
T Wave	Amplitude msec	0.17	0.17	0.09

135

TABLE 2. NORMAL VALUES FOR ECG OF COLWORTH WISTAR MALE RATS MAINTAINED ON STOCK
PELLETED DIET (SPITAL)

*Mean values for duration and amplitude of ECG components and heart rate
in male rats on Spital diet for 9 months*

| | | Duration (msec) | | | Amplitude (mV) | | | Heart rate/min |
		P	QRS	P–R	Q–T	P	QRS	T	
Spital Diet	Mean	14.3	16.7	45.6	56.0	0.133	0.995	0.116	423.7
9 months	S.D.	3.8	4.0	7.5	10.7	0.022	0.194	0.046	40.3

In a parallel study groups of 20 male and 20 female rats were maintained from weaning on the stock diet and on a purified powdered diet which is used in feeding trials in this laboratory. Heart rates were recorded from restrained unanaesthetized animals at 4-weekly intervals over a 2-year period and ECG recordings were made as described above from 7 animals in each group after 2 years on the diets (Table 3). The heart rates in the two groups showed significant differences after 1 month on the diet, the animals on the purified diet having a faster heart rate. This difference was maintained throughout the study up to week 97 (Fig. 2). Data derived from measurements of systolic blood pressure (tail cuff method) throughout the 2-year study are shown in Fig. 3.

ECG data (Tables 2 and 3) suggest that the prolongation with age of the Q–T interval in the Spital-fed animals could be attributed to the progressive change in heart rate.

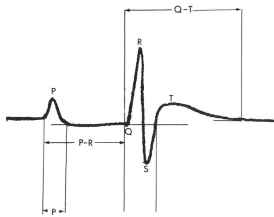

Fig. 1. ECG wave form (traced from actual recording) showing reference points for measurements. Note shift in isoelectric line. The end of the T wave is taken where the trace becomes parallel to the isoelectric line of the PR segment—this line is used for all amplitude measurements.

TABLE 3. COMPARISON OF ECG OF RATS MAINTAINED ON A CONVENTIONAL PELLETED STOCK DIET (SPITAL) AND ON A POWDERED PURIFIED DIET MIXTURE (USED IN OUR LABORATORY FOR ALL LONG-TERM FEEDING TRIALS)

24 *months*
Test of significant difference between mean values in males and females and combined groups on Spital and purified diet

		Duration (msec)			Amplitude (mV)				Heart rate/min
		P	QRS	P–R	Q–T	P	QRS	T	
Spital	Male	13.6	28.5	62.4	103.7	0.140	0.939	0.134	360.6
	Female	14.4	26.7	59.5	99.6	0.207**	0.879	0.179	403.4
Combined		14.0	27.6	61.0	101.7	0.174†	0.909	0.156	382.0
Purified Diet	Male	14.7	27.1	63.9	105.6	0.111	1.114	0.149	334.5
	Female	15.4*	21.4	56.5	96.3	0.168	1.205	0.188	399.7
Combined		15.1	24.2	60.2	100.9	0.140	1.160	0.168	367.1

* P wave duration significantly longer in females on purified diet.
** P wave amplitude significantly higher in females on Spital diet.
† P wave amplitude significantly higher in group on Spital diet.

Under our experimental conditions, particularly in rats under barbiturate anaesthesia, when recording at very fast paper speeds (80 cm/sec) and at high gain (8 cm/mV) a downgoing deflexion was observed prior to the commencement of the R-wave. This we have regarded as a Q-wave; it was not seen when recording a calibrating triangular wave form of 10 msec duration and 1 mV amplitude at 100 msec intervals and hence was not a

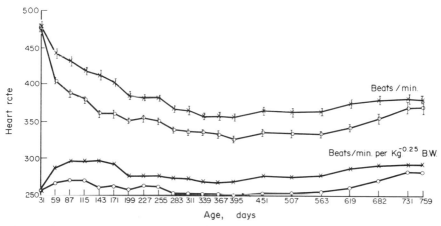

Fig. 2. Effect of diet on heart rate of rats fed Spital (O) or Purified Diet (×) for 105 weeks. Each point represents the mean result of values from male and female rats together with the standard error (I). Upper graphs show actual heart rate in beats/min. Lower graphs show derived value with respect to body weight:beats/min/kg$^{-0.25}$ body weight.

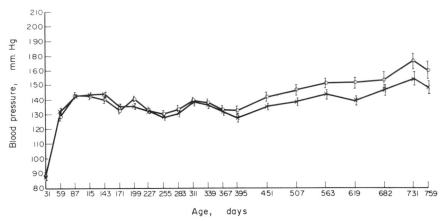

Fig. 3. Effect of diet on indirectly measured systolic blood pressure of rats fed Spital (O) or Purified Diet (×) for 105 weeks. Each point represents the mean result of values from male and female rats together with the standard error (I).

recording artefact. The duration of the downward deflexion was approximately 0.8 msec and its amplitude 0.05 mV and thus for practical purposes, with conventional pen recording systems it would not be detected and thus the measurement of the complex can be considered to be equivalent to the RT interval reported by other workers.

Relationship between Arterial Pressure and ECG Wave Form in Rats. Experiments carried out on Spontaneously Hypertensive (SHR) and Normotensive (NR) Control Rats

G. V. MARCHETTI, E. BALDOLI, A. NAVA, M. CAPELLINI,
G. BIANCHI AND G. F. Di FRANCESCO

In rats with genetic hypertension (SHR) the systolic arterial pressure is normal at birth, begins to increase after about 20 days, reaches about 200–260 mm Hg after 70–80 days and remains at this level for life[1].

In these rats stress represented by arterial hypertension leads to cardiac hypertrophy.

This model thus offers a unique possibility to study the morphological and electrophysiological changes that occur in the myocardium in response to arterial hypertension.

The present investigation is intended to ascertain the level and time-course of cardiac hypertrophy and modifications of ECG time intervals and wave forms that appear in hypertensive rats of various ages, ranging between 30 days and 550 days.

METHOD

Arterial pressure was measured at the tail using an indirect method[2]. Cardiac hypertrophy was evaluated by calculating the heart weight/body weight and left ventricle weight/right ventricle weight ratios and ratios of the weight of left ventricle, right ventricle and septum versus body weight and total heart.

The ECG was recorded in rats after light anaesthesia with pentobarbital and urethane. Six standard leads (I, II, III, aVL, aVR, aVF) and two precordial leads (right and left) were recorded.

The following ECG indices were calculated: heart rate, P wave duration in lead II, P-Q interval in lead II, QRS and QT duration in lead II,

G. V. Marchetti et al.

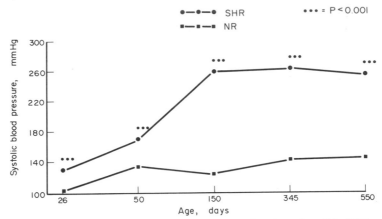

Fig. 1. Time-course of systolic blood pressure measured indirectly at the tail in SHR and NR rats of various ages.

intrinsecoid deflection in V_5, height of R wave in V_5 and depth of S wave in V_1, voltage of T wave in lead II, the frontal electric axis was calculated by the method of Goldman[3] and T wave abnormalities were considered[4].

RESULTS

Arterial pressure is normal in 26-day-old SHR and NR and in NR of all ages. It is above normal in all other groups of SHR reaching values of about 260 mm Hg (Fig. 1). Table 1 shows that there is a significant cardiac hypertrophy in young and old SHR.

The body weight is noticeably different in SHR and NR (Table 2) and therefore the heart weight/body weight ratio cannot be considered as a reliable index of cardiac hypertrophy.

TABLE 1. HEART WEIGHT (mg)/BODY WEIGHT (g)

Age (days)	SHR Number	SHR Average ± S.E.	NR Number	NR Average ± S.E.	P
26	15	4.6 ± 0.1	15	3.9 ± 0.1	<0.001
50	10	3.8 ± 0.1	16	3.2 ± 0.0	<0.001
150	5	4.1 ± 0.1	10	2.4 ± 0.0	<0.001
345	8	4.0 ± 0.1	12	2.6 ± 0.1	<0.001
550	7	4.6 ± 0.1	8	2.1 ± 0.2	<0.001

Comparison between the averages of SHR groups <0.001.
Comparison between the averages of NR groups <0.001.
Comparison between the averages of SHR and NR groups <0.001.

TABLE 2. BODY WEIGHT (g)

Age (days)	SHR Number	Average ± S.E.	NR Number	Average ± S.E.	P
26	15	56 ± 1	15	74 ± 2	N.S.
50	10	175 ± 5	16	181 ± 4	N.S.
150	5	314 ± 8	10	370 ± 7	<0.001
345	8	392 ± 15	12	541 ± 8	<0.001
550	7	380 ± 7	8	605 ± 25	<0.001

Comparison between the averages of SHR groups <0.001.
Comparison between the averages of NR groups <0.001.
Comparison between the averages of SHR and NR groups <0.001.

A more correct approach for evaluating hypertrophy is to measure left ventricle weight/right ventricle weight and left ventricle weight/total heart weight ratios.

The ratios are similar in 26-day-old SHR and NR whereas they are increasingly higher in older SHR (Tables 3, 4). Therefore the heart is normal in 26-day-old SHR whereas from 50 days on, the left ventricle in SHR becomes clearly hypertrophic in respect to NR.

TABLE 3. LEFT VENTRICULAR WEIGHT (mg)/RIGHT VENTRICULAR WEIGHT (mg)

Age (days)	SHR Number	Average ± S.E.	NR Number	Average ± S.E.	P
26	15	2.64 ± 0.11	15	2.45 ± 0.10	N.S.
50	10	2.71 ± 0.13	16	1.96 ± 0.06	<0.001
150	5	3.60 ± 0.28	10	2.33 ± 0.06	<0.001
345	8	3.64 ± 0.17	12	2.95 ± 0.12	<0.001
550	7	4.17 ± 0.31	8	2.88 ± 0.17	<0.001

Comparison between the averages of SHR groups <0.001.
Comparison between the averages of NR groups <0.001.
Comparison between the averages of SHR and NR groups <0.001.

TABLE 4. LEFT VENTRICULAR WEIGHT (mg)/HEART WEIGHT (mg)

Age (days)	SHR Number	Average ± S.E.	NR Number	Average ± S.E.	P
26	15	0.55 ± 0.013	15	0.54 ± 0.012	N.S.
50	10	0.58 ± 0.014	16	0.51 ± 0.011	<0.01
150	5	0.62 ± 0.016	10	0.55 ± 0.008	<0.05
345	8	0.68 ± 0.056	12	0.58 ± 0.093	<0.001
550	7	0.65 ± 0.015	8	0.59 ± 0.009	<0.05

Comparison between the averages of SHR groups <0.01.
Comparison between the averages of NR groups <0.05.
Comparison between the averages of SHR and NR groups <0.001.

G. V. Marchetti et al.

TABLE 5. ECG HEIGHT OF R WAVE V_5 (mvolt)

Age (days)	Number	SHR Average ± S.E.	Number	NR Average ± S.E.	P
26	15	0.75 ± 0.06	15	0.46 ± 0.08	<0.01
50	20	0.39 ± 0.05	17	0.38 ± 0.05	N.S.
150	9	0.67 ± 0.08	17	0.30 ± 0.03	<0.001
345	8	0.95 ± 0.09	12	0.39 ± 0.05	<0.001
550	12	1.00 ± 0.13	9	0.34 ± 0.04	<0.001

Comparison between the averages of SHR groups <0.001.
Comparison between the averages of NR groups N.S.
Comparison between the averages of SHR and NR groups <0.001.

TABLE 6. ECG DEPTH OF S WAVE V_1 (mvolt)

Age (days)	Number	SHR Average ± S.E.	Number	NR Average ± S.E.	P
26	15	0.28 ± 0.04	15	0.21 ± 0.09	N.S.
50	20	0.39 ± 0.04	17	0.04 ± 0.02	<0.001
150	9	0.39 ± 0.10	17	0.06 ± 0.01	<0.01
345	8	1.68 ± 0.10	12	0.35 ± 0.06	<0.001
550	12	1.17 ± 0.19	9	0.17 ± 0.07	<0.001

Comparison between the averages of SHR groups <0.001.
Comparison between the averages of NR groups N.S.
Comparison between the averages of SHR and NR groups <0.001.

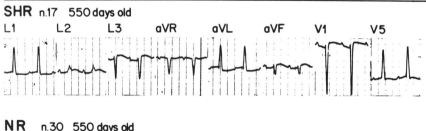

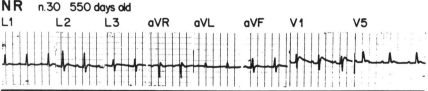

Fig. 2. Example of ECG recorded in 550-day-old SHR and NR. In SHR, R wave is very tall in aVL, D_1 and V_5 whereas S wave is considerably deep in L_3 and V_1. ST interval is virtually absent in NR electrocardiograms whereas in SHR it is shifted downwards in aVL, D_1 and V_5.

We can thus conclude that myocardial hypertrophy accompanies the development of hypertension and does not seem to precede it as affirmed by Sen *et al.*[5].

PQ, QRS and QT duration increase in proportion with age and pressure in SHR (P < 0.001). A smaller increase is also observed in NR. QT duration is longer in old SHR than in matched NR.

The voltage of R wave in V_5 and S wave in V_1 is higher in SHR than NR (Tables 5 and 6).

There is a significant difference in ECG time intervals only between the groups of old SHR and NR (Fig. 2). These data show, in conclusion, that it is difficult to identify the early stage of cardiac hypertrophy on the basis of ECG only.

REFERENCES

1. Okamoto, K. and Aoki, K. (1963) Development of a strain of spontaneously hypertensive rats. *Japan. Circul. J.* **27**, 282.
2. Friebel, H. and Vreden, E. (1958) Ein Gerät zur Blutdruckmessung an der Ratte. *Arch. exp. Path. Pharmak.* **232**, 419.
3. Goldman, M. J. (1973) *Principles of Clinical Electrocardiography.* 8th edition. Lange Medical Pub., Los Altos, CA.
4. Dunn, F. G., Pfeffer, M. A. and Frohlich, E. D. (1978) ECG alterations with progressive left ventricular hypertrophy in spontaneous hypertension. *Clin. exp. Hypertens.* **1**, 67.
5. Sen, S., Tarazi, R. C., Khairallah, Ph. A. and Bumpus, F. M. (1975) Cardiac hypertrophy in spontaneously hypertensive rats. *Circul. Res.* **35**, 775.

Comparison of ECG and Morphological Parameters in Male and Female Spontaneously Hypertensive Rats (SHR)

R. MÜLLER-PEDDINGHAUS, U. G. KÜHL AND
G. BUSCHMANN

ABSTRACT

The experiments were performed in spontaneously hypertensive rats (SHR) and normotensive Wistar rats (NR) of either sex. The animals were divided into six groups:

Groups 1 and 2 (old SHR), consisting of 8 males (13 months, 340–420 g) and 11 females (15 months 220–280 g), were anesthetized with 1.25 g urethane/kg intraperitoneally for ECG recording and sacrificed at the end of the experiment for determination of relative heart weights and for histopathological examination of hearts and kidneys.

Groups 3 and 4 (growing SHR) were 6 males (9 to 25 weeks, 150–325 g) and 5 females (9 to 25 weeks, 130–205 g), groups 5 and 6 (growing NR) were 8 males (6 to 18 weeks, 120–370 g) and 8 females (7 to 19 weeks, 120–220 g). In these animals, ECG recordings were performed at biweekly intervals under pentobarbital-anesthesia (50 mg/kg intraperitoneally).

In all animals the ECG was taken by a lead in the direction of the heart axis and evaluated by on-line biosignal processing.

In growing NR as well as in growing SHR heart rate decreased with age, whereas PR, QRS and RαT intervals increased with age in SHR, but not in NR.

In contrast to both NR and young SHR marked alterations were observed in QRS and T wave configurations of old SHR. QRS complexes longer than 20 ms appeared to be more frequent in male (5/8) than in female (3/11) old SHR.

No sex differences were found for the relative heart weights of the old SHR. In males as well as in females left ventricular hypertrophy was present, and 7 out of 8 males showed histological signs of hypertensive arteriopathy in the heart and/or the kidneys compared to 4 out of 11 females.

The apparent sex difference in the prevalence of hypertensive arteriopathy and of QRS complexes of more than 20 ms in the SHR is in agreement with the hypothesis that a prolongation of QRS may be indicative of myocardial lesions in the rat.

1. INTRODUCTION

Hypertension in rats is known to be associated with morphological alterations such as hypertensive arteriopathy and left ventricular hypertrophy (Dimitrov and Kiprov, 1974; Yamori et al., 1976; Limas et al., 1980).

Electrocardiographic changes related to hypertension in rats have been reported by Sambhi and White (1960), Dimitrov and Kiprov (1974), and Yamori et al. (1976). The aim of our study was to determine possible age and sex dependencies of ECG changes in spontaneously hypertensive rats using the method of on-line biosignal processing (Schumacher et al., page 171 of this volume) for the evaluation of rat electrocardiograms with an abnormal configuration.

2. METHODS

Normotensive Wistar rats (NR Han: Wistar) and spontaneously hypertensive rats (SHR, Okamoto-NIH-Montreal-Boehringer-Ingelheim-Kißlegg) of either sex were used. The animals were divided into six groups:

Groups 1 and 2 (old SHR) consisted of 8 males (group 1; 13 months, 340–420 g body weight) and 11 females (group 2; 15 months, 220–280 g) with an already high spontaneous mortality rate. They were anesthetized with 1.25 g urethane/kg intraperitoneally for ECG recording and sacrificed at the end of the experiment for determination of relative heart weights and for histopathological examination of hearts and kidneys.

TABLE 1

Group	Age (weeks)	n	Prevalence of hypertensive arteriopathy Heart	Kidney	Heart rate (1/min)	Pr int. (ms)	QRS (ms)	RαT int. (ms)
Male SHR	9	6	—	—	397 ±15 }**	43 ±2.2	13 ±1.3 }*	26 ±5.8
	25	5	—	—	326 ±27	48 ±4.5	17 ±3.5	32 ±6.3
	83	8	7/8	6/8	295 ±49	54 ±6.4	23.5 ±5.7	39 ±11.2
Female SHR	9	5	—	—	362 ±27	42 ±1.9	12 ±1.3	23 ±1.6
	25	2	—	—	328	41	17	22
	91	11	4/11	2/11	314 ±39	55 ±5.6	19.8 ±3.5	33 ±15.9
Male NR	6	8	—	—	429 ±34 }***	44 ±3.0	13 ±1.1	21 ±2.2
	18	8	—	—	359 ±26	44 ±2.2	14 ±0.6	24 ±4.2
Female NR	7	8	—	—	441 ±20	42 ±1.2 }**	14 ±1.6 }*	28 ±7.8
	18	8	—	—	372 ±22	44 ±3.1	15 ±1.0	25 ±2.4

— Not measured.   Means ± SD.

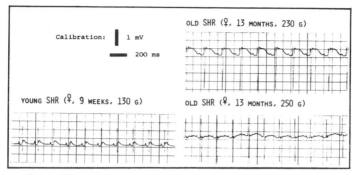

Fig. 1. Electrocardiogram of young and old SHR (lead heart axis).

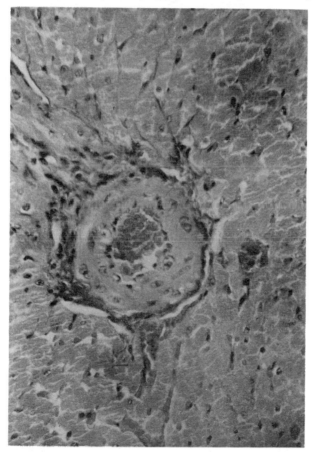

Fig. 2. Moderate severe diffuse medial hypertrophy of medium size artery; polymorph, highly activated nuclei of arterial smooth muscle cells which lost their characteristic elongated form (15-month-old female SHR; rel. heart weight 0.50%; van Gieson's stain; paraffin embedding; 100:1).

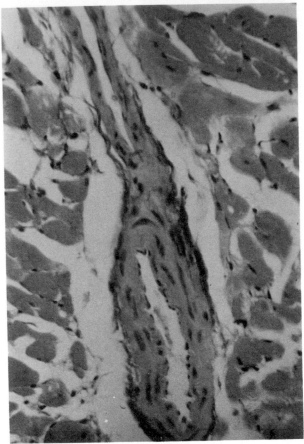

Fig. 3. Unchanged medium size artery with normal width and characteristic elongated smooth muscle nuclei (15-month-old female SHR; rel. heart weight 0.51%; van Gieson's stain; paraffin embedding; 100:1).

Groups 3 and 4 (growing SHR) consisted of 6 males (group 3; 9 to 25 weeks, 150–325 g) and 5 females (group 4; 9 to 25 weeks, 130–205 g).

Groups 5 and 6 (growing NR) were 8 males (group 5; 6 to 18 weeks, 120–370 g) and 8 females (group 6; 7 to 19 weeks, 120–220 g).

In groups 3, 4, 5 and 6 ECG recordings were performed at biweekly intervals under pentobarbital-anesthesia (50 mg/kg intraperitoneally).

In all animals the ECG was taken by a lead in the direction of the heart axis (Spörri, 1944). The measurement of the ECG parameters was done by on-line biosignal processing (Schumacher et al., page 171 of this volume).

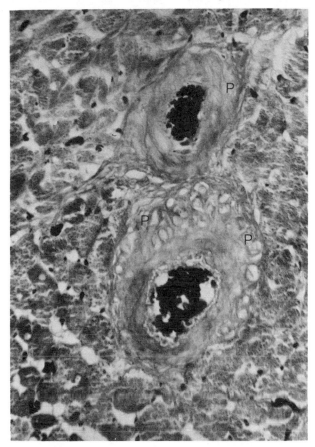

Fig. 4. Severe diffuse medial hyperplasia (P) of medium size artery; marked increase in width and loss of normal architecture (13-month-old male SHR; rel. heart weight 0.63%. Azan's stain; paraffin embedding; 100:1).

3. RESULTS

In growing NR as well as in growing SHR the heart rate decreased with age (Table 1, Fig. 8), whereas PR, QRS and RαT intervals increased with age in SHR (Fig. 9), but not in NR.

In contrast to both NR and young SHR, marked alterations were observed in QRS and T wave configurations of old SHR (Fig. 1). QRS changes consisted in high voltage with a deep S wave, the T waves were either enlarged or flattened. There were no obvious sex differences in the configuration of the ECG or in the duration of the PR and RαT intervals (Table 1). In old SHR, QRS complexes longer than 20 ms appeared to be more frequent in males (5/8) than in females (3/11).

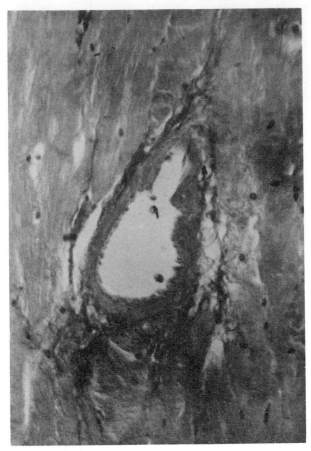

Fig. 5. Unchanged medium size artery of normal width with slightly increased perivascular connective tissue (blue) (15 month old female SHR; rel. heart weight 0.75%. Azan's stain; paraffin embedding; 100:1).

No sex differences were found for the relative heart weights in the old SHR (0.57 ± 0.08 in males, and 0.60 ± 0.08 in females). The histopathological findings in these hearts consisted of diffuse hypertensive arteriopathy and medial hypertrophy and hyperplasia. Hypertensive arteriopathy was more frequent and more severe in male than in female SHR (Table 1, Figs. 2–7).

In the kidneys, medial hypertrophy of renal arteries (not depicted) was less marked than in the heart. In some animals focal lesions such as severe proliferation of smooth muscle cells in small renal arteries and fibrinoid necrosis of medium size renal arteries (1 male, 1 female) were found (Fig. 7). The latter changes were not seen in the heart.

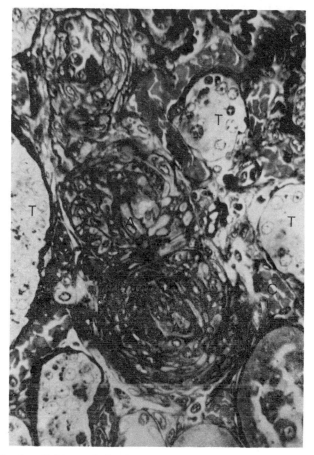

Fig. 6. Severe focal medial hyperplasia of a small renal artery (A); capillaries (C); tubuli (T) (13-month-old male SHR; rel. heart weight 0.56%; Movat's stain; methacrylate embedding; 160:1).

4. DISCUSSION

The observed ECG and histopathological alterations in SHR are in agreement with published data. Dimitrov and Kiprov (1974) described ECG changes in rats with spontaneous hypertension corresponding to ECG changes seen in humans with arterial hypertension. The authors found enlarged, high voltage QRS complexes and an increased relative duration of the QT intervals, but normal PQ intervals and normal heart rates as compared with the control group. No alterations of the T waves were seen, but some of the SHR showed a depression of ST due to disturbed repolarization in the hypertrophied left ventricle. Using vectorcar-

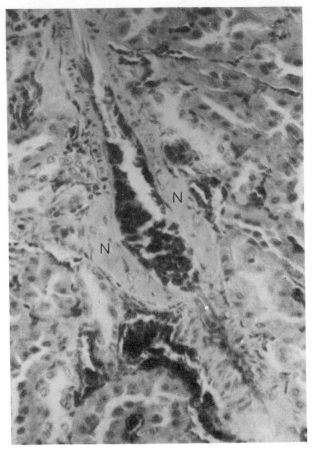

Fig. 7. Local fibrinoid necrosis (N) of a medium size renal artery (13-month-old male SHR; rel. heart weight 0.60%; Hematoxylin-Eosin-stain; paraffin embedding; 100:1).

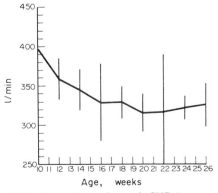

Fig. 8. Heart rate in growing male SHR (mean ± S.D.).

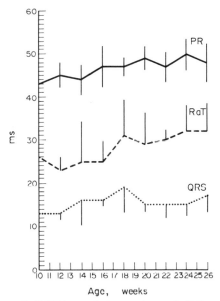

Fig. 9. Changes in ECG intervals in growing male SHR (mean ± S.D.).

diography, Yamori *et al.* (1976), too, found a widening of the QRS complexes and a prolongation of the QT intervals in SHR in comparison to control rats of the Wistar–Kyoto strain.

Histopathological alterations similar to those found in our experiments have also been extensively described by Limas *et al.* (1980).

The apparent sex differences in the prevalence of hypertensive arteriopathy and, to a lesser degree, in the presence of QRS complexes of more than 20 ms in the old SHR is in agreement with the hypothesis that a prolongation of QRS may be indicative of myocardial lesions in the rat (Buschmann *et al.*, 1980).

5. REFERENCES

Buschmann, G., Schumacher, W., Budden, R. and Kühl, U. G. (1980) Evaluation of the effect of dopamine and other catecholamines on ECG and blood pressure in rats using on-line biosignal processing. *J. Cardiovasc. Pharmacol.* (in press).

Dimitrov, T. and Kiprov, D. (1974) Electrocardiographic changes in rats with spontaneous hypertension. *Eksp. Med. Morfol.* **13**, 173–180.

Limas, C., Westrum, B. and Limas, C. J. (1980) The evolution of vascular changes in the spontaneously hypertensive rat. *Am. J. Pathol.* **98**, 357–369.

Sambhi, M. P. and White, F. N. (1960) The electrocardiogram of the normal and hypertensive rat. *Circul. Res.* **8**, 129–134.

Schumacher, W., Budden, R., Buschmann, G. and Kühl, U. G. (1980) A new method for the evaluation of ECG and blood pressure parameters in anesthetized rats by on-line biosignal processing. *International Workshop on the Rat Electrocardiogram in Acute and Chronic Pharmacology and Toxicology*, July 14–15, 1980, Hannover.

Spörri, H. (1944) Der Einfluß der Tuberkulose auf das Elektrokardiogramm—Untersuchungen an Meerschweinchen und Rindern. *Arch. Wiss. Prakt. Tierheilk.* **79**, 1–57.

Yamori, Y., Ohtaka, M. and Nara, Y. (1976) Vectorcardiographic study on left ventricular hypertrophy in spontaneously hypertensive rats. *Jpn. Circ. J.* **40**, 1315–1329.

Measurement of the Cardiodynamics, Hemodynamics and the ECG in the Anesthetized Rat. Effects of Catecholamines (dopamine and isoproterenol)

G. SCHROEDER, B. MAASS, D. BARTELS AND
G. MANNESMANN

ABSTRACT

For many years rats have been used routinely for pharmacological and toxicological studies. For cardiovascular investigations we established a test-model using anaesthetized rats with implanted catheters which allows the measurement or calculation of the following parameters:

Systolic, diastolic and mean arterial blood pressure, the amplitude of arterial blood pressure, the left-ventricular end-diastolic pressure, the maximal rate of rise of left-ventricular pressure, heart rate, cardiac output, peripheral vascular resistance, myocardial O_2-consumption and the evaluation of the ECG as described by Buschmann, G. et al. (Evaluation of the effect of Dopamine and other catecholamines on ECG and blood pressure in rats using on-line biosignal processing; in print).

Using this experimental model the effects of continuous intravenous Dopamine and Isoproterenol infusion were investigated. Infusion of Dopamine resulted in an increase of blood pressure, heart rate, heart contractility and peripheral vascular resistance and caused a reduction in cardiac output. The Isoproterenol infusion lowered blood pressure and peripheral vascular resistance and increased heart contractility, heart rate and cardiac output.

The results were in accordance with the known cardiovascular effects of Dopamine and Isoproterenol. It could therefore be concluded that the model, being relatively simple and inexpensive, can be used routinely for investigations on the cardiovascular effects of pharmacological compounds.

STATEMENT OF PROBLEM

For the investigation of cardiovascular drug effects we established a test-model using anaesthetized rats which allows the measurement or calculation of the following cardiovascular parameters:

Ps   systolic blood pressure
PD   diastolic blood pressure

155

P_M	mean arterial blood pressure
ΔP	amplitude of arterial blood pressure
LVEDP	left-ventricular end-diastolic pressure
$LVdp/dt_{max}$	max. rate of rise of left ventricular pressure
HR	heart rate
CO	cardiac output
W	peripheral vascular resistance
I_{O_2}	myocardial oxygen consumption
ECG	electrocardiogram

CONCLUSION

The results we obtained in our experiments confirm the well-known cardiovascular effects of the investigated catecholamines Dopamine and Isoproterenol.

Therefore it is concluded that the described test-model, which is relatively simple and inexpensive, can be used routinely for cardiovascular investigations.

MATERIALS AND METHODS

Animals

♂, Wistar-SPF-Rats, 280–350 g b.w.

Anaesthesia

1.25 g/kg b.w. urethane i.p.

Calculation of the Cardiovascular Parameters

After completion of the preparation, pre-application values were obtained during a thirty min. equilibration period. The mean values of systolic and diastolic blood pressure, ΔP, left-ventricular end-diastolic blood pressure and the maximal rate of rise of left-ventricular pressure were calculated from ten consecutive pulse waves per time point. Mean arterial blood pressure, peripheral vascular resistance and myocardial

O_2-consumption were calculated as follows:

$$P_M = P_D + 0.42 \times \Delta P$$

$$W = \frac{\dfrac{P_M}{10} \times 800 \text{ mm Hg}}{CO \ (ml/min/100 \text{ g b.w.})}$$

$$I_{O_2} = HR \times P_M$$

The ECG data were evaluated by continuous on-line biosignal processing.

Experiments

The effects of continuous intravenous infusion of Dopamine-HCl (Dopamin®, Guilini-Pharma) and Isoproterenol-Sulfate (Aludrin®, Boehringer Ingelheim) at an initial dose of 0.01 μmol kg⁻¹ min⁻¹ and 0.001 μmol kg⁻¹ min⁻¹ respectively were investigated. Every ten minutes (10 min, 20 min and 30 min) the drug concentration was increased tenfold without changing the infusion volume (0.1 ml/min/animal).

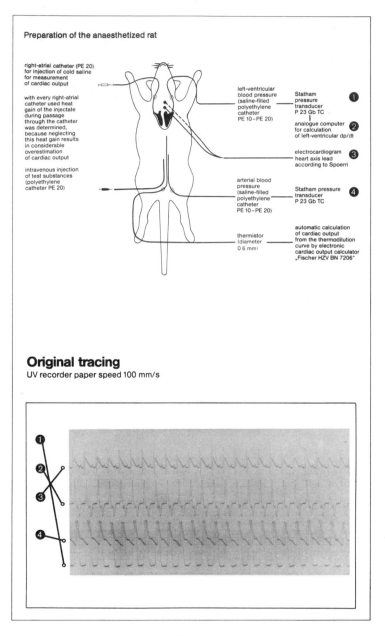

Fig. 1.

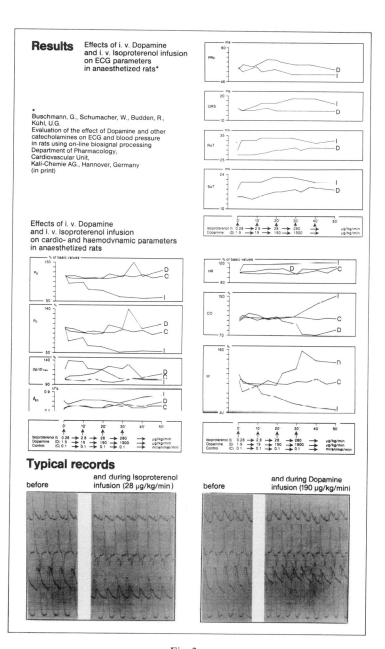

Fig. 2.

Graphical Representation of the Time Evolution of ECG Data using a Computer Data Storage and Plot Package

J. ELSNER AND R. KNUTTI

ABSTRACT

A general computer data storage, analysis, and plot scheme, usable for any type of data structure, is presented. The time evolution of the subacute effect of emetine on heart rate, PR-interval, QRS-interval, R:S wave voltage ratio and on the T-voltage is shown as an example for the usefulness of this program package. The concept of the significance limit is introduced.

INTRODUCTION

The visual inspection of the qualitative and quantitative properties of the experimental data is a very important, but often ignored step in the process of scientific data analysis. The main reason why data are rarely represented graphically is the fact that the work involved for plotting data is considerable.

The computer program package presented here provides a tool to scientific research, for fast data storage, retrieval, analysis, and graphical representation. The data are stored in a structured way, either manually through a data editor, or with the help of standardized procedures. The data are referenced for editing, retrieval, and analysis by hierarchically ordered user defined labels. Data stored in this way are accessible for any kind of analysis by programs using the appropriate data access scheme.

Five general purpose programs exist today for assistance to the user:

DSD: the Data Structure Definition program creates a preformatted file, interpreting a user provided Data Structure Definition file written in a comprehensive PASCAL-like language.

DED: the Data Editor follows the given data structure, by prompting each data element for manual input. Several instructions provide for an editor-like flexibility for deleting, correcting, and locating the data.

DLS: the Data List program lists the whole data file creating automatically an appropriate layout.

DUP: the Data Update program copies data of existing files into new files having a different (extended or restricted) structure.

DPL: the Data Plot program plots the data according to a user supplied Data Plot Description File. This file is a sequence of keywords, some with arguments, supplying the program with the data identification and plot format information.

These programs were developed in FORTRAN on a PDP11/34 minicomputer running under the RSX11M operating system, using a modified VERSAPLOT software from VERSATEC, and a VERSATEC 1200 Printer/Plotter.

THE EXPERIMENT

The experiment has been described in detail by Zbinden et al.[1]. Three groups of 8 female rats, ZUR:SIV-Z strain, were treated by subcutaneous injections on 5 days per week. The low dose group got 1 mg/kg emetine dihydrochloride in 2 ml/kg per injection during 7 weeks and the high dose group 5 mg/kg per injection during $3\frac{1}{2}$ weeks. The control group was given equal volume of 0.9% NaCl.

The ECG was recorded before the daily treatment from the restrained, unanaesthetized rats with needle electrodes placed at lead D^2. These measures were performed two times per week during the respective treatment period.

PR- and QRS-intervals and R-, S- and T-wave voltages were measured manually on the paper recordings in 10 consecutive heart cycles, and the heart rate was calculated from RR-intervals.

The results are shown in Figures 1 and 2 exhibiting a dose- and time-related effect of emetine on the PR-interval, the QRS-interval, and the T-voltage, but none on the heart rate and the R:S wave voltage ratio.

Figure 3 shows the parameter distributions pooled over the whole time of the experiment for the three groups. The widening of the PR- and QRS-interval and the T-voltage distributions of the treated groups may be attributed to the change of these values over time. The bimodal distribution of the R:S voltage ratio results from the fact that the S wave vanishes in certain cases, resulting in a ratio of 100%.

The normality of the distribution is examined in Figure 4, where the cumulative relative frequency distribution is plotted with a normal probability scale as the ordinate. The expected frequencies (i.e. the frequencies

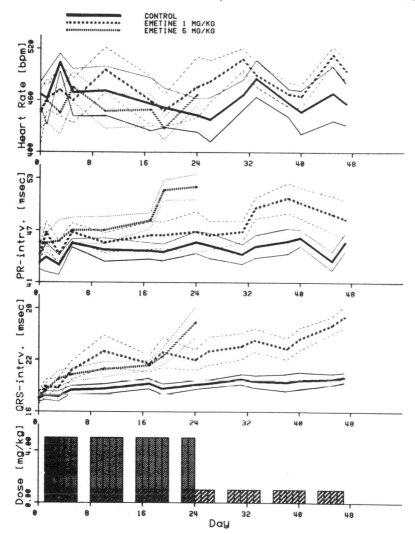

Fig. 1. The cumulative relative frequency distributions of the same values as in Fig. 3, plotted with the normal probability scale as the ordinate. The straight lines are regression lines of the points.

from a normal distribution) would fall on the regression lines of the points shown. It can be seen that the distributions are sufficiently normal to allow the use of parametric statistics.

The following sections describe the process by which these plots could be obtained.

J. Elsner and R. Knutti

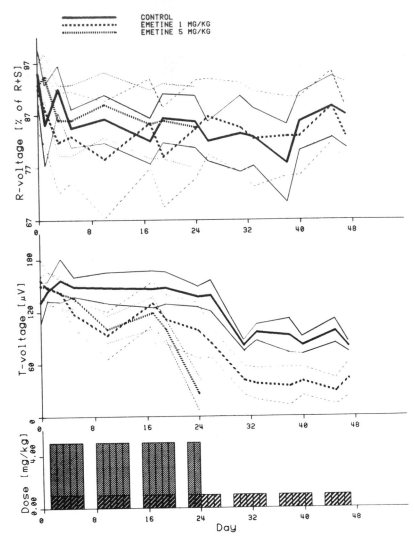

Fig. 2. The distributions of the five ECG parameters pooled over the whole time of the
experiment for the three experimental groups.

THE DATA STRUCTURE DEFINITION

The definition of the data structure is a critical step in the process of the
graphical data analysis. A chosen structure determines all following steps,
i.e., the data input, the listing format, and all subsequent references to the
individual data or sets of data. The factors which determine the appro-

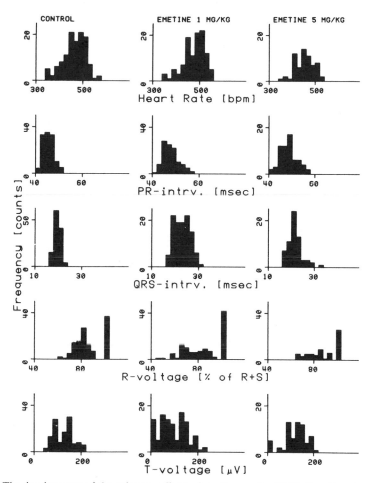

Fig. 3. The development of the subacute effects of emetine on the ECG: R-voltage in percent of (R + S)-voltage and the T-voltage. Progressive flattening of T-wave, no effect on R:S wave voltage ratio.

priate choice of the data structure are:

—the form in which the data were originally recorded,
—the desired prompting of the data editor,
—the desired access to the data as sets,
—global and local characteristics of the data.

The data structure has to be defined in a hierarchic fashion in which a key-label at a specific level points to sets of key-labels at a deeper level. The natural method for representing hierarchic structures is by a tree of nodes. Figure 1 shows such a tree we chose for the data of the emetine experi-

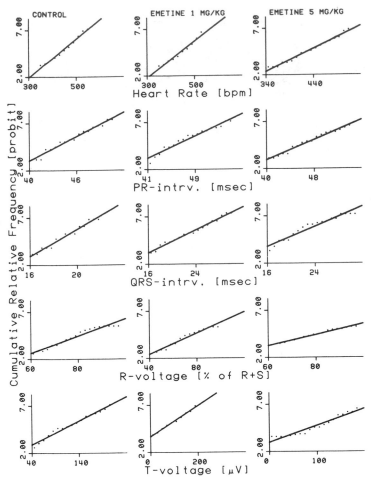

Fig. 4. The development of the subacute effects of emetine on the ECG: heart rate, PR-interval, and QRS-interval. Progressive prolongation of PR and QRS interval, no effect on heart rate.

ment. Two arrays of values contain the treatment days on one hand, and the measure days on the other. They are valid for all three animal groups. Each animal group contains an identification, the dosage for each treatment day, and five ECG parameters. Each parameter contains values for each measure day and for each of eight animals.

This diagram is translated into a Data Structure Definition file as shown below.

```
data:   Day: ARRAY [1, .48] of integer;
        Measure Day: ARRAY [1..15] of integer;
        Group: ARRAY [1..3] of gr;
```

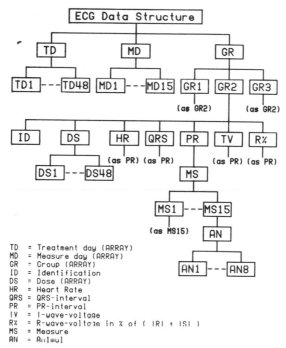

Diagram 1. The hierarchical data structure used for the storage of the ECG parameters represented as a node-tree.

gr: Group Identification: name;
           Dose: ARRAY [1..48] of real;
           Heart Rate [bpm]: meas;
           QRS-intrv. [msec]: meas;
           PR-intrv. [msec]: meas;
           T-voltage ['my' V]: meas;
           R-voltage [% of R + S]: meas;
meas: Measure: ARRAY [1..15] of anim;
anim: Animal: ARRAY [1..8] of integer.

The names "data", "gr", "meas" and "anim" are auxiliary labels for internal references; the names "Day", "Measure Day", "Group" etc. are the actual labels used for editor prompting and data references.

THE DATA EDITOR

The data may be input using the data editor DED. This program allows insertion of the data in a sequence indicated by the data structure: lower levels of the data hierarchy have precedence; successive nodes of higher levels get active only when all ramifications of the actual node are satisfied. The scheme of the ECG data structure above results in the following sequence:

—Treatment Days 1 to 48,
—Measure Days 1 to 15,
—Group 1/Group Identification,
—Group 1/Dose 1 to 48,
—Group 1/Heart Rate/Measure 1/Animal 1 to 8,
—Group 1/Heart Rate/Measure 2/Animal 1 to 8,
etc.

This typing can be made in one complete or in several partial sessions. Simple instructions allow one to step back to the last data item, to the first item of a set or of the file, to search specific nodes or the next empty data item, to delete data (data may be nil), or to modify the data or the node names.

THE DATA PLOT DESCRIPTION

The edited data may be represented graphically in various ways through a Data Plot Definition (DPD) file. This file consists of a sequence of keywords with arguments, giving information to the program DPL about which data to plot and in which format. A large set of keywords is available to plot text, to adjust the linewidth, to scale the data, to plot families of lines and bar graphs, and for other features. Two DPD file segments are shown here as illustration.

The instructions to plot the upper graph of Fig. 1 are shown below. The keywords are the first item of each line, followed by arguments. This plot represents the means and upper and lower significance limits of the heart rate values of all three groups.

x-data:
variable:　　　　　　　Measure Day

y-data:
minmax:　　　　　　　6.75, 9.
node:　　　　　　　　Heart Rate [bpm]
parameter:　　　　　　Group
variable:　　　　　　　Measure
l-significance:　　　　　Animal
linewidth:　　　　　　1

new data:

y-data:
node: Heart Rate [bpm]
parameter: Group
variable: Measure
u-significance: Animal

new data:

y-data:
node: Heart Rate [bpm]
parameter: Group
variable: Measure
mean: Animal
linewidth: 8

The DPD file segment contains the instructions to plot the upper left graph of Fig. 4 representing the cumulative relative frequency distribution of the heart rate values of group 1, the control group, with a normal probability scale as the ordinate and a linear regression line.

x-minmax: 0.,2.
y-minmax: 6.,8.5
point plot:
linreg:
relative:
cumulative:
frequency: 20
probit:
node: Heart Rate [bpm]
node: Group
index: 1
parameter: Measure
variable: Animal

THE SIGNIFICANCE LIMIT

The significance limit of a set of data is defined as a value having the following properties:

—the difference between it and the mean is proportional to the standard deviation;
—it is equal to the corresponding significance limit of another set of data with an identical degree of freedom and distribution, having a significantly different mean at the level of 0.05.

The two significance limits sl($+$) and sl($-$) may be calculated from these constraints as follows:

$$sl(+) = \overline{X} + sd$$

$$sl(-) = \overline{X} - sd$$

sd being the significance difference:

$$sd = t_{0.05(2),(2n)} - \sqrt{\frac{\overline{X^2} - \overline{X}^2}{2n}}$$

t is the critical value of the t-distribution and n the degree of freedom.

Thus, two sets of data on the plots at a specific point in time may be considered to be different if the two corresponding significance intervals do not overlap. At the same time these intervals are a measure for the variance of the data.

It is understood that the 0.05-significance of the difference between two sets is warranted by these limits only if the two sets of data are normally distributed and have the same degree of freedom and standard deviation. Otherwise other statistical tests need to be performed to confirm this preliminary result.

REFERENCES

1. Zbinden, G., Kleinert, R. and Rageth, B. (1980) Assessment of emetine cardiotoxicity in a subacute toxicity experiment in rats. *J. Cardiovasc. Pharmacol.* **2,** 155–164.
2. Grauwiler, J. (1965) *Herz und Kreislauf der Saeugetiere.* Birkhaeuser Verlag, Basel.

A New Method for the Evaluation of ECG and Blood Pressure Parameters in Anesthetized Rats by On-line Biosignal Processing*

W. SCHUMACHER, R. BUDDEN, G. BUSCHMANN
AND U. G. KÜHL

ABSTRACT

A method for the on-line evaluation of ECG and blood pressure signals in anesthetized rats is presented. The accuracy of the method was verified by the comparison of conventional and computerized results. In order to find the most suitable ECG lead for the computer evaluation, different leads were processed simultaneously from the same rats. The dependence of ECG intervals and segments on the heart rate was examined, and a formula was derived for the correction of the PR interval.

1. INTRODUCTION

Until now the electrocardiogram has only rarely been evaluated in acute as well as in chronic pharmacological and toxicological experiments with small laboratory animals. This may partly be due to the fact that—as a rule—a substantial number of animals is used in these experiments, resulting in a high expense of technical and personal facilities.

We therefore developed a method for the computerized on-line evaluation of rat ECG and blood pressure biosignals. The establishment of a rapid and reliable method for the measurement of rat ECG parameters might lead to a more frequent incorporation of the ECG in rat experiments and thus augment the usability of this species.

2. EXPERIMENTAL DESIGN

The experiments were performed in male rats (Han:Wistar, 300–360 g), anesthetized with urethane (1.25 g/kg i.p.). The animals were fixed in the

* Part of the contents of this paper has been published elsewhere (Buschmann et al., 1980).

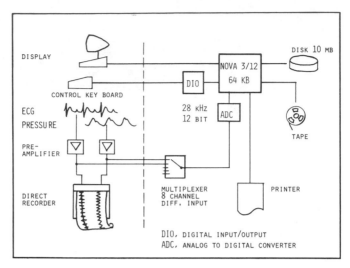

DISPLAY

DISK 10 MB

NOVA 3/12
64 KB

DIO

CONTROL KEY BOARD

ECG
PRESSURE

28 kHz
12 BIT

ADC

TAPE

PRE-
AMPLIFIER

DIRECT
RECORDER

MULTIPLEXER
8 CHANNEL
DIFF. INPUT

PRINTER

DIO, DIGITAL INPUT/OUTPUT
ADC, ANALOG TO DIGITAL CONVERTER

Fig. 1. System design for the on-line analysis of ECG and blood pressure signals in anesthetized rats.

supine position; ECG (lead: heart axis, Spörri, 1944) and the blood pressure (left carotid artery) of four rats were recorded simultaneously on a
direct recorder (Hellige). In parallel the analog signals were fed into a
process computer (NOVA 3/12, Data General) (Fig. 1).

These computer-evaluated parameters were stored on a magnetic disk
for further statistical calculations.

3. SIGNAL PROCESSING

The *evaluation cycles* of the experiment were 30 s (Fig. 2A). At the beginning of each evaluation cycle a 5 s period of every analog signal is digitized
at a rate of 1 kHz and stored (Fig. 2B). Initially, the 5 s ECG *signal period*
is checked for the fastest positive to negative movement (dU/dt_{min}). This
value is used for the determination of the point of dU/dt_{min} within the
single ECG complexes. The interval between the preceding and the actual
point of dU/dt_{min} is taken for the RR interval. ECG complexes are
accepted for signal averaging, if the actual RR interval does not exceed the
individual tolerance limits. ECG *signal segments* of 512 ms distributed cen-
trally around the point of dU/dt_{min} are averaged. For the respective pressure signal a segment of 512 ms, beginning at the point of dU/dt_{min} of the
ECG signal, is averaged, too (Fig. 2C). This procedure is repeated until five
comparable signal segments are averaged.

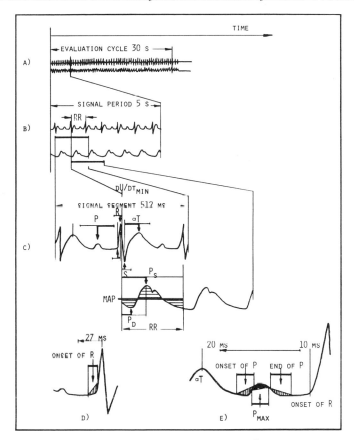

Fig. 2. Steps of evaluation, recognition and definition of the significant signal points.

Within these *signal segments* the following points are localized:

(a) R_{max}: a region of 24 ms before dU/dt_{min} is scanned for the point of the highest voltage.

(b) Onset of R: starting at the point of R_{max} a "window" (12 ms width) is moved "backward" over a 27 ms region. The discrete point, where the area between the signal curve and the straight line between the section points of the window limbs and the signal curve is a maximum, is defined as the onset of R (Fig. 2D). If present, the minimum of Q is found as the onset of R.

(c) S_{min}: this is the point of the lowest voltage in a region up to 24 ms "forward" from the point dU/dt_{min}.

(d) $\alpha T'$ is the point of the maximum voltage within an interval of 50 ms starting at S_{min}. The signal period between $S_{min} + 2$ ms and $\alpha T' + 10$ ms is

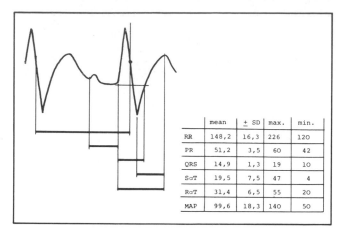

	mean	± SD	max.	min.
RR	148,2	16,3	226	120
PR	51,2	3,5	60	42
QRS	14,9	1,3	19	10
SαT	19,5	7,5	47	4
RαT	31,4	6,5	55	20
MAP	99,6	18,3	140	50

Fig. 3. Definitions of the measured ECG intervals and segments and pre-drug values of 132 animals.

smoothed by the moving average method. This region is again scanned for the point of the highest voltage ($= \alpha T$). Only if the T wave is positive, is αT found exactly.

(e) The P wave is the most pronounced sequence of a concave to convex to concave signal movement in the region between the onset of $R - 10$ ms and the point of αT of the preceding ECG complex $+ 20$ ms. This sequence is found by the "moving window" method, too (compare 3b). The sum of the absolute values of the three resulting areas must be a maximum for the scanned region. The onset of P, P_{max} and the end of P are indicated by the middle point of the window at the points of local maximum/minimum (Fig. 2E).

(f) The voltage of the isoelectric line is calculated by the mean of five signal points, placed in the middle between the end of P and the onset of R. All amplitude values are corrected by this value.

(g) The onset and the end of the S wave are the intersection points of the isoelectric line and the S wave.

(h) Systolic blood pressure is the highest amplitude value of the averaged pressure curve within the first RR interval (Fig. 2C).

(i) Diastolic blood pressure is the lowest value between the point of dU/dt_{min} of the ECG signal segment and P_s.

The mean arterial blood pressure (MAP) is calculated by integration of the averaged pressure signal for the period of one "RR interval".

From these characteristic points ECG intervals and segments are determined. The definitions of the measured ECG intervals and the pre-drug values of 132 animals are given in Fig. 3.

TABLE 1. CORRELATION COEFFICIENTS BETWEEN COMPUTERIZED AND CONVEN-TIONAL RESULTS (N = 28) (**p < 0.01; ***p < 0.001)

| | Investigator | | | | |
	1	2	3	4	5
RR	0.998***	0.996***	0.997***	0.998***	0.997***
PR	0.958***	0.940***	0.931***	0.940***	0.853***
QRS	0.026	−0.172	0.186	−0.183	0.002
SαT	0.597***	0.638***	0.552**	0.613***	0.632***
P_s	0.958***	0.920***	0.949***	0.944***	0.950***
P_b	0.975***	0.965***	0.954***	0.973***	0.974***

4. CONTROL OF THE METHOD

(a) Comparison of Computer and Conventional Evaluation

Five investigators evaluated the ECG and blood pressure tracings from the direct recorder. Measurements were taken from signal periods corresponding to the evaluation cycles of the computer. The comparison of the computer and the conventional results was performed by linear regression analysis or by the Wilcoxon test for difference pairs (Table 1). Only for QRS was no correlation present; this was due to the small variation within the QRS value population. For QRS duration no significant differences were found between the computer and four out of the five investigators; in one case the mean QRS duration was longer than the computer values (1.1 ms, p < 0.025). PR intervals were 1.57–3.5 ms longer in four out of five investigators (p < 0.001). This difference is due to the fact that the onset of P is found earlier by manual measurements.

All investigators determined shorter SαT segments than the computer (3.1–4.2 ms; p < 0.005 and <0.001) caused probably by a signal distortion by the direct recorder. The simultaneous registration of ECG curves on the direct recorder and on an oscilloscope shows that the direct recorder in part produced N waves (Heering, 1970) which are not present on the oscilloscope (Fig. 4).

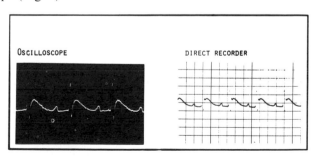

Fig. 4. Demonstration of a signal distortion by the direct recorder.

TABLE 2. CORRELATION COEFFICIENTS (PR INTERVAL)
BETWEEN THE SINGLE "INVESTIGATORS" (N = 28)

	Investigator				
	1	2	3	4	5
Computer investigator	0.958	0.946	0.931	0.940	0.853
5	0.793	0.769	0.840	0.803	
4	0.950	0.941	0.934		
3	0.921	0.938			
2	0.935				

Taking the PR interval as an example, it can be shown that the correlations between the computer evaluation and the conventional ones were even better than the correlations between the individual conventional evaluations (Table 2).

(b) Different ECG Leads

Comparing the results of the computer evaluation of different simultaneously evaluated ECG leads (I, II, III, J, A, D; Nehb, 1938; Spörri, 1944) in the same rat, it was found that the leads II and A offer the best coinciding results, and are both the best for reproduction (Table 3). All other leads produced either small amplitudes (I, III, D) or fairly severe configuration changes (I, J, D) (Fig. 5). For our method, lead A was chosen because it is less sensitive to changes in electrode position than lead II.

HEART RATE DEPENDENCE OF DIFFERENT ECG INTERVALS

The relation of the measured ECG intervals to heart rate was studied in a series of experiments with hypothermia-induced heart rate variations

TABLE 3. RESULTS (MEANS ± SD, N = 13) FROM DIFFERENT ECG LEADS IN THE SAME ANIMAL.
TWO EXPERIMENTS AT DIFFERENT TIME

	Experiment 1				Experiment 2			
	I	III	II	A	A	II	D	J
RR	169.2	169.1	168.5	169.0	153.6	153.6	153.5	153.6
	±3.11	±3.04	±3.10	±3.37	±1.12	±1.12	±1.27	±1.33
PR	54.8	47.5	48.1	48.3	47.2	47.0	44.7	46.8
	±1.17	±1.05	±0.49	±0.65	±0.90	±0.82	±7.40	±1.09
QRS	11.0	14.9	16.9	15.7	15.5	16.9	18.5	15.5
	±0.0	±0.28	±0.28	±0.48	±0.52	±0.28	±5.53	±0.52
SαI	2.4	13.3	19.2	14.1	18.4	19.2	10.8	18.2
	±0.51	±3.43	±4.26	±0.76	±3.95	±4.63	±3.00	±4.65

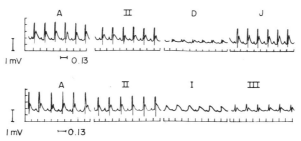

Fig. 5. Simultaneous recordings of four different ECG leads in one rat (A, II, D, J and A, II, I, III resp.).

between 197 and 441 beats/min (RR intervals 305–136 ms). A close correlation was only found between RR and PR intervals (R = 0.61–0.99; p < 0.001). A formula for the individual correction of the PR interval is derived from this model (Fig. 6):

$$PR_{c(i)} = PR_{(i)} + (RR_{(0)} - RR_{(i)} \times 0.2$$

$PR_{c(i)}$ corrected PR interval at the time i
$PR_{(i)}$ measured PR interval at the time i
$RR_{(0)}$ RR interval at the time o (pre-drug value)
$RR_{(i)}$ RR interval at the time i.

PR_c is a derived value supplying information about the extent of a change in the duration of the PR interval at a constant heart rate.

6. CONCLUSION

The method presented supplies correct data for the evaluation of ECG and blood pressure parameters in anesthetized rats. It may be well suited for the routine assessment of drug actions in this model.

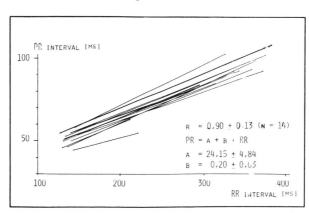

Fig. 6. Correlations between PR and RR intervals in experiments with hypothermia-induced heart rate variations.

7. REFERENCES

Buschmann, G., Schumacher, W., Budden, R. and Kühl, U. G. (1980) Evaluation of the effect of dopamine and other catecholamines on ECG and blood pressure in rats using on-line biosignal processing. *J. Cardiovasc. Pharmacol.* (in press).

Heering, H. (1970a) Das Elektrokardiogramm der wachen und narkotisierten Ratte. *Arch. Int. Pharmacodyn. Ther.* **185**, 308–328.

Nehb, W. (1938) Zur Standardisierung der Brustwandableitungen des Elektrokardiogramms. *Klin. Wochenschr.* **17**, 1807–1811.

Spörri, H. (1944) Der Einfluß der Tuberkulose auf das Elektrokardiogramm—Untersuchungen an Meerschweinchen und Rindern. *Arch. Wiss. Prakt. Tierheilk.* **79**, 1–57.

Computer-assisted Analysis of Arrhythmias in the Rat

P. W. MACFARLANE, K. A. KANE, M. PODOLSKI
AND E. WINSLOW

The technique of ambulatory monitoring has been available for some time to permit the study of cardiac rhythm in humans over extended periods, e.g. 24 hr. However, the equipment used to date is not suitable, without modification, for application to analysis of ECGs recorded from rats in view of the increased heart rate in the latter. For this reason a new method has been developed for analysis of cardiac rhythm in the rat with the intention of facilitating the tedious task of counting the incidence of aberrant beats in the experimental situation.

METHODS

A single ECG lead (in our case either lead 1 or lead 2) is recorded on magnetic tape (RACAL Store-7) at a speed of 7.5 in per second. With the particular experiment undertaken, it was necessary to record the ECG for only 40 min although the method permits recording for up to 6 hr. The ECG was obtained under anaesthesia following coronary artery ligation. At the end of the experiment the ECG is replayed at a speed of 1.875 in per second on to a Medilog I cassette tape recorder manufactured by Oxford Medical Limited (Fig. 1). The 40 min recording is therefore transformed into a 2.66 hr recording on the cassette.

The system used for analysis of the ECG is similar to that previously described for the human ECG (Macfarlane et al., 1979). It consists of an Oxford Replay System (PB2), a Reynolds Medical Highspeed ECG analyser (Pathfinder) and a PDP8A computer system as shown in Fig. 2. The ECG signal is fed from the cassette replay unit directly into the Pathfinder at 60 times the cassette recording speed so that the 2.66 hr recording is replayed for analysis in 2.6 min.

The Pathfinder has a facility for learning the "normal" QRS configuration of the ECG under study. When this is effectively stored in the Pathfinder memory, all incoming beats are then compared with this so called "normal" beat in order to detect any significant difference in morphology.

179

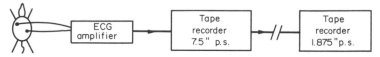

Fig. 1. A scheme of the recording technique used. The ECG replayed at 1.875 per second is transferred to an Oxford cassette recorder.

Thus the ECG recording must first of all be replayed to the Pathfinder in a learning phase. Thereafter the tape is rewound and restarted for analysis proper to commence.

When the Pathfinder detects a QRS complex, it decides whether it is normal or abnormal and produces various logic pulses. In our system, these pulses are linked to a PDP8A computer which can store details of every QRS complex detected. Basically, a record is kept of whether the beat is normal or abnormal together with a measurement of the RR interval between the preceding and present QRS complex under study. In addition for each cycle, an estimate of the "ST segment deviation" can be stored but in the experimental rat, this is of little meaning. A record is also kept of the time from commencement of the analysis to each beat.

In addition to storing details of each beat, the computer continually digitizes the ECG at an effective rate of 500 samples per second with respect to the original recording. In practice the A-D conversion rate of the

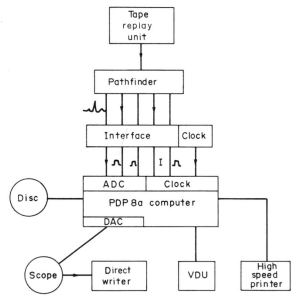

Fig. 2. The hardware used for 24-hr ECG analysis.

computer is 7500 samples/sec. This means that effectively a 2 sec cyclic buffer of rat ECG is contained in the system and if a simple PDP8A computer program itself detects any arrhythmias, the buffered data is transferred to disc for storage and subsequent display. In addition to this, the Pathfinder itself can be initialized to display any arrhythmias detected and these can be printed out directly on the Pathfinder itself. Thus, there are two methods of capturing arrhythmias.

The interface (see Fig. 2) between the Pathfinder and the computer serves two purposes. Firstly it removes any high frequency noise from the ECG before it is input to the PDP8 computer and secondly it contains logic for widening the square wave logic pulses produced by the Pathfinder. A clock is also included in the interface to control sampling of the ECG as the PDP8 clock is used to handle interrupts via Schmitt triggers and for measuring the RR interval.

OUTPUT

The output from the computer consists of details of heart rate averaged for each 15-sec interval of the original recording, the number of aberrant beats in this period, whether they be early or late, the number of premature normal beats, etc. Because the recording was replayed at a reduced rate it is necessary for the computer program to compensate for this fact. The estimate of ST deviation can also be output as can the presence or absence of tachycardia, bradycardia and ventricular tachycardia. Any of these parameters can be output individually in graphical trend form.

There is also an arrhythmia section of the computer program which allows samples (Fig. 3) captured by the computer as described above to be printed out on a direct writer. A program option provides a list of all times when the rhythm strip has been stored either because the computer detected an abnormality or because a facility for recording samples at a regular interval is available.

Thus the output from the system consists of a detailed printout of the heart rate for each 15-sec interval together with the incidence of abnormalities during the corresponding period. In addition regular samples of the ECG together with arrhythmias captured by the system can also be output.

DISCUSSION

The technique of effectively reducing the heart rate of a rat by a factor of four in order to allow it to be analyzed by the Pathfinder is a simple but effective solution to the problem of dealing with the high heart rate of the rat. Because the Pathfinder will normally accommodate heart rates of up to

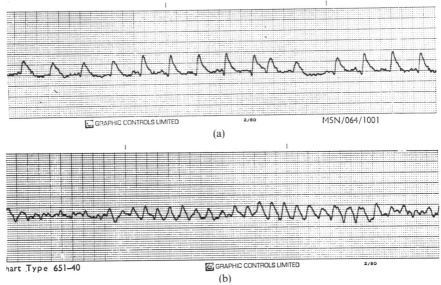

(a)

(b)

Fig. 3.(a) An arrhythmic event in a rat ECG printed effectively at 100 mm/sec (the actual writer speed was 25 mm/sec). (b) Ventricular flutter/fibrillation in a rat ECG printed at an effective rate of 100 mm/sec.

220 per minute, the technique can theoretically cope with heart rates of up to 880 per minute in the rat. This is certainly well in excess of the normal rate for the anaesthetized rat. Heart rates higher than 880 would necessitate a greater reduction in the replay recording ratio tending to create problems with the increased width of the QRS complex. Fortunately, the normal QRS complex of the rat has a duration in the approximate range 15 to 20 msec so that when slowed by a factor of four, it corresponds with the human QRS complex which has a normal average duration of 80 msec in the adult.

The method used whereby the ECG is transferred from one tape recorder to another is more cumbersome than is necessary but was adopted by way of experiment to evaluate the feasibility of the technique. It would be perfectly straightforward to tape record on the RACAL Store-7 or equivalent and replay directly into the Pathfinder. However, because the Pathfinder expects ECGs to be replayed at 60 times recording speed, the required replay speed would be 15 times the recording speed to achieve a reduction of the order of four. This can be achieved with good quality instrumentation tape recorders and is a much neater solution to the problem. This approach is likely to be adopted in future now that the method has been proved feasible.

The accuracy of the technique is fully dependent on the accuracy of the Pathfinder and the quality of the recording. Various studies have reported that the sensitivity of the Pathfinder in the detection of ectopic beats is high, up to 97% (Moller, 1978) with the specificity being very much higher although this is inevitable if it is related to the number of beats present in the recording. However, in the rat it has been found from the limited number of tapes studied so far that there can be difficulty in differentiating QRS complexes with a high "ST junction" from aberrantly conducted complexes which have an apparent bundle branch block type configuration when compared with the human ECG. On the other hand the occurrence of such complexes in our experiments has been associated with a tachycardia and it is feasible for the computer to detect the tachycardia and count the number of beats in the paroxysm, so obviating this particular difficulty.

Another factor which may be of some importance is the appropriate choice of lead. From the limited experience to date it would appear that lead 2 gives a better differentiation between the ectopic beats and normal beats than does lead 1. However, this particular point requires further study.

In summary it has been shown that a computer-assisted method for the calculation of the rate of occurrence of aberrant beats in arrhythmias in the experimental rat is a feasible technique. There is no doubt, however, that further refinements to the method could be made in order to improve the technique.

REFERENCES

Macfarlane, P. W., McClung, J., Irving, A., Watts, M. P., Taylor, T. P. and Lawrie, T. D. V. (1979) Computer Assisted Analysis of Dynamic (24 hour) Electrocardiograms. In: *Progress in Electrocardiology* (P. W. Macfarlane, ed). pp 123–126. Pitman Medical, Tunbridge Wells.

Moller, M. (1978) Reliability of quantitative analysis of ambulatory ECG tape recordings *Trans. European Soc. Cardiology* 1.

Development of ECG Changes during the Infusion of Beta-blockers in Anesthetized Rats

G. BUSCHMANN, U. G. KÜHL AND R. BUDDEN

ABSTRACT

The experiments were performed in male rats (Han:Wistar, 300–360 g) anesthetized with urethane (1.25 g/kg i.p.). The animals were fixed in the supine position and prepared for recording of ECG (lead: heart axis) and blood pressure (left carotid artery). The unspecific beta-receptor blocking drug propranolol and the cardioselective beta-blockers metoprolol, practolol and talinolol were infused intravenously at a basal rate of $0.01 \, \mu$mol kg^{-1} min^{-1}. Every ten minutes the infusion rate was increased tenfold up to 10 μmol kg^{-1} min^{-1}, which was given until death or until the end of the experiment (50 min). The infusion volume was maintained constant at 0.1 ml min^{-1}. The ECG and blood pressure parameters were evaluated by on-line biosignal processing.

All drugs tested induced a continuous fall in heart rate. At the highest infusion rate propranolol and talinolol caused A-V block and ventricular bradycardia, whereas metoprolol and practolol produced a marked bradycardia without disturbing the sinus rhythm.

Except for practolol all drugs prolonged the PR interval in a dose-related manner, the prolongation being most prominent with propranolol, weaker with talinolol and only slight with metoprolol. Practolol did not induce an appreciable alteration of PR up to a cumulated dose of 211 μmol/kg. After correction of the PR values for heart changes (PR$_c$) an increase was found only for the highest infusion rates of propranolol and talinolol.

Whereas metoprolol and practolol were without significant effects on the duration of the QRS complex throughout the experiment, high doses of talinolol and propranolol caused a significant widening of QRS.

The RαT interval (αT indicates the apex of T) was slightly shortened by practolol and lower doses of propranolol, but significantly prolonged by high doses of propranolol. Metoprolol and talinolol did not affect RαT.

Therapeutic doses of all beta-blockers induced an increase in mean arterial blood pressure (MAP), which with the cardioselective beta-blockers metoprolol, practolol and talinolol was exclusively due to an increase of the diastolic values. With 1.0 μmol kg^{-1} min^{-1} (propranolol) or 10 μmol kg^{-1} min^{-1} (metoprolol, practolol, talinolol) a continuous decline of MAP was observed, terminating in death of the animals during propranolol and talinolol infusions.

The results presented demonstrate that there is a good correspondence of the ECG changes observed with those expected by theoretical considerations, and that the on-line evaluation of rat ECG and blood pressure used in the present studies provides rapid and reliable information in the pharmacological screening of drug effects.

1. INTRODUCTION

Beta-receptor blocking agents are characterized by their competitive antagonism to adrenergic beta-receptor stimulating agents. But although the

185

TABLE 1. PHARMACODYNAMIC PROPERTIES OF THE BETA-
RECEPTOR BLOCKING AGENTS TESTED

Drug	Cardioselectivity	MSA*	ISA**
Propranolol	−	+	−
Metoprolol	+	−	−
Practolol	+	−	+
Talinolol	+	(+)	(+)

* Membrane Stabilizing Activity.
** Intrinsic Sympathomimetic Activity.
+ Present.
− Not present.
(+) Weak action.

general picture of their cardiovascular actions is determined by the beta-sympatholysis, variations in the effects produced by the individual antagonists may be found due to distinct differences in the pattern of pharmacodynamic as well as pharmacokinetic properties.

Regarding the pharmacodynamics, the cardiovascular profile of a beta-blocker may not only be influenced by differences in its affinity to adrenergic β_1- and β_2-receptors ("cardioselectivity") but also by an additional action as a partial agonist due to stimulation of beta-receptors ("intrinsic sympathomimetic activity", ISA). Moreover, at higher doses some beta-blockers have non-specific, "membrane-stabilizing" effects (MSA) appearing as "quinidine-like", antiarrhythmic, or local anesthetic actions in animal experiments.

The present investigations were intended:

(a) to establish a method for the rapid screening of drugs with regard to their cardiovascular profile, applying under practical conditions the method of computerized ECG and blood pressure evaluation described by Schumacher *et al.* (p. 171 of this book), and

(b) to try to characterize different types of β-blocking agents (Table 1) on the basis of their electrocardiographic and blood pressure effects.

2. METHODS

The experimental and biometrical procedures were the same as described elsewhere (Budden *et al.* and Schumacher *et al.*, this book).

The drugs tested and the respective infusion rates are given in Table 2. Stock solutions were prepared with water except for talinolol, which was dissolved in 6% 1 N HCl + 94% H_2O, and from these the dilutions used for infusion were made with isotonic saline. Neither saline (cf. Budden *et al.*, this book) nor 6% 1 N HCl, both infused at a rate of 0.1 ml/min, caused significant alterations of the parameters under investigation.

TABLE 2. DRUGS AND INFUSION RATES TESTED

Drugs	n	0–10	10–20	20–30	Infusion period (min) 30–50
Propranolol	4	0.01	0.1	1.0	$10.0 \ \mu mol \ kg^{-1} \ min^{-1}$
Metoprolol**	4	0.01	0.1	1.0	$10.0 \ \mu mol \ kg^{-1} \ min^{-1}$
Practolol†	4	0.01	0.1	1.0	$10.0 \ \mu mol \ kg^{-1} \ min^{-1}$
Talinolol‡	4	0.01	0.1	1.0	$10.0 \ \mu mol \ kg^{-1} \ min^{-1}$

* d.1-propranolol hydrochloride (Bonapace, Milano).
** d.1-metoprolol tartrate (Ciba-Geigy GmbH).
† d.1-practolol hydrochloride.
‡ d.1-talinolol (VEB Arzneimittelwerk Dresden).

3. RESULTS

All drugs tested exerted a significant negative chronotropic action at therapeutic dosages (propranolol > metoprolol > talinolol ∼ practolol), the fall in heart rate progressing with increasing doses (Tables 3–6). At the highest infusion rate propranolol and talinolol caused A–V block and ventricular bradycardia, whereas metoprolol and practolol produced a marked bradycardia without disturbing the sinus rhythm (Fig. 1).

Except for practolol all drugs induced a dose-dependent prolongation of the PR interval. This effect was already seen at low dosages including the therapeutic dose range. With increasing doses, the prolongation of PR was most prominent with propranolol (Table 3), weaker with talinolol (Table 6), and only slight with metoprolol (Table 4). Practolol, on the other hand, did not induce an appreciable alteration of PR up to a cumulated dose of 211 μmol/kg (Table 5). Correcting the PR values for heart rate changes, a dose-dependent shortening of PR_c was calculated for metoprolol, practolol and the three lower infusion rates of propranolol, and an increase for the highest dosages of propranolol and talinolol (Tables 3–6).

Whereas metoprolol and practolol were without significant effects on the duration of the QRS complex throughout the experiment (Tables 4 and 5), talinolol and particularly propranolol caused a significant widening of QRS at high doses (Tables 3 and 6).

The RαT interval was slightly shortened by practolol (Table 5) as well as by low and medium doses of propranolol, but significantly prolonged by high doses of the latter antagonist (Table 3). Metoprolol and talinolol did not appreciably affect RαT.

Therapeutic doses of all drugs tested induced an increase in mean arterial blood pressure (MAP) (propranolol ∼ metoprolol ∼ talinolol > practolol; Tables 3–6). With the cardioselective beta-blockers metoprolol, practolol and talinolol the elevation of MAP was exclusively due to an increase of the diastolic values, whereas the systolic pressures were unaffected or

TABLE 3. EFFECTS OF AN INTRAVENOUS INFUSION OF PROPRANOLOL (mol. wt. 296) ON HEART RATE, ECG PARAMETERS AND ON MEAN ARTERIAL BLOOD PRESSURE (MAP) IN ANESTHETIZED MALE WISTAR RATS (1.25 URETHANE/kg INTRAPERITONEALLY)

Experimental time (min)	Cumulated dose (μmol kg^{-1})	n	Heart rate (min^{-1})	PR interval (ms)	PRc interval (ms)	QRS (ms)	RαT interval (ms)	MAP* (mm Hg)
0	0	4	409 ± 16	52 ± 3.2	52 ± 3.2	15 ± 0.9	31 ± 2.2	112 ± 19
10	0.1	4	342 ± 18†	54 ± 2.6	48 ± 3.8**	15 ± 0.0	27 ± 2.5**	141 ± 18†
13	0.4‡	4	319 ± 17†	55 ± 2.4**	46 ± 3.2†	15 ± 0.8	26 ± 2.7**	139 ± 16†
20	1.1	4	293 ± 15†	55 ± 2.6†	43 ± 3.7†	14 ± 0.9†	25 ± 2.9**	138 ± 20†
30	11	4	240 ± 33†	64 ± 3.0†	42 ± 8.0**	16 ± 0.9	28 ± 3.5	95 ± 40
33.5	46	4	203 ± 20†	94 ± 12.5†	64 ± 13.0	35 ± 7.0**	47 ± 6.3**	49 ± 18†
36	71	3	98 ± 9†	131 ± 9.5†	—	34 ± 3.0**	47 ± 2.6**	29 ± 11**

Infusion rates were 0.01; 0.1; 1.0; 10.0 μmol kg^{-1} min^{-1}; they were increased at 10, 20, and 30 min after the start of the lowest infusion rate. ECG lead: heart axis (Spörri, 1944). Cumulated lethal dose: 114 ± 13 μmol kg^{-1}. Means ± SD.
* MAP: Mean arterial pressure (mm Hg) × 0.1333 = (kPa).
**,† $p < 0.05$ and $p < 0.01$ to predrug value (Student's t-test for paired observations).
‡ Therapeutic dose range (0.1 mg/kg i.v. = 0.35 μmol/kg).

TABLE 4. EFFECTS OF AN INTRAVENOUS INFUSION OF METOPROLOL (mol. wt. 399) ON HEART RATE, ECG PARAMETERS AND ON MEAN ARTERIAL BLOOD PRESSURE (MAP) IN ANESTHETIZED MALE WISTAR RATS (1.25 URETHANE/kg INTRAPERITONEALLY)

Experimental time (min)	Cumulated dose (μmol kg^{-1})	n	Heart rate (min^{-1})	PR interval (ms)	PR$_c$ interval (ms)	QRS (ms)	RαT interval (ms)	MAP* (mm Hg)
0	0	4	420 ± 12	51 ± 1.9	51 ± 1.9	16 ± 1.8	28 ± 10.5	112 ± 15
9	0.09	4	353 ± 18†	54 ± 1.9†	49 ± 1.3**	16 ± 2.5	25 ± 3.4	135 ± 7**
14	0.5‡	4	344 ± 23†	56 ± 2.6†	50 ± 2.8	17 ± 2.9	27 ± 3.4	138 ± 12†
18	0.9	4	338 ± 27†	55 ± 2.3**	49 ± 2.5	16 ± 2.8	25 ± 2.9	137 ± 10**
22.5	3.6	4	327 ± 29†	55 ± 2.9**	47 ± 2.4**	17 ± 2.7	27 ± 6.5	138 ± 5**
33	41.1	4	280 ± 30†	57 ± 2.0†	43 ± 2.4**	17 ± 3.1	26 ± 4.6	117 ± 11
41	121	4	243 ± 33†	60 ± 2.0†	39 ± 3.9**	18 ± 3.4	29 ± 6.9	64 ± 7**

Infusion rates were 0.01; 0.1; 1.0; 10.0 μmol kg^{-1} min^{-1}; they were increased at 10, 20, and 30 min after the start of the lowest infusion rate. ECG lead: heart axis (Spörri, 1944). Cumulated lethal dose: >211 μmol kg^{-1}.

Means ± SD.

* MAP: Mean arterial pressure (mm Hg) × 0.1333 = (kPa).

**,† $p < 0.05$ and $p < 0.01$ to predrug value (Student's t-test for paired observations).

‡ Therapeutic dose range (0.2 mg/kg i.v. = 0.5 μmol/kg).

TABLE 5. EFFECTS OF AN INTRAVENOUS INFUSION OF PRACTOLOL (mol. wt. 303) ON HEART RATE, ECG PARAMETERS AND ON MEAN ARTERIAL BLOOD PRESSURE (MAP) IN ANESTHETIZED MALE WISTAR RATS (1.25 URETHANE/kg INTRAPERITONEALLY

Experimental time (min)	Cumulated dose (μmol kg^{-1})	n	Heart rate (min^{-1})	PR interval (ms)	PR$_c$ interval (ms)	QRS (ms)	RαT interval (ms)	MAP* (mm Hg)
0	0	4	389 ± 14	52 ± 2.5	52 ± 2.5	15 ± 1.0	30 ± 1.7	101 ± 17
2	0.02	4	363 ± 4**	51 ± 4.1	50 ± 3.0**	15 ± 1.2	27 ± 2.1†	87 ± 20
10	0.1	4	352 ± 8†	52 ± 3.2	49 ± 3.8	14 ± 0.9	27 ± 2.3**	102 ± 16
20	1.1‡	4	327 ± 9†	52 ± 4.3	46 ± 4.2**	15 ± 1.4	26 ± 1.6†	110 ± 14
30	11	4	313 ± 26†	53 ± 3.7	46 ± 4.2**	15 ± 1.9	25 ± 1.2†	118 ± 9
50	211	4	303 ± 28†	52 ± 3.0	43 ± 2.8†	15 ± 1.2	26 ± 2.3**	62 ± 9**

Infusion rates were 0.01; 0.1; 1.0; 10.0 μmol kg^{-1} min^{-1}; they were increased at 10, 20, and 30 min after the start of the lowest infusion rate. ECG lead: heart axis (Spörri, 1944). Cumul. lethal dose: >211 μmol kg^{-1}.

Means ± SD.

* MAP: Mean arterial pressure (mm Hg) × 0.1333 = (kPa).

**,† p < 0.05 and p < 0.01 to predrug value (Student's t-test for paired observations).

‡ Therapeutic dose range (0.3 mg/kg i.v. = 1.0 μmol/kg).

TABLE 6. EFFECTS OF AN INTRAVENOUS INFUSION OF TALINOLOL (mol. wt. 368) ON HEART RATE, ECG PARAMETERS AND ON MEAN ARTERIAL BLOOD PRESSURE (MAP) IN ANESTHETIZED MALE WISTAR RATS (1.25 URETHANE/kg INTRAPERITONEALLY)

Experimental time (min)	Cumulated dose (μmol kg^{-1})	n	Heart rate (min^{-1})	PR interval (ms)	PR$_c$ interval (ms)	QRS (ms)	RαT interval (ms)	MAP* (mm Hg)
0	0	4	408 ± 14	51 ± 2.3	51 ± 2.3	15 ± 1.7	28 ± 6.2	113 ± 17
1.5	0.015	4	404 ± 16**	51 ± 2.6	51 ± 2.5	16 ± 1.8	30 ± 5.9	114 ± 17
11.5	0.25	4	367 ± 20†	53 ± 3.1	50 ± 3.2	16 ± 1.9	30 ± 8.4	128 ± 13
14	0.5‡	4	346 ± 23†	54 ± 1.4	49 ± 1.9	15 ± 3.4	28 ± 7.1	138 ± 13**
21.5	2.6	4	331 ± 23†	55 ± 1.2**	49 ± 1.5	16 ± 2.3	29 ± 6.6	137 ± 13**
29.5	10.6	4	300 ± 16†	62 ± 1.7†	52 ± 2.3**	17 ± 3.4	28 ± 5.3	136 ± 18**
34	51.1	4	258 ± 13†	77 ± 0.5†	60 ± 2.2†	25 ± 2.9†	36 ± 4.0	88 ± 28

Infusion rates were 0.01; 0.1; 1.0; 10.0 μmol kg^{-1} min^{-1}; they were increased at 10, 20, and 30 min after the start of the lowest infusion rate. ECG lead: heart axis (Spörri, 1944). Cumulated lethal dose: 174 ± 35 μmol kg^{-1}.

Means ± SD.

* MAP: Mean arterial pressure (mm Hg) × 0.1333 = (kPa).

**,† $p < 0.05$ and $p < 0.01$ to predrug value (Student's t-test for paired observations).

‡ Therapeutic dose range (0.2 mg/kg i.v. = 0.54 μmol/kg).

G. Buschmann, U. G. Kühl and R. Budden

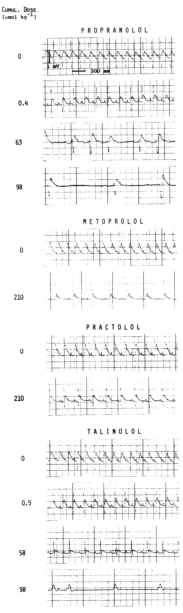

Fig. 1. ECG changes (lead: heart axis) in anesthetized rats during intravenous infusion of increasing doses of different beta-receptor blocking agents. Infusion rates 0.01/0.1/1.0/10.0 μmol kg^{-1} min^{-1}, increased, 10, 20 and 30 min after the start of the lowest rate.

slightly reduced. Propranolol, on the other hand, increased both systolic ($+13\%$) and diastolic ($+28\%$) blood pressures. With 1.0 μmol kg^{-1} min^{-1} (propranolol) or 10 μmol kg^{-1} min^{-1} (metoprolol, practolol, talinolol) the hypertensive effect turned to a continuous decline of MAP, terminating in death of the animals during propranolol and talinolol infusions (cumulated lethal doses 114 $\pm$ 13 and 174 $\pm$ 35 μmol/kg, respectively), whereas metoprolol and practolol were not lethal within the dose range tested (cumulated lethal doses > 211 μmol/kg).

4. DISCUSSION

The significant reduction in heart rate seen with therapeutic doses of all drugs tested can be attributed to the beta-adrenergic blockade exerted by low doses of beta-blocking agents, since in clinically relevant doses these drugs have no direct depressant effect on the sinus node (Wit *et al.*, 1975; Gettes and Chen, 1978). The clear fall in heart rate appears to be due to a high sympathetic tone present in our experimental animals, as the basal values are rather high, and the degree of heart rate slowing is usually related to existing sympathetic tone (Wit *et al.*, 1975).

With propranolol, metoprolol and talinolol, the negative chronotropic effect was accompanied by a slowing of A–V conduction as evidenced by the prolongation of the PR interval. Our findings with propranolol confirm the results of Doherty and Aviado (1975) after a single intravenous administration (0.5 mg/kg) and those of Farmer and Levy (1968) after repeated subcutaneous injections. With talinolol, a PQ prolongation was observed after i.v. injections in anesthetized dogs (Femmer *et al.*, 1975) and in man (Assmann *et al.*, 1977). Beta-blocking doses of propranolol have been shown to prolong A–V conduction in man (Berkowitz *et al.*, 1969; Smithen *et al.*, 1971; Seides *et al.*, 1974) and dog (Whitsitt and Lucchesi, 1968; Priola, 1973) even when heart rate is maintained constant by atrial pacing. These findings suggest that the formula used in our experiments to correct the PR interval for changes in heart rate (PR$_c$) tends to "overcorrection" of PR towards too short PR$_c$ values (cf. Budden *et al.*, 1980).

Whereas the prolongation of PR normally seen with low, clinically-used doses of beta-blockers is due to their beta-blocking action, higher doses may have an additional effect by a direct depression of A–V transmission (Whitsitt and Lucchesi, 1968; Gettes and Chen, 1978). The degree of PR prolongation induced by increasing doses of propranolol, metoprolol and talinolol in our rat experiments is in good agreement with this concept, as the prolongation was most prominent with propranolol, the drug with the strongest membrane effect, whereas on the other hand metoprolol, which is devoid of MSA, induced only slight changes.

In contrast to the three other beta-blocking agents, practolol did not affect the PR interval up to a dose of 211 μmol/kg. This might partially be explained by the relatively strong intrinsic sympathomimetic action of this drug counteracting the slowing of A–V conduction, as postulated by Smithen *et al.* (1971), who also did not find an effect of low doses of practolol on the PR interval in man during atrial pacing. The same results were obtained by Gleichmann *et al.* (1973) and Thormann *et al.* (1975). A decrease in heart rate without any observable prolongation of the PR interval was observed by Baumgartl *et al.* (1971) in man (10 mg) and by Barrett (1975) in anesthetized dogs (0.25–4.0 mg/kg) after intravenous injections of practolol.

The lack of an effect of therapeutic doses of the four beta-blockers on the duration of the QRS complex is in agreement with the well-known absence of a significant action of beta-blocking doses on conduction in the ventricular muscle (Wit *et al.*, 1975). On the other hand, at higher doses the QRS durations show an obvious relation to the membrane stabilizing potencies of these drugs, quite similar to what has been demonstrated for the PR interval.

The significant shortening of the RαT interval with therapeutic doses of propranolol and practolol may indicate some acceleration of ventricular muscle repolarization, since the duration of the QRS complex is unaltered. The difference to metoprolol and talinolol in this respect cannot be explained on the basis of our data. In man a slight shortening of the QT interval, corrected for heart rate (QT_c), has been found with propranolol (Stern and Eisenberg, 1969; Seides *et al.*, 1974).

In contrast to the changes in heart rate and ECG the increase in MAP seen during infusion of low doses of all 4 blockers is somewhat surprising. In normotensive as well as in spontaneously hypertensive and metacorticoid hypertensive rats Glavaš *et al.* (1976) observed a rise in systolic blood pressure after low intravenous doses of propranolol and practolol. Yamamoto and Sekiya (1969, 1974), and Yamamoto *et al.* (1975) also reported a sustained pressor action of low i.v. doses of propranolol and practolol in urethane-anesthetized rats, whereas in the guinea pig propranolol was without appreciable blood pressure effect. They assumed that in the rat the β-adrenergic vasodilator tone in the peripheral vessels is stronger than in other species.

Our results support the view of Yamamoto *et al.* (1975) that not only propranolol but also, though to a lesser extent, "cardioselective" β-blockers, too, may block β_2-receptors in the peripheral vascular bed of the anesthetized rat, yielding a relative preponderance of the alpha-receptors with an increase in vascular resistance (Sannerstedt *et al.*, 1970; Brunner, 1977). In addition, the findings of Yamamoto and Sekiya (1974) with propranolol indicate that the reduction in cardiac output as a factor in the hypotensive effect of β-receptor blockade (Brunner, 1977) may be weaker in the rat than in other species.

Whether the sole increase in diastolic pressure with unchanged or even slightly decreased systolic values observed with metoprolol, practolol and talinolol is related to the cardioselectivity of these drugs cannot be decided on the basis of our findings.

From the results presented the following conclusions may be drawn:

(a) There is a good correspondence of the ECG changes observed with those expected by theoretical considerations concerning additional intrinsic sympathomimetic or membrane stabilizing activities of the antagonists.

(b) The on-line evaluation of rat ECG and blood pressure used in the present studies provides rapid and reliable information in the pharmacological screening of drug effects.

5. REFERENCES

Assmann, I., Fiehring, H., Dittrich, P. and Oltmanns, G. (1977) Wirkung des Beta$_1$-Rezeptorenblockers Cordanum® auf das Reizbildungs- und Reizleitungssystem des Herzens. *Dtsch. Gesundh.-Wesen* **32**, 1081–1084.

Barrett, A. M. (1975) A survey of the pharmacological properties of adrenergic beta-receptor antagonists. In: *Kardiale Sympathikolyse als Therapeutisches Prinzip* (H. Lydtin and W. Meesmann, eds.) pp. 1–23. Georg Thieme Verlag, Stuttgart.

Baumgartl, P., Knapp, E., Raas, E. and Aigner, A. (1971) Hämodynamische Wirkungen von Practolol (ICI 50 172). *Med. Klin.* **66**, 597–601.

Berkowitz, W. D., Wit, A. L., Lau, S. H., Steiner, C. and Damato, A. N. (1969) The effects of propranolol on cardiac conduction. *Circulation* **40**, 855–862.

Brunner, H. (1977) The antihypertensive effect of β-blockers. *Contrib. Nephrol.* **8**, 171–181.

Budden, R., Buschmann, G. and Kühl, U. G. (1980) The rat ECG in acute pharmacology and toxicology. *International Workshop on the Rat Electrocardiogram in Acute and Chronic Pharmacology and Toxicology*, July 14–15, 1980, Hannover.

Doherty, R. E. and Aviado, D. M. (1975) Toxicity of aerosol propellants in the respiratory and circulatory systems. VI. Influence of cardiac and pulmonary vascular lesions in the rat. *Toxicology* **3**, 213–224.

Farmer, J. B. and Levy, G. P. (1968) A comparison of some cardiovascular properties of propranolol, MJ 1999 and quinidine in relation to their effects in hypertensive animals. *Br. J. Pharmacol.* **34**, 116–126.

Femmer, K., Bartsch, R., Leonhardt, U., von Littrow, C. and Riedel, H. (1975) Zur Pharmakologie von (±)-1-[4-Cyclohexylureidophenoxy]-2-hydroxy-3-tert.-butylaminopropan (Talinolol, Cordanum®, 02-115) *Pharmazie* **30**, 642–651.

Gettes, L. S. and Chen, C.-M. (1978) Mechanisms and efficacy of beta-blocking agents in the treatment of arrhythmias. In: *Neural Mechanisms in Cardiac Arrhythmias* (P. J. Schwartz, A. M. Brown, A. Malliana and A. Zanchetti, eds.) pp. 377–399. Raven Press, New York.

Glavaš, E., Gudeska, S., Stojanova, D. and Nikodijević, B. (1976) Comparative action of beta-adrenergic blocking agents on the blood pressure, ECG and noradrenaline level in normotensive and hypertensive rats. *God. Zb. Med. Fak. Skopje* **22**, 11–18.

Gleichmann, U., Seipel, L. and Loogen, F. (1973) Der Einfluß von Antiarrhythmika auf die intrakardiale Erregungsleitung (His-bündel-elektrographie) und Sinusknotenautomatie beim Menschen. *Dtsch. Med. Wochenschr.* **98**, 1487–1494.

Priola, D. V. (1973) Effects of beta receptor stimulation and blockade on A–V nodal and bundle branch conduction in the canine heart. *Am. J. Cardiol.* **31**, 35–40.

Sannerstedt, R., Julius, S. and Conway, J. (1970) Hemodynamic responses to tilt and beta-adrenergic blockade in young patients with borderline hypertension. *Circulation* **42**, 1057–1064.

Schumacher, W., Budden, R., Buschmann, G. and Kühl, U. G. (1980) A new method for the evaluation of ECG and blood pressure parameters in anesthetized rats by on-line bio-signal processing. *International Workshop on the Rat Electrocardiogram in Acute and Chronic Pharmacology and Toxicology*, July 14–15, 1980, Hannover.

Seides, S. F., Josephson, M. E. Batsford, W. P., Weisfogel, G. M., Lau, S. H. and Damato, A. N. (1974) The electrophysiology of propranolol in man. *Am. Heart J.* **88**, 733–741.

Smithen, C. S., Balcon, R. and Sowton, E. (1971) Use of bundle of His potentials to assess changes in atrioventricular conduction produced by a series of beta-adrenergic blocking agents. *Br. Heart J.* **33**, 955–961.

Stern, S. and Eisenberg, S. (1969) The effect of propranolol (Inderal) on the electrocardiogram of normal subjects. *Am. Heart J.* **77**, 192–195.

Thormann, J., Schwarz, F. and Zimmermann, H. (1975) Effects of practolol on A–V conduction during atrial stimulation in 50 patients with and without coronary heart disease. *Basic Res. Cardiol.* **70**, 299–306.

Whitsitt, L. S. and Lucchesi, B. R. (1968) Effects of beta-receptor blockade and glucagon on the atrioventricular transmission system in the dog. *Circul. Res.* **23**, 585–595.

Wit, A. L., Hoffman, B. F. and Rosen, M. R. (1975) Electrophysiology and pharmacology of cardiac arrhythmias IX. Cardiac electrophysiologic effects of beta adrenergic receptor stimulation and blockade. Part C. *Am. Heart J.* **90**, 795–803.

Yamamoto, J. and Sekiya, A. (1969) On the pressor action of propranolol in the rat. *Arch. Int. Pharmacodyn.* **179**, 372–380.

Yamamoto, J. and Sekiya, A. (1974) Differences in the cardiac and pressor responses to propranolol of rats and guinea pigs. *Jpn. J. Pharmacol.* **24**, 253–259.

Yamamoto, J., Sekiya, A. and Maekawa, H. (1975) Effects of several β-blockers on blood pressure in the rat. *Jpn. J. Pharmacol.* **25**, 465–471.

Development of ECG and Blood Pressure Changes in Anesthetized Rats during the Infusion of Antiarrhythmic Compounds

U. G. KÜHL, G. BUSCHMANN AND R. BUDDEN

ABSTRACT

Using on-line biosignal evaluation (Schumacher *et al.*, this book, p. 171) the antiarrhythmic agents N-n-propyl-ajamaline bitartrate (NPAB) propafenon HCl, lidocaine HCl, sparteine and verapamil HCl were tested in anesthetized rats (urethane 1.25 g/kg i.p.). The effects of a stepwise increasing continuous infusion of the test compounds on the ECG (lead heart axis) and blood pressure (carotid artery) were analysed and compared to the effects, which could be expected according to their electrophysiological mode of action (Vaughan Williams, 1970, 1979; Singh and Hauswirth, 1974).

Whereas NPAB and propafenon at therapeutic concentrations increased PR and QRS duration, this was not seen with lidocaine, sparteine and verapamil.

1. INTRODUCTION

One category of drugs, where ECG analysis is of special interest not only in the characterization of the side effects but also in the analysis of the mode of action, is the group of antiarrhythmic agents.

Among the cardiac side effects of antiarrhythmic drugs, their effects on the conduction velocity play an important role in therapy because a reduction in conduction velocity may favor re-entry (Chung, 1973) and thus produce ventricular fibrillation (Bleifeld, 1971).

In the screening of new antiarrhythmic compounds it should be desirable to assess their effects on the ECG intervals in small laboratory animals like rats in order to select compounds not only on the basis of their antiarrhythmic activity but also on the basis of their effects on the conduction velocity.

197

TABLE 1

CLASS*	MODE OF ACTION	DRUGS	EXPECTED ECG CHANGES			
			RR	PR	QRS	RαT
1a	MEMBRANE STABILISATION AND REDUCED CONDUCTION VELOCITY	QUINIDINE, AJMALINE, NPAB [1]	(↑)	↑	↑	↑
1b	MEMBRANE STABILISATION AND UNCHANGED CONDUCTION VELOCITY	LIDOCAINE	(↑)	∅	∅	∅
2′	ANTI-SYMPATHETIC	PROPRANOLOL	↑	∅	∅	∅
3	UNIFORM PROLONGATION OF ACTION POTENTIAL DURATION	AMIODARONE	∅	∅	∅	↑
4	CALCIUM ANTAGONISTIC	VERAPAMIL	↑	∅	∅	∅

↑ increase
∅ unchanged

*classification according to Vaughan Williams 1970, 1979 and Singh and Hauswirth 1974

[1] N-Propyl-Ajmaline Bitartrate

According to the classification of Vaughan Williams (1970, 1979) and Singh and Hauswirth (1974) four classes of antiarrhythmic action may be defined (Table 1).

In our experiments typical representatives of class 1a (NPAB: N-propyl-ajmaline bitartrate), class 1b (lidocaine), and class 4 were examined. Some of the class 2 drugs are the subject of another paper (Buschmann *et al.*, p. 185).

The aims of the present study were:

(a) to compare the measured ECG changes induced by the representative compounds with the expected ones (Table 1).

(b) to apply the method of computerized ECG and blood pressure evaluation presented by Schumacher *et al.* (p. 171) under practical conditions, and

(c) to compare the effects of sparteine sulfate and propafenon with those of the other compounds tested.

2. METHODS

The experimental and biometrical procedures were the same as described elsewhere (Budden *et al.*, 1981; Schumacher *et al.*, this book, p. 171).

The drugs tested and the respective infusion rates are given in Table 2. Stock solutions were prepared with water, further dilutions were made with isotonic saline. No significant alterations of the parameters under investigation were caused by the infusion of isotonic saline (0.1 ml/min).

TABLE 2. DRUGS AND INFUSION RATES OF THE COMPOUNDS TESTED

Drug	Infusion period (min)			
	0–10	10–20	20–30	30–50
NPAB[1]	0.01	0.032	0.1	$0.32 \, \mu\text{mol kg}^{-1} \text{min}^{-1}$
Lidocaine[2]	0.02	0.2	2.0	$20.0 \, \mu\text{mol kg}^{-1} \text{min}^{-1}$
Sparteine[3]	0.01	0.1	1.0	$10.0 \, \mu\text{mol kg}^{-1} \text{min}^{-1}$
Propafenon[4]	0.032	0.1	0.32	$1.0 \, \mu\text{mol kg}^{-1} \text{min}^{-1}$
Verapamil[5]	0.032	0.1	0.32	$1.0 \, \mu\text{mol kg}^{-1} \text{min}^{-1}$

[1] N-propyl-ajmaline bitartrate, Giulini Pharma GmbH.
[2] Lidocaine HCl, Xylocaine®, Astra Chemicals.
[3] Sparteine sulfate, Giulini Pharma GmbH.
[4] Propafenon HCl, Knoll AG.
[5] Verapamil HCl, Knoll AG.

3. RESULTS

Whereas NPAB produced a marked prolongation of A–V conduction (Table 3, Fig. 1) at very low dosages, this was not seen with lidocaine (Table 4, Fig. 1) and verapamil (Table 5). Propafenon, too, caused an increase in the PR interval (Table 7); during sparteine infusion an appreciable prolongation of PR was only seen at rather high dosages (Table 6, Fig. 1). All drugs tested exerted a dose-dependent bradycardiac action of different degree (Tables 3–7). As can be seen from Fig. 1, the decrease in heart rate by lidocaine and sparteine was mainly due to an increase in the αTP segment. In contrast, the αTP segment was shortened with NPAB (Fig. 1), indicating that the decrease in heart rate was caused by a prolongation of the excitation cycle of the heart and not by a prolongation of the electrical diastole.

Whereas the QRS duration and the RαT interval remained unchanged during the infusion of lidocaine and verapamil, these parameters were prolonged at the higher infusion rates by NPAB, sparteine and propafenon (Tables 3–7).

Both sparteine and propafenon produced a significant increase in the mean arterial pressure at lower infusion rates (Tables 6 and 7) due to an increase of the diastolic values. The hypertensive effect of sparteine, however, was much more pronounced than with propafenon.

At the highest infusion rate NPAB caused complete A–V block and ventricular rhythm in all animals, whereas lidocaine and sparteine, in spite of a pronounced bradycardia, did not disrupt sinus rhythm (Fig. 1).

4. DISCUSSION

In general, the effects of the tested drugs in our model were in good agreement with published data as well as with clinical experience.

TABLE 3. EFFECTS OF AN INTRAVENOUS INFUSION OF N-PROPYL-AJMALINE BITARTRATE (NPAB) (mol. wt. 518) ON HEART RATE, ECG PARAMETERS AND ON MEAN ARTERIAL BLOOD PRESSURE (MAP) IN ANESTHETIZED MALE WISTAR RATS (1.25 URETHANE/kg INTRAPERITONEALLY)

Experimental time (min)	Cumulated dose (μmol kg⁻¹)	n	Heart rate (min⁻¹)	PR interval (ms)	PR_c interval (ms)	QRS (ms)	RαT interval (ms)	MAP* (mm Ng)
0	0	4	442 ± 7	51 ± 4.9	51 ± 4.9	14 ± 0.8	27 ± 2.9	101 ± 6
10	0.1	4	429 ± 7	53 ± 5.1	52 ± 5.1	14 ± 1.5	27 ± 3.3	113 ± 10
20	0.416‡	4	400 ± 20**	60 ± 4.0**	57 ± 4.5**	15 ± 1.0**	28 ± 4.1	103 ± 13
29.5	1.37	4	389 ± 15†	71 ± 3.5†	66 ± 3.8†	19 ± 1.0†	34 ± 2.8***	97 ± 14
32.5	2.21	4	385 ± 24**	76 ± 5.2**	72 ± 5.1***	24 ± 2.6†	42 ± 6.4**	93 ± 13
39, 5–41.5	4.4–5.1	1/1	350–317	92–108	85–96	26–41	51–57	71–57

Infusion rates were 0.01; 0.032; 0.1; 0.316 μmol kg⁻¹ min⁻¹; they were increased at 10, 20, and 30 min after the start of the lowest infusion rate. ECG lead: heart axis (Spörri, 1944). Cumulated lethal dose: > 7.7 μmol kg⁻¹ min⁻¹.
Means ± SD.
* MAP: Mean arterial pressure (mm Hg) × 0.1333 = (kPa).
**, †, *** p < 0.05, 0.01 and 0.001 to predrug value (Student's paired t-test).
‡ Therapeutic dose range in man (20 mg/man p.o. = 0.55 μmol/kg).

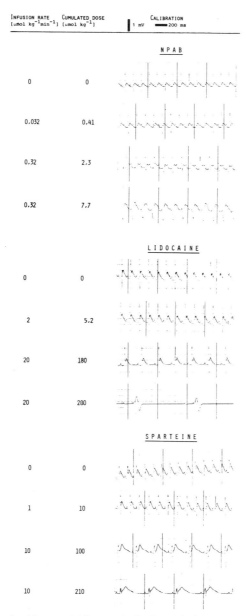

Fig. 1. ECG changes (lead heart axis) in anesthetized rats during the intravenous infusion of increasing doses of N-propyl-ajmaline-bitartrate (NPAB), lidocaine and sparteine.

TABLE 4. EFFECTS OF AN INTRAVENOUS INFUSION OF LIDOCAINE HCl (XYLOCAIN®) (mol. wt. 271) ON HEART RATE, ECG PARAMETERS AND ON MEAN ARTERIAL BLOOD PRESSURE (MAP) IN ANESTHETIZED MALE WISTAR RATS (1.25 URETHANE/kg INTRAPERITONEALLY)

Experimental time (min)	Cumulated dose (μmol kg^{-1})	n	Heart rate (min^{-1})	PR interval (ms)	PR$_c$ interval (ms)	QRS (ms)	RαT interval (ms)	MAP* (mm Hg)
0	0	4	433 ± 33	52 ± 4.6	52 ± 4.6	15 ± 1.7	29 ± 9.4	111 ± 14
9	0.18	4	425 ± 36	52 ± 3.6	50 ± 1.4	15 ± 1.2	32 ± 2.9	113 ± 19
19.5	2.1	4	409 ± 37†	52 ± 4.6	50 ± 2.7	15 ± 1.5	29 ± 3.3	111 ± 16
21.5	5.2‡	4	406 ± 35**	53 ± 5.1	50 ± 4.2	15 ± 1.2	29 ± 3.8	109 ± 11
24	10.2	4	377 ± 26†	54 ± 5.0	50 ± 3.6	16 ± 1.4	27 ± 5.5	96 ± 11**
28	18.2	4	349 ± 45**	54 ± 4.3	47 ± 6.0	15 ± 2.6	31 ± 5.1	91 ± 18

Infusion rates were 0.02; 0.2; 2.0; 20.0 μmol kg^{-1} min^{-1}; they were increased at 10, 20, and 30 min after the start of the lowest infusion rate. ECG lead: heart axis (Spörri, 1944). Cumul. lethal dose: 211 ± 24 μmol kg^{-1}.

Means ± SD.

* MAP: Mean arterial pressure (mm Hg) × 0.1333 = (kPa).

**,† p < 0.05 and p < 0.01 to predrug value (Student's t-test for paired observations).

‡ Therapeutic dose range in man (100 mg/man i.v. = 5.3 μmol/kg).

TABLE 5. EFFECTS OF AN INTRAVENOUS INFUSION OF VERAPAMIL (mol. wt. 491) ON HEART RATE, ECG PARAMETERS AND ON MEAN ARTERIAL BLOOD PRESSURE (MAP) IN ANESTHETIZED MALE WISTAR RATS (1.25 URETHANE/kg INTRAPERITONEALLY)

Experimental time (min)	Cumulated dose (μmol kg^{-1})	n	Heart rate (min^{-1})	PR interval (ms)	PRc interval (ms)	QRS (ms)	RαT interval (ms)	MAP* (mm Hg)
0	0	4	440 ± 14	50 ± 3.8	50 ± 3.8	15 ± 0.8	32 ± 4.9	101 ± 15
1	0.032	4	437 ± 15	50 ± 3.7	50 ± 3.6	15 ± 2.3	28 ± 7.8	107 ± 21
7.5	0.24‡	4	395 ± 27**	50 ± 3.0	46 ± 3.7	15 ± 0.9	33 ± 3.0	107 ± 26
14.5	0.77	4	345 ± 19†	49 ± 3.5	41 ± 4.6	15 ± 1.2	29 ± 4.7	82 ± 17**
20	1.32	4	319 ± 11***	50 ± 4.2	39 ± 3.5	15 ± 0.9	26 ± 5.3	78 ± 17**
23.5	2.42	4	286 ± 20***	50 ± 6.0	35 ± 4.4	15 ± 1.3	33 ± 12.2	64 ± 12†

Infusion rates were 0.0316; 0.1; 0.316; 1.0 μmol kg^{-1} min^{-1}; they were increased at 10, 20, and 30 min after the start of the lowest infusion rate. ECG lead: heart axis (Spörri, 1944). Cumulated lethal dose: 25 ± 5.0 μmol kg^{-1}.
Means ± SD.
* MAP: Mean arterial pressure (mm Hg) × 0.1333 = (kPa).
,†,* p < 0.05, p < 0.01 and p < 0.001 to predrug value (Student's paired t-test).
‡ Therapeutic dose range in man (5–10 mg/h i.v. = 0.15–0.29 μmol/kg).

TABLE 6. EFFECTS OF AN INTRAVENOUS INFUSION OF SPARTEINE SULFATE (mol. wt. 423) ON HEART RATE, ECG PARAMETERS AND ON MEAN ARTERIAL BLOOD PRESSURE (MAP) IN ANESTHETIZED MALE WISTAR RATS (1.25 URETHANE/kg INTRAPERITONEALLY)

Experimental time (min)	Cumulated dose (μmol kg^{-1})	n	Heart rate (min^{-1})	PR interval (ms)	PR$_c$ interval (ms)	QRS (ms)	RαT interval (ms)	MAP* (mm Hg)
0	0	3	428 ± 19	50 ± 1.7	50 ± 1.7	15 ± 1.1	33 ± 3.5	102 ± 8
8	0.08	3	366 ± 19***	52 ± 3.8	45 ± 3.2**	15 ± 1.2	28 ± 4.5	138 ± 4**
18.5	0.95	3	358 ± 29**	51 ± 2.6	45 ± 0.6**	15 ± 1.5	26 ± 2.1	130 ± 11
29	10.1‡	3	377 ± 22†	53 ± 2.5**	49 ± 2.0	15 ± 1.5	32 ± 3.0	130 ± 8
39	101	3	224 ± 20†	65 ± 4.5***	37 ± 9.0	36 ± 3.0†	71 ± 5.1**	97 ± 13
49	201	3	149 ± 46***	72 ± 5.1†	—	38 ± 3.7†	90 ± 3.5†	81 ± 12

Infusion rates were 0.01; 0.1; 1.0; 10.0 μmol kg^{-1} min^{-1}; they were increased at 10, 20, and 30 min after the start of the lowest infusion rate. ECG lead: heart axis (Spörri, 1944). Cumulated lethal dose: >211 μmol kg^{-1}.

Means ± SD.

* MAP: Mean arterial pressure (mm Hg) × 0.1333 = (kPa).

,†,* $p < 0.05$, $p < 0.01$ and $p < 0.001$ to predrug value (Student's paired t-test).

‡ Therapeutic dose range in man (200 mg/man i.v. = 6.8 μmol/kg).

TABLE 7. EFFECTS OF AN INTRAVENOUS INFUSION OF PROPHAFENON HCl (mol. wt. 378) ON HEART RATE, ECG PARAMETERS AND ON MEAN ARTERIAL BLOOD PRESSURE (MAP) IN ANESTHETIZED MALE WISTAR RATS (1.25 URETHANE/kg INTRAPERITONEALLY)

Experimental time (min)	Cumulated dose (μmol kg^{-1})	n	Heart rate (min^{-1})	PR interval (ms)	PR$_c$ interval (ms)	QRS (ms)	RαT interval (ms)	MAP* (mm Hg)
0	0	4	419 ± 18	50 ± 3.0	50 ± 3.0	15 ± 0.5	28 ± 2.9	100 ± 8
10	0.316	4	413 ± 27	51 ± 2.8	52 ± 2.2	15 ± 0.8	28 ± 2.3	111 ± 8
20	1.32	4	380 ± 43	55 ± 2.8	53 ± 2.9	16 ± 1.9	27 ± 2.6	113 ± 8**
30	4.48²	4	346 ± 38**	59 ± 1.0†	54 ± 4.5	18 ± 2.4	28 ± 4.1	111 ± 14
40	14.5	4	299 ± 17†	69 ± 3.7†	59 ± 5.2**	22 ± 5.5	36 ± 7.5	106 ± 6
49.5	24.0	3	278 ± 24**	73 ± 3.7†	60 ± 7.4	25 ± 5.0	40 ± 8.5	87 ± 21

Infusion rates were 0.0316; 0.1; 0.316; 1.0 μmol kg^{-1} min^{-1}; they were increased at 10, 20, 30 min after the start of the lowest infusion rate. ECG lead: heart axis (Spörri, 1944). Cumul. lethal dose: >24.5 μmol kg^{-1}.

Means ± SD.

* MAP: Mean arterial pressure (mm Hg) × 0.1333 = (kPa).

**,† p < 0.05 and p < 0.01 to predrug value (Student's paired t-test).

‡ Therapeutic dose range in man (70 mg/man i.v. = 2.6 μmol/kg).

At clinically effective doses the class 1a drug NPAB produced a marked prolongation of A–V conduction in our experiments. After peroral administration of 4 mg NPAB/kg, v. Philipsborn (1973) found a prolongation of PR without changes in heart rate and QT in awake rats. However, comparing the effects of the drug in awake and in thiobutabarbital anesthetized rats, the initially prolonged PR interval showed a continuous regression starting at 30 minutes after the administration in awake, but a continuous increase in anesthetized animals. In addition, the basal heart rate was significantly higher in the anesthetized than in the awake animals. The heart rate decreased with NPAB in the anesthetized, but remained unchanged in the awake animals. According to these results it cannot be excluded that, as it is true for other drugs, the effects of anesthesia on basal physiological conditions or an interaction of the anesthetic agent with NPAB has influenced our results. Clinically, as demonstrated by the results of Seipel *et al.* (1974), NPAB prolongs A–V conduction, too, mainly by increasing the HV interval of the His-bundle-electrogram.

The newer antiarrhythmic agent propafenon caused an increase of PR, PR_c and QRS in therapeutic doses. This agrees with the clinical results of Seipel *et al.* (1977) who found a prolongation of all parts of the His-bundle-electrogram in man.

In our experiments lidocaine, representing the group of membrane stabilizing drugs without a marked effect on conduction velocity (Vaughan Williams, 1979; Singh and Hauswirth, 1974), did not change any of the measured ECG parameters at therapeutic dosages except for a moderate decrease in heart rate. In contrast to our results, Valle *et al.* (1975) found a significant increase in the PR interval in rats, whereas QRS and QT remained unchanged.

With verapamil, a representative of class 4 action, no changes in the measured ECG parameters were observed except for a marked reduction in heart rate. As expected, the mean arterial blood pressure was significantly decreased by the calcium antagonistic drug. However, the dose producing a significant bradycardia was about three times smaller than the dose causing a significant hypotension. The lack of an effect of verapamil on A–V conduction is consistent with the report of Bleifeld (1971). However, Seipel *et al.* (1974) found a significant prolongation of the AH interval of the His-bundle-electrogram at therapeutic dose levels in man (0.1–0.15 mg/kg).

After peroral administration of 33.3 mg/kg sparteine sulfate to rats, v. Philipsborn (1973) found a moderate decrease in heart rate and a slight increase in PR whereas the QT interval was not changed. At a corresponding intravenous dose range we observed, in addition to the bradycardia and the increase in PR, a marked prolongation of QRS and RαT. Seipel *et al.* (1974) did not find any prolongation of A–V conduction after intravenous sparteine sulfate in man, either.

From the results presented the following conclusions may be drawn:

(a) There is a good correspondence between the observed ECG changes induced by the representative antiarrhythmic agents NPAB, lidocaine, and verapamil and the expected ones.

(b) As far as the effects on the conduction velocity are concerned, sparteine is rather "lidocaine-like" than "quinidine-like", and propafenon is rather "quinidine-like" than "lidocaine-like".

(c) The computerized ECG and blood pressure evaluation used in the presented studies (Schumacher *et al.* p. 171) provides reliable data for the biological assessment of drug effects in anesthetized rats.

5. REFERENCES

Bleifeld, W. (1971) Side effects of antiarrhythmic drugs. *Naunyn-Schmiedeberg's Arch. Pharmacol.* **269**, 282–297.

Chung, E. K. (1973) *Principles of Cardiac Arrhythmias.* pp. 159–161, 318–319. The Williams & Wilkins Company, Baltimore.

von Philipsborn, G. (1973) Zur Wirkung von N-Propyl-ajmaliniumhydrogentartrat (NPAB), Sparteinsulfat (Spartein) und NPAB + Spartein auf das Eledrokardiogramm und auf Aconitinarrhythmien von SIV-Ratten. *Arzneim.-Forsch. (Drug Res.)* **23**, 1729–1733.

Seipel, L., Both, A., Breithardt, G., Gleichmann, U. and Loogen, F. (1974) Action of antiarrhythmic drugs on His-bundle-electrogram and sinus node function. *Acta Cardiol.* [*Suppl*] XVIII, 251–267.

Seipel, L., Breithardt, G., Both, A. and Wiebringhaus, E. (1977) Wirkung von Propafenon auf den Sinusknoten und die intrakardiale Erregungsleitung beim Menschen. In: *Fortschritte in der Pharmakotherapie von Herzrhythmusstörungen,* (H. Hochrein, H.-J. Hapke, O. A. Beck eds.). Gustav Fischer Verlag, Stuttgart, New York.

Singh, B. N. and Hauswirth, O. (1974) Comparative mechanism of action of antiarrhythmic drugs. *Am. Heart J.* **87**, 367–382.

Valle, L. B. S., Oliveira-Filho, R. M., Armonia, P. L., Nassif, M. and Saraceni, G. J. (1975) Sensibilisation de la bradycardie pendant l'hypotension finale déclenchée par la sérotonine chez le rat: Effect de la lidocaine. *Arch. Int. Physiol. Biochim.* **83**, 647–657.

Vaughan Williams, E. M. (1970) Classification of anti-arrhythmic drugs. In: *Symposium on Cardiac Arrhythmias* (E. Sandoe, E. Flenstedt-Jensen, K. H. Olesen eds.). A. B. Astra, Sodertalje, Sweden.

Vaughan Williams, E. M. (1979) Characterisation of new antiarrhythmic drugs. *Prog. Pharmacol.* **2** (4), 13–23.

Computer Control of a Modified Langendorff Perfusion Apparatus and Assessment of the Isolated Heart Viability by Fourier Analysis

C. G. ADEM, F. I. CHAUDHRY AND J. B. HARNESS

This paper illustrates the construction of an isolated rat heart cryopreservation apparatus which is interfaced to a process control computer. The computer control program allows interactive calibration of the instruments, accurate control of variables and modifications of parameters during the experiments. The flexibility of the equipment is demonstrated by running two isolated perfused hearts under four combinations: same or different temperature with same or different perfusates. Each of these combinations can be checked with identical or different perfusate flows, thus increasing the experimental choice. A simplified diagram of the cryopreservation system is shown in Fig. 1. The perfusate (Krebs solution) is pumped

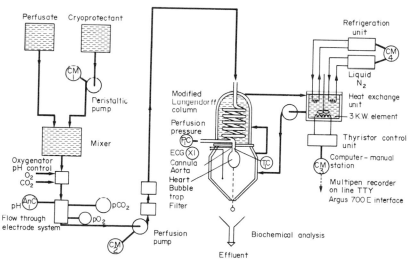

Fig. 1. Simplified diagram of existing cryopreservation process.

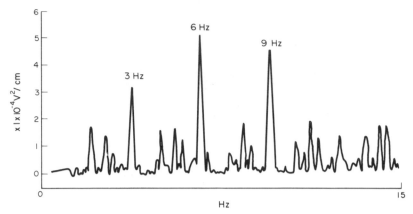

Fig. 2. Spectrum of frequency components after autocorrelation of normal ECGs of a heart at 36°C.

into the organ and can be mixed to a specified concentration with the cryoprotectant (CPA), ethylene glycol. Gas consisting of 95% oxygen and 5% carbon-dioxide is bubbled into the perfusate which is then pumped through a pulse suppressor (bubble trap) and filtered to the column at approximately 0.05 ml sec^{-1}. The column allows a cannulated heart to be suspended on the outlet of a glass perfusion coil and the temperature of the surrounding jacket is regulated by the circulation of water/glycol mixture from a stirred bath. Hearts are cooled at 1°C per minute from 37°C to the lowest temperature; when the temperature falls below 23.5°C, ethylene glycol is slowly added to the perfusate until it reaches 3 molar concentration and the heart is further cooled to −22°C and held at this tempera-

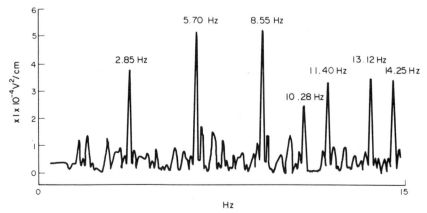

Fig. 3. Spectrum of frequency components after autocorrelation of ECGs of a heart at 36°C after ethanediol administration and removal.

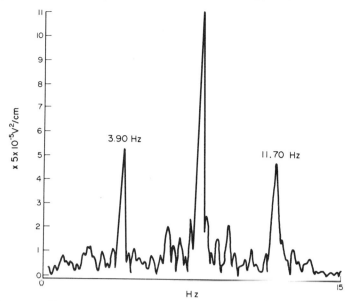

Fig. 4. Spectrum of frequency components after autocorrelation of normal ECGs of a heart at 35°C after cooling to −22°C.

ture for a predetermined period. It is removed upon warming and before toxic effects are visible, thus leading to good recovery.

Electrocardiogram (ECG) collection and analyses were done both on line and off-line. ECG signals of rat hearts before and after cooling were analysed by a technique called "Fast Fourier". The frequency spectrum of the ECG wave will change if it is damaged. The frequency spectrum of a good heart being "retrograde perfused" at 37°C contains 3 peaks (Fig. 2). The fundamental frequency corresponds to the heart rate, with the second harmonic dominant in power. A damaged heart developed higher frequency harmonics and displayed non-harmonic peaks as well (Figs. 3 and 4).

Fourier analyses of the ECG signals undertaken are consistent and seem quite promising, thus leading to an instantaneous analysis of the state of the heart.

The Effects of Antiadrenergic and Antihistaminic Drugs on ECG Alterations induced by Anthracyclines in Rats

G. SOLDANI, M. DEL TACCA, L. GIOVANNINI
AND A. BERTELLI

INTRODUCTION

Among anthracycline antibiotics, daunorubicin and doxorubicin are important antitumor drugs whose long-term administration in man is compromised by the development of a dose-related cardiomyopathy[1]. Toxicological studies have shown that treatment of experimental animals with daunorubicin was followed by tachycardia, arrhythmias and electrocardiographical alterations[2]. In particular, early widening of the QRS complex appeared to be the most sensitive indicator of cardiotoxicity in rats[3]. ECG alterations in guinea-pigs which had been given a single high dose of daunorubicin corresponded to a significant increase in the catecholamine content of the heart, but treatment with α- and β-blockers failed to protect cardiac function[4,5]. Recently, Bristow et al.,[6] have suggested that renal and cardiac lesions in rabbits and dogs might be due to an increased level of both histamine and catecholamines as a result of the administration of the anthracyclines.

The aim of the present study was to investigate the general and cardiac toxicity of daunorubicin, doxorubicin and new derivatives 4-demethoxy-daunorubicin and 4'-epidoxorubicin in the rat, as well as the effect of pretreatment with H_1, H_2, α- and β-blockers.

MATERIALS AND METHODS

Four groups of 10 male Wistar rats (200–250 g) were given 5 injections of 4 mg/kg i.p. of daunorubicin (mol. wt. 563.98), doxorubicin (mol. wt. 579.98), 4'-epidoxorubicin (mol. wt. 579.98) and 4-demethoxydaunorubin

213

(mol. wt. 533.97) respectively and were compared with control rats receiving NaCl 0.9% (0.2 ml/kg i.p., 5 injections; 30 animals). In addition, the same experimental procedure was applied to 4 groups of 10 rats pretreated daily with chlorpheniramine (10 mg/kg), plus cimetidine (10 mg/kg), plus phentolamine (2 mg/kg), plus metoprolol (2.5 mg/kg). These drugs were administered to the rats dissolved in saline solution by means of stomach probe, 30 min before the injections.

General and cardiac toxicity of anthracyclines was estimated by evaluating the number of animals which died during treatment, the mean body weight changes, the development of ascites and the extent of ECG modifications. An OTE Biomedical ECG C1m model (Montedison Florence) was used for recording ECGs. Needle electrodes were inserted under light ether anesthesia under the skin for the limb lead at position 2 and the paper speed was 10 cm/sec. ECG recordings were performed after the animal showed signs of recovery from anesthesia.

RESULTS AND DISCUSSION

The main parameters of general toxicity of the four compounds examined are reported in Table 1. The body weights of rats treated with all the compounds became lower than those of the controls. A high percentage of mortality was observed in the case of demethoxydaunorubicin, doxorubicin and daunorubicin, while the animals treated with epidoxorubicin survived 100% (Table 1).

TABLE 1. GENERAL TOXICITY OF ANTHRACYCLINE ANTIBIOTICS

Drugs	Dose (mg/kg)	No of injections	No of deaths/ total number of animals*	Mean change in body weight** (g ± S.E.)	Ascites***
Daunorubicin	4	5	8/10	−43.8 ± 4.3	+ +
Daunorubicin + $H_1H_2\alpha\beta$	4	5	4/10	−25.1 ± 4.0	+
Doxorubuicin	4	5	8/10	−36.2 ± 8.5	+
Doxorubicin + $H_1H_2\alpha\beta$	4	5	9/10	−35.0 ± 2.8	+
4-Demethoxydaunorubicin	4	5	10/10	−32.5 ± 6.2	+ +
4-Demethoxydaunorubicin + $H_1H_2\alpha\beta$	4	5	10/10	−27.0 ± 7.1	+ +
4'-Epidoxorubicin	4	5	0	−13.4 ± 1.7	—
4'-Epidoxorubicin + $H_1H_2\alpha\beta$	4	5	0	+9.3 ± 3.4	—
0.9% NaCl	0.2†	5	0	+27.2 ± 6.8	—

* During treatment and up to 10 days after treatment.
** During first week of treatment.
*** + = Moderate; + + = Marked.
† ml/kg.

As far as cardiac toxicity is concerned, previous observations demonstrated that repeated administration of anthracycline derivatives to rats caused significant widening of the QRS complex[3,7].

In this study the mean duration of the QRS complex determined in 30 ECGs from control rats prior to treatment was 13.2 msec $\pm$ 0.68 S.E. After 3 injections of demethoxydaunorubicin 4 mg/kg, the QRS mean value was 17.9 msec $\pm$ 0.85 (10 expts; P < 0.001). While in the case of doxorubicin the QRS widening was significant after the fourth injection (18.6 msec $\pm$ 0.73, P < 0.001; 10 expts). Daunorubicin caused a significant widening of the QRS interval at the fifth injection (16.9 msec $\pm$ 0.69, P < 0.005; 10 expts). Epidoxorubicin did not produce significant changes in the QRS complex during treatment or during the 10 days following treatment. The P–R interval was found to be not significantly modified in treated rats. These results indicate that, while intraventricular conduction is altered early on, the A–V conduction system appears to be less susceptible to the toxicity of these drugs. No reduction in the QRS voltage was observed.

In our experiments pretreatment with H_1, H_2, α- and β-blockers did not modify the general and cardiac toxicity either of demethoxydaunorubicin or doxorubicin, but protected animals treated with daunorubicin (Table 1; Fig. 1). The signs of toxicity consisting in mortality percentages or alter-

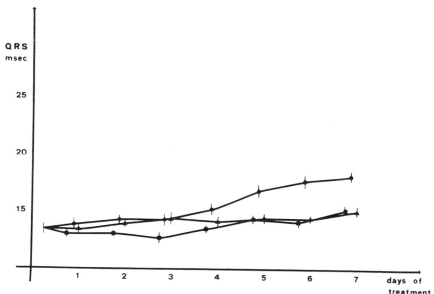

Fig. 1. Graphic representation of the QRS widening (including S-wave trough) in groups of 10 rats treated with daunorubicin (●) 5 × 4 mg/kg i.p.; daunorubicin (■) 5 × 4 mg/kg i.p. + H_1 + H_2 + α + β; and 0.9% NaCl (▲) 5 × 0.2 ml/kg. Each value represents the mean $\pm$ S.E. (vertical lines).

ations of the QRS complex were significantly reduced when daunorubicin was administered in association with H_1, H_2, α- and β-blockers.

The overall results indicate that epidoxorubicin appeared to possess the lowest degree of toxicity. In addition, pretreatment with antihistaminic and antiadrenergic drugs was effective against the toxic effects of daunorubicin. The failure of pretreatment in preventing toxicity in the case of doxorubicin and demethoxydaunorubicin might be due either to a higher release of histamine and catecholamines produced by such drugs or to an earlier involvement of other toxic factors.

ACKNOWLEDGEMENTS

The authors wish to thank Farmitalia–Carlo Erba for the gift of daunomicin, doxorubicin, 4-demethoxydaunorubicin and 4′-epidoxorubicin. The technical assistance of Mr. A. Giacomelli is gratefully acknowledged.

REFERENCES

1. Ghione, M. (1978) Cardiotoxic effects of antitumor agents. *Cancer Chemother. Pharmacol.* **1**, 25.
2. Herman, E. H., Schein, P. and Farmar, R. M. (1969) Comparative cardiac toxicity of daunomycin in three rodent species. *Proc. Soc. Exp. Biol. Med.* **130**, 1098.
3. Zbinden, G. and Brändle, E. (1975) Toxicologic screening of daunorubicin (NSC-82151), Adriamycin (NSC-123127) and their derivatives in rats. *Cancer Chemother. Rep.* **59**, 707.
4. Del Tacca, M., Soldani, G., Paparelli, A., Breschi, M. C. and Mazzanti, L. (1979) Morphological and functional studies on the cardiac neurotoxicity of daunomycin. *Intern. Congr. Neurotoxicol.*, Varese 27–30 Sept., 1979, Abs. 86 bis.
5. Soldani, G., del Tacca, M. and Bernardini, C. (1980) Noradrenaline and adrenergic blockers in daunomycin cardiotoxicity. *Clin. Toxicol.* (in press).
6. Bristow, M. R., Billingham, M. E. and Daniels, G. R. (1979) Histamine and catecholamines mediate adriamycin cardiotoxicity. *Proc. Am. Ass. Cancer Res.*, Fifteenth Meet. 20, 477.
7. Choe, J. Y., Combs, A. B. and Folkers, K. (1979) Prevention by coenzyme Q10 of the electrocardiographic changes induced by adryamicin in rats. *Res. Comm. Chem. Pathol. Pharmacol.* 23, 199.

Drug-induced Alterations in Electrical, Mechanical and Biochemical Activity of the Isolated Perfused Rat Heart

CARL E. ARONSON

Chlorpromazine[1], Disophenol[2] and Bunamidine[3], drugs reported to produce electrocardiographic changes *in vitro*, were examined at various concentrations in isolated rat hearts perfused by the Langendorff technique[4] for periods ranging up to 60 min.

Chlorpromazine (50–5000 ng/ml) prolonged PR and QT intervals (Table 3) and at 5000 ng/ml, it caused electrical alternation with high and low beats, ventricular aberration and ventricular ectopic beats (Fig. 1). In addition, it decreased spontaneous heart rate and isometric systolic tension (Table 1). Chlorpromazine altered tissue concentrations of several glycoly-

TABLE 1. EFFECTS OF CHLORPROMAZINE ON MECHANICAL ACTIVITY OF THE ISOLATED PERFUSED RAT HEART[a]

Drug and concentration[b]	Perfusion time[c] (min)	M[d]	Heart rate (bpm)	Coronary flow (ml/min)	Isometric systolic tension (g)
None	0	7	291 ± 8.6	9.0 ± 1.0	15.9 ± 1.2
	30		274 ± 4.3[e]	9.6 ± 0.9	15.6 ± 1.5
	60		261 ± 10.8	9.0 ± 1.2	13.4 ± 2.0
Chlorpromazine	0	8	281 ± 9.7	8.0 ± 0.6	16.2 ± 0.7
(50 ng/ml)	30		266 ± 10.5	8.4 ± 0.6	15.3 ± 1.0
	60		255 ± 15.0	7.4 ± 0.6	12.4 ± 1.4[e]
Chlorpromazine	0	8	278 ± 11.0	7.8 ± 0.6	15.4 ± 1.0
(500 ng/ml)	30		274 ± 8.9	8.6 ± 0.5	14.7 ± 0.7
	60		266 ± 8.9	8.2 ± 0.6	12.4 ± 0.7[e]
Chlorpromazine	0	9	280 ± 14.1	8.0 ± 0.6	16.1 ± 0.7
(5000 ng/ml)	30		240 ± 17.3[e]	10.2 ± 0.9[e]	9.8 ± 1.1[e]
	60		190 ± 21.2[e]	8.8 ± 0.5	7.3 ± 1.0[e]

[a] Hearts obtained from untreated normal male animals (220–250 g).
[b] Calculated and expressed as the hydrochloride salt.
[c] Duration of perfusion time after initial 15-min equilibration period.
[d] Number of hearts in each group.
[e] Significant (P ≤ 0.05) compared to 0 perfusion time within each group by paired variate *t* test.

217

218

C. E. Aronson

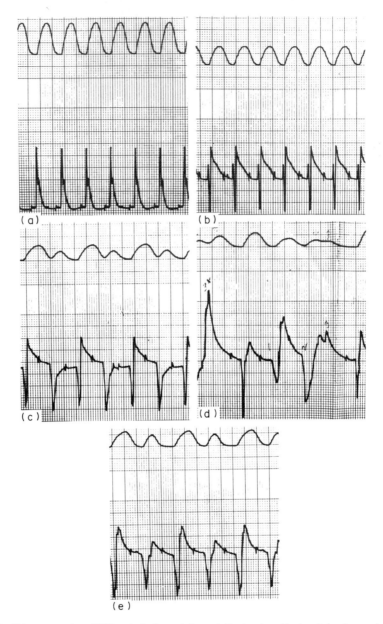

Fig. 1. Chlorpromazine (5000 ng/ml). Isometric systolic tension (1 g/mm) is shown in the upper part of each tracing, while electrical activity (2 mV/cm) is shown below. The first recording (A, 0-time) was made after 15-min of drug-free perfusion before switching to chlorpromazine. Subsequent recordings were made at 15-min (B), 30-min (C), 45-min (D) and 60-min (E). PR and QT interval prolongation, electrical and mechanical alternations, ventricular aberration and ectopic ventricular beats can be seen.

TABLE 2. EFFECTS OF CHLORPROMAZINE ON BIOCHEMICAL ACTIVITY OF THE ISOLATED PERFUSED RAT HEART[a]

Metabolite[b]	n[c]	Concentration of chlorpromazine in perfusion medium (ng/ml)[d]						
		0	n[c]	50	n[c]	500	n[c]	5000
Glycogen	6	11.65 ± 0.98	6	10.99 ± 0.61	6	12.05 ± 0.05	7	11.85 ± 0.78
D-fructose 1,6-di PO_4	6	0.0102 ± 0.0018	6	0.0426 ± 0.0030e	6	0.0234 ± 0	7	0.0372 ± 0.0037e
Dihydroxyacetone PO_4	6	0.0447 ± 0.0088	6	0.0305 ± 0.0171	6	0.0475 ± 0	7	0.0145 ± 0.0053e
D-glyceraldehyde-3-PO_4	6	0.0420 ± 0.0048	6	0.0486 ± 0.0040	6	0.0478 ± 0.004	7	0.0744 ± 0.0084e
L-(−)-Glycerol-1-PO_4	6	0.0238 ± 0.0690	6	0.1153 ± 0.0195	6	0.1137 ± 0.0399	7	0.0220 ± 0.0092e
Pyruvate	6	0.0083 ± 0.0052	6	0.0348 ± 0.0107e	6	0.0796 ± 0.0040b	7	0.0778 ± 0.0084e
L-(+)-Lactate	6	0.5032 ± 0.0684	6	0.3308 ± 0.0333	6	0.4661 ± 0.0917	7	0.4495 ± 0.0366
Adenosine-5'-tri PO_4	6	2.2311 ± 0.1624	6	2.4170 ± 0.1250	6	2.0063 ± 0.0711	7	2.3921 ± 0.1344
Adenosine-5'-di PO_4	6	0.2343 ± 0.0488	6	0.2046 ± 0.0294	6	0.2148 ± 0.0476	7	0.1542 ± 0.0302
Adenosine-5'-mono PO_4	6	0.0667 ± 0.0063	6	0.0740 ± 0.0040	6	0.0513 ± 0.0070	7	0.0480 ± 0.0037
Creatine PO_4	6	1.9245 ± 0.1235	6	1.5056 ± 0.1568	6	1.9608 ± 0.1005	7	2.0461 ± 0.1938

[a] Hearts obtained from untreated normal male animals (220–250 g).

[b] Values expressed as μm/g of tissue (wet weight) after 60 min of perfusion (post-equilibration).

[c] Number of hearts in each group.

[d] Calculated and expressed as the hydrochloride salt. Hearts were perfused with drug-free or chlorpromazine-containing medium for 60 min after the initial 15-min equilibration period.

[e] Significant ($P \leq 0.05$) compared to control (0 drug level) by an independent t test.

TABLE 3. EFFECTS OF CHLORPROMAZINE ON ELECTRICAL ACTIVITY OF THE
ISOLATED PERFUSED RAT HEART[a]

Drug and concentration[b]	Perfusion time[c] (min)	N[d]	PR interval (msec)	QT interval (msec)
None	0	7	42 ± 1.2	73 ± 3.3
	30		42 ± 1.1	73 ± 2.1
	60		41 ± 0.8	74 ± 2.2
Chlorpromazine	0	8	42 ± 0.9	70 ± 0
(50 ng/ml)	30		43 ± 1.2	72 ± 1.3
	60		44 ± 0.9	74 ± 1.6[e]
Chlorpromazine	0	8	44 ± 1.8	69 ± 1.8
(500 ng/ml)	30		43 ± 1.9	73 ± 2.7
	60		44 ± 2.3	74 ± 2.8[e]
Chlorpromazine	0	9	40 ± 0.8	70 ± 1.3
(5000 ng/ml)	30		65 ± 6.1[e]	127 ± 5.8[e]
	60		87 ± 5.3[e,f]	165 ± 12.6[e]

[a] Hearts obtained from untreated normal male animals (220–250 g).
[b] Calculated and expressed as the hydrochloride salt.
[c] Duration of perfusion time after initial 15-min equilibration period.
[d] Number of hearts in each group.
[e] Significant ($P \leq 0.05$) compared to 0 perfusion time with each group by paired variate t test.
[f] N = 8.

tic intermediates (Table 2), however, it had no effect on adenine nucleotides (ATP, ADP and AMP) and creatine phosphate.

At the highest concentration tested, disophenol (1000 ng/ml) caused severe conduction disturbances (Table 6, Fig. 2), decreased spontaneous rate (Table 4) and cardiac arrest occurred frequently within 5 min after exposure to the drug. Ectopic ventricular beats, ventricular tachycardia and ventricular aberrations were recorded (Fig. 2). At 1000 ng/ml, disophenol decreased tissue glycogen and ATP content markedly, and produced a metabolite profile consistent with an inhibition of mitochondrial function (Table 5).

Bunamidine (Table 7), a drug associated with sudden death in dogs, has been reported, *in vivo* to sensitize the myocardium to endogenous catacholamines and to precipitate ventricular fibrillation. In the isolated perfused rat heart, bunamidine (2500 ng/ml)-induced alterations in electrical activity were evident within 1–3 min after exposure to the drug. QRS and T wave forms were altered by 2–1 AV block developed. Subsequently fusion of the QRS and T waves occurred and a 3–2 AV block accounted for the mechanical bigeminy observed. When mechanical activity ceased at 5 min, only P waves accompanied by low amplitude deflections bearing no temporal relationship to the P waves were evident (Fig. 3).

Bunamidine also decreased tissue content of glycogen, adenine nucleotides and creatine phosphate (Table 8), and it produced a metabolite profile

TABLE 4. EFFECTS OF DISOPHENOL ON MECHANICAL ACTIVITY OF THE ISOLATED PERFUSED RAT HEART[a]

Drug and concentration	Perfusion time[b] (min)	n[c]	Heart rate (b.p.m.)	Coronary flow (ml/min)	Isometric systolic tension (g)	Diastolic tension[d] (g)
None	0	11	286 ± 6.2	10.1 ± 0.7	16.1 ± 0.9	4.9 ± 0.1
	30		267 ± 4.9[e]	9.7 ± 0.7	15.7 ± 1.0	4.6 ± 0.1[e]
	60		256 ± 8.5[e]	8.3 ± 0.8	13.2 ± 1.3[e]	4.9 ± 0.4
Disophenol (10 ng/ml)	0	7	283 ± 12.9	7.3 ± 0.2	15.0 ± 0.4	5.0 ± 0
	30		253 ± 6.1	7.4 ± 0.4	16.9 ± 0.7[e]	4.1 ± 0.1[e]
	60		257 ± 8.9	7.5 ± 0.6	14.2 ± 0.6	4.2 ± 0.2
Disophenol (100 ng/ml)	0	7	296 ± 12.1	8.1 ± 1.1	13.2 ± 1.0	5.2 ± 0.3
	30		257 ± 14.4[e]	8.3 ± 1.1	12.1 ± 1.4	5.6 ± 0.5
	60		249 ± 12.6[e]	8.0 ± 1.4	8.9 ± 1.1	6.1 ± 0.5
Disophenol (1000 ng/ml)	0	7	291 ± 8.6	8.5 ± 0.7	15.9 ± 0.6	5.0 ± 0
	30		77 ± 38.1[e]	6.3 ± 1.6	1.8 ± 1.4[e]	15.5 ± 1.9[e]
	60		49 ± 21.9[e]	3.0 ± 0.5[e]	0.6 ± 0.2[e]	16.5 ± 0.7[e]

[a] Hearts obtained from untreated normal male animals (220–250 g).
[b] Duration of perfusion after initial 15-min equilibration period.
[c] Number of hearts in each group.
[d] Initial diastolic tension was imposed on each heart at the start of the 15-min equilibration period.
[e] Significant (P ≤ 0.05) compared to 0 perfusion time within each group by paired variate t-test.

TABLE 5. EFFECTS OF DISOPHENOL ON BIOCHEMICAL ACTIVITY OF THE ISOLATED PERFUSED RAT HEART[a]

Metabolite[b]	n[e]	0	n[c]	10	n[c]	100	n[c]	1000	n[d]
				Concentration of disophenol in perfusion medium (ng/ml)[d]					
Glycogen	9	12.06 ± 0.99	5	12.03 ± 1.04	5	0.91 ± 0.64[e]	5	1.48 ± 0.21[e]	5
D-Glucose-6-PO$_4$	9	0.0497 ± 0.0033	5	0.0432 ± 0.0049	5	0.0422 ± 0.0032	5	0.0724 ± 0.0072[e]	5
D-Fructose-1,6-di PO$_4$	9	0.0114 ± 0.0013	5	0.0140 ± 0	5	0.0244 ± 0.0058[e]	5	0.0284 ± 0.0075[e]	5
D-Glyceraldehyde-3-PO$_4$	9	0.0362 ± 0.0057	5	0.0362 ± 0.0074	5	0.0194 ± 0.0077	5	0.0248 ± 0.0095[e]	5
L-(−)-Glycerol-1-PO$_4$	9	0.1662 ± 0.0485	5	0.0564 ± 0.0167	5	0.1112 ± 0.0188	5	0.3522 ± 0.0418[e]	5
Pyruvate	9	0.0177 ± 0.0094	5	0.0556 ± 0.0146[e]	5	0.0480 ± 0.0094	5	0.0338 ± 0.0112	5
L-(+)-Lactate	9	0.4294 ± 0.0643	5	0.2430 ± 0.0569	5	0.5148 ± 0.1068	5	0.9336 ± 0.1546[e]	5
Adenosine-5'-tri PO$_4$	9	2.0650 ± 0.1429	5	2.3898 ± 0.1507	5	1.9532 ± 0.1359	5	0.6814 ± 0.1223[e]	5
Adenosine-5'-di PO$_4$	9	0.2131 ± 0.0331	5	0.1326 ± 0.0264	5	0.1434 ± 0.0141	5	0.1114 ± 0.0282	5
Adenosine-5'-mono PO$_4$	9	0.0782 ± 0.0100	5	0.1086 ± 0.0295	5	0.0770 ± 0.0191	5	0.2580 ± 0.0296[e]	5
Creatine PO$_4$	9	1.8450 ± 0.0892	5	1.6768 ± 0.1585	5	1.8704 ± 0.2014	5	1.1708 ± 0.1106[e]	5

[a] Hearts obtained from untreated normal male animals (220–250 g).
[b] Values expressed as μm/g of tissue (wet weight) after 60 min of perfusion (post-equilibration).
[c] Number of hearts in each group.
[d] Hearts were perfused with drug-free or disophenol-containing medium for 60 min after the initial 15-min equilibration period.
[e] Significant ($P \leq 0.05$) compared to control (0 drug level) by an independent t test.

TABLE 6. EFFECTS OF DISOPHENOL ON ELECTRICAL ACTIVITY OF THE ISOLATED PERFUSED RAT HEART[a]

Drug and concentration	Perfusion time[b] (min)	N[c]	PR interval (msec)	QT interval (msec)
None	0	11	41 ± 0.8	72 ± 2.1
	30		41 ± 0.7	72 ± 1.4
	60		41 ± 0.6	73 ± 1.5
Disophenol	0	7	40 ± 0.9	69 ± 1.6
(10 ng/ml)	30		42 ± 2.0	75 ± 3.3
	60		43 ± 2.0	73 ± 2.8
Disophenol	0	7	39 ± 0.6	71 ± 1.1
(100 ng/ml)	30		41 ± 1.6	78 ± 2.5[d]
	60		42 ± 2.0	81 ± 3.4[d]
Disophenol	0	7	40 ± 0	70 ± 0
(1000 ng/ml)	30		45 ± 5[e]	85 ± 5.0[e]
	60		40[f]	80[f]

[a] Hearts obtained from untreated normal male animals (220–250 g).
[b] Duration of perfusion time after initial 15-min equilibration period.
[c] Number of hearts in each group.
[d] Significant ($P \leq 0.05$) compared to 0 perfusion time within each group by paired variate t test.
[e] $N = 2$.
[f] $N = 1$.

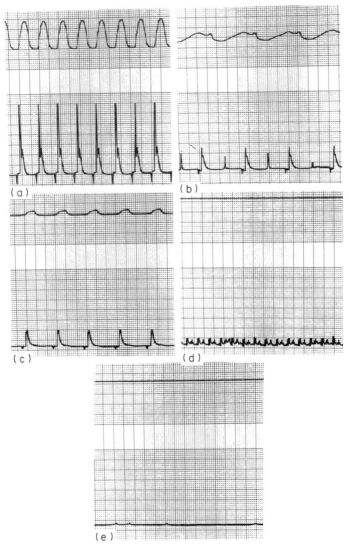

Fig. 2. Disophenol (1000 ng/ml). Isometric systolic tension (1 g/mm) is shown in the upper part of each tracing while electrical activity (2 mV/cm) is shown below. The first recording (A, 0-time) was made after 15-min or drug-free perfusion before switching to disophenol. Subsequent recordings were made at 15-min (B), 30-min (C), 42-min (D) and 60-min (E). Ectopic ventricular beats, a sinus rhythm followed by ventricular tachycardia, and a series of very small ectopic ventricular beats can be seen.

TABLE 7. EFFECTS OF BUNAMIDINE ON MECHANICAL ACTIVITY OF THE ISOLATED PERFUSED RAT HEART[a]

Drug and concentration[b]	Perfusion time[c] (min)	n[d]	Heart rate (b.p.m.)	n[d]	Coronary flow (ml/min)	n[d]	Isometric systolic tension (g)	n[d]	Diastolic tension[e] (g)
None	0	9	270 ± 11.2	9	8.3 ± 0.6	9	18.4 ± 0.9	9	4.5 ± 0.2
	30	9	250 ± 10.0	9	8.6 ± 0.9	9	18.7 ± 1.6	9	4.2 ± 0.3
	60	9	227 ± 11.3[f]	9	9.1 ± 0.8	9	17.1 ± 1.5	9	4.2 ± 0.4
Bunamidine (100 ng/ml)	0	7	274 ± 12.1	7	8.3 ± 0.3	7	18.4 ± 1.3	7	4.5 ± 0.1
	30	7	244 ± 15.3[f]	7	10.5 ± 0.6[f]	7	18.2 ± 1.1	7	3.8 ± 0.2[f]
	60	7	223 ± 18.4[f]	7	11.4 ± 0.5[f]	7	16.5 ± 1.6[f]	7	3.6 ± 0.3[f]
Bunamidine (1000 ng/ml)	0	7	261 ± 8.6	7	8.6 ± 0.9	7	19.1 ± 1.6	7	4.6 ± 0.1
	30	7	210 ± 11.3[f]	7	11.5 ± 1.3[f]	7	15.9 ± 1.2[f]	7	3.9 ± 0.1[f]
	60	4	195 ± 15.0[f]	4	9.1 ± 0.9	4	8.4 ± 0.7[f]	7	5.5 ± 0.9
Bunamidine (2500 ng/ml)	0	9	263 ± 8.3	9	8.3 ± 0.5	9	17.3 ± 0.9	9	4.9 ± 0.1
	30	7	227 ± 8.9[f]	7	8.5 ± 1.1	7	12.1 ± 2.0	9	6.7 ± 1.0
	60	3	220 ± 10.0	3	6.5 ± 1.2	3	13.3 ± 0.9	9	8.4 ± 1.2[f]
Bunamidine (10,000 ng/ml)	0	7	266 ± 12.1	7	8.0 ± 0.9	7	15.2 ± 0.9	7	4.9 ± 0.1
	30	1	180	7	4.1 ± 0.8[f]	1	2.0	7	12.3 ± 0.7[f]
	60	0	—	7	2.9 ± 0.4[f]	0	—	7	12.0 ± 0.6[f]

[a] Hearts obtained from untreated normal male animals (220–250 g).
[b] Calculated and expressed as the free base.
[c] Duration of perfusion time after initial 15-min equilibration period.
[d] Number of hearts from which measurements were obtained.
[e] An initial diastolic tension was imposed on each heart at the start of the 15-min equilibration period.
[f] Significant (P ≤ 0.05) compared to 0 perfusion time within each group by paired variate t test.

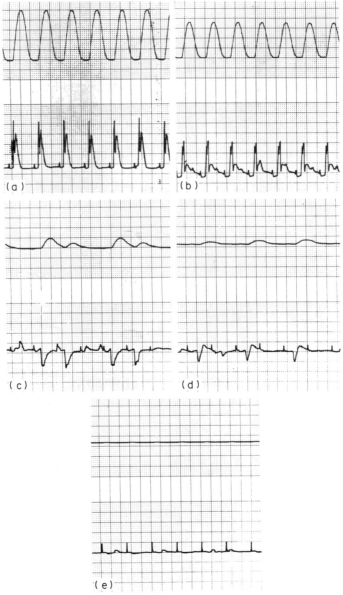

Fig. 3. Bunamidine (2500 ng/ml). Isometric systolic tension (1 g/mm) is shown in the upper part of each tracing while electrical activity (2 mV/cm) is shown below. The first recording (A, 0-time) was made after 15-min of drug-free perfusion before switching to bunamidine. Subsequent recordings were made at 2-min (B), 3-min (C), 4-min (D) and 5-min (E). QRS and T wave alterations, PR prolongation, 2–1 AV block, QRS and T wave fusion, 3–2 AV block and mechanical bigeminy, variable AV block with dropped beats, and P waves at regular intervals can be seen.

TABLE 8. EFFECTS OF BUNAMIDINE ON BIOCHEMICAL ACTIVITY OF THE ISOLATED PERFUSED RAT HEART[a]

Metabolite[b]	n[c]	0	n[c]	Concentration of bunamidine in perfusion medium (ng/ml)[d] 1000	n[c]	2500	n[c]	10,000
Glycogen	7	11.48 ± 0.40	5	6.24 ± 0.35[e]	6	6.86 ± 0.65[e]	5	4.26 ± 0.63[e]
D-Glucose-6-PO$_4$	7	0.0342 ± 0	5	0.0536 ± 0.0077[e]	6	0.0737 ± 0.0134[e]	5	0.0602 ± 0.0057[e]
Dihydroxyacetone PO$_4$	7	0.0457 ± 0.0069	5	0.0376 ± 0.0077[e]	6	0.0280 ± 0.0050	5	0.0780 ± 0.0103[e]
D-Glyceraldehyde-3-PO$_4$	7	0.0376 ± 0.0134	5	0.0416 ± 0	6	0.0238 ± 0.0013	5	0.0332 ± 0.0044
L-(−)-Glycerol-1-PO$_4$	7	0.1430 ± 0.0148	5	0.2804 ± 0.0534[e]	6	0.2208 ± 0.0187[e]	5	0.3386 ± 0.0319[e]
L-(+)-Lactate	7	0.3130 ± 0.0352	5	0.4720 ± 0.0178[e]	6	0.4917 ± 0.0825[e]	5	0.8002 ± 0.0521[e]
Adenosine-5'-tri PO$_4$	7	2.0551 ± 0.1125	5	1.5112 ± 0.1414[e]	6	1.1337 ± 0.2035[e]	5	0.4640 ± 0.0885[e]
Adenosine-5'-di PO$_4$	7	0.3056 ± 0.0278	5	0.5358 ± 0.0299	6	0.1772 ± 0.0345[e]	5	0.0920 ± 0.0128[e]
Adenosine-5'-mono PO$_4$	7	0.0774 ± 0.0069	5	0.2324 ± 0.0118[e]	6	0.0838 ± 0.0115	5	0.1498 ± 0.0139[e]
Creatine PO$_4$	7	2.170 ± 0.1360	5	1.6262 ± 0.1970[e]	6	1.3877 ± 0.2476[e]	5	0.7158 ± 0.1237[e]

[a] Hearts obtained from untreated normal male animals (220–250 g).
[b] Values expressed as μm/g of tissue (wet weight) after 60 min of perfusion (post-equilibration).
[c] Number of hearts in each group.
[d] Hearts were perfused with drug-free or bunamidine-containing medium for 60 min after the initial 15-min equilibration period.
[e] Significant (P ≤ 0.05) compared to control (0 drug level) by an independent t-test.

TABLE 9. EFFECTS OF BUNAMIDINE ON ELECTRICAL ACTIVITY OF THE ISOLATED PERFUSED RAT HEART[a]

Drug and concentration[b]	Perfusion time[c] (min)	N[d]	PR interval (msec)	QT interval (msec)
None	0	9	46 ± 1.2	72 ± 1.5
	30	9	45 ± 1.4	72 ± 1.5
	60	9	47 ± 1.8	74 ± 1.8
Bunamidine	0	7	47 ± 2.5	73 ± 1.8
(100 ng/ml)	30	7	63 ± 6.4^e	106 ± 8.7^e
	60	7	79 ± 14.3^e	113 ± 11.7^e
Bunamidine	0	7	45 ± 1.6	73 ± 1.8
(1000 ng/ml)	30	7	80 ± 9.3^e	117 ± 9.4
	60	7	85 ± 15.5	138 ± 25.3
Bunamidine	0	9	42 ± 1.1	76 ± 1.8
(2500 ng/ml)	30	7	70 ± 3.8^e	140 ± 9.8^e
	60	3	83 ± 14.5	160 ± 17.3
Bunamidine	0	7	42 ± 1.5	76 ± 1.8
(10,000 ng/ml)	30	1	80	140
	60	0	—	—

[a] Hearts obtained from untreated normal male animals (220–250 g).

[b] Calculated and expressed as the free base.

[c] Duration of perfusion time after initial 15-min equilibration period.

[d] Number of hearts from which measurements were obtained.

[e] Significant ($P \leq 0.05$) compared to 0 perfusion time within each group by paired variate t test.

TABLE 10. EFFECTS OF EPINEPHRINE AND BUNAMIDINE ON GLYCOGEN CONTENT AND PHOSPHORYLASE ACTIVITY IN THE ISOLATED PERFUSED RAT HEART[a]

Drug in medium	Agonist	N[b]	Glycogen[g] (μm/g)	% Phosphorylase a[h]
None[c]	PSS[e]	5	10.56 ± 0.27	12.4 ± 1.3
None[c]	Epinephrine[f]	6	12.71 ± 1.18	49.9 ± 3.5^i
Bunamidine[d]	PSS[e]	5	10.93 ± 0.82	13.2 ± 2.0^j
Bunamidine[d]	Epinephrine[f]	6	10.89 ± 0.62	$47.9 \pm 2.8^{i,k}$

[a] Hearts obtained from normal male rats (220–250 g).

[b] Number of hearts in each group.

[c] Hearts perfused for a total of 20 min with drug-free K–R buffer.

[d] Hearts perfused for 15 min with drug-free K–R buffer, then switched to bunamidine (100 ng/ml) containing K–R medium for 5 min.

[e] 0.1 ml physiological saline solution (0.9% NaCl) + 0.5 ml drug-free K–R buffer injected as a bolus at 20 min. Hearts were frozen approximately 15 sec after injection of PSS.

[f] 0.1 ml epinephrine (0.5 μg total dose) in PSS + 0.5 ml K–R buffer injected as a bolus at 20 min (15 control + 5 bunamidine). Hearts were frozen at the peak of the epinephrine-induced positive inotropic response (approximately 15 sec after injection).

[g] Calculated on basis of tissue wet weight.

[h] Phosphorylase a = Cori Units Phosphorylase a/Total Cori Units Phosphorylase $(b + a) \times 100$.

[i] Significant ($P \leq 0.05$) compared to none-PSS by Student's t test.

[j] Significant ($P \leq 0.05$) compared to none-epinephrine by Student's t test.

[k] Significant ($P \leq 0.05$) compared to bunamidine-PSS by Student's t test.

TABLE 11. EFFECTS OF EPINEPHRINE AND BUNAMIDINE ON ISOMETRIC SYSTOLIC TENSION IN THE ISOLATED PERFUSED RAT HEART[a]

Drug in medium	Agonist	N[b]	Isometric systolic tension (g)		
			Pre	Post	Δ (Pre-post)
None[c]	PSS[e]	5	17.1 ± 1.5	15.4 ± 1.6	−1.7 ± 0.5
None[c]	Epinephrine[f]	6	17.2 ± 0.9	20.9 ± 1.3	3.7 ± 1.3[g]
Bunamidine[d]	PSS[e]	5	15.2 ± 1.8	14.9 ± 1.7	−0.3 ± 0.4[h]
Bunamidine[d]	Epinephrine[f]	6	17.9 ± 1.0	22.2 ± 1.0	4.3 ± 0.3[g,i]

[a] Hearts obtained from normal male rats (220–250 g).
[b] Number of hearts in each group.
[c] Hearts perfused for a total of 20 min with drug-free K–R buffer.
[d] Hearts perfused for 15 min with drug-free K–R buffer, then switched to bunamidine (100 ng/ml) containing medium for 5 min.
[e] 0.1 ml physiological saline solution (0.9% NaCl) + 0.5 ml drug-free K–R buffer injected as a bolus at 20 min. Hearts were frozen approximately 15 sec after injection of PSS.
[f] 0.1 ml epinephrine (0.5 μg total dose) in PSS + 0.5 ml drug-free buffer injected as a bolus at 20 min (15 control + 5 bunamidine). Hearts were frozen at the peak of the epinephrine-induced positive inotropic response (approximately 15 sec after injection).
[g] Significant (P ≤ 0.05) compared to none-PSS by Student's *t* test.
[h] Significant (P ≤ 0.05) compared to none-epinephrine by Student's *t* test.
[i] Significant (P ≤ 0.05) compared to bunamidine-PSS by Student's *t* test.

similar to that of disophenol (Table 5). At the lowest concentration found to alter electrical activity (100 ng/ml) (Table 9), bunamidine did not change the sensitivity of our preparation to epinephrine, using isometric systolic tension development and the conversion of phosphorylase *b* to *a* as indicators (Tables 10 and 11).

REFERENCES

1. Aronson, C. E. and Serlick, E. R. (1977) *Toxicol. Appl. Pharmacol.* **39,** 157–176.
2. Aronson, C. E. and Serlick, E. R. (1977) *Biochem. Pharmacol.* **26,** 2297–2305.
3. Aronson, C. E. and Hanno, E. R. S. (1978) *Gen. Pharmacol.* **9,** 101–112.
4. Aronson, C. E. and Serlick, E. R. (1976) *Toxicol. Appl. Pharmacol.* **38,** 479–488.

The Surface ECG and Cardiac Histopathology during Chronic Administration of Anthracycline Antitumor Agents in the Rat

J. P. BUYNISKI AND R. S. HIRTH

The recent development of analogs of adriamycin (ADM) has resulted in a need for an animal system to evaluate the cardiac effects of the newer analogs. It appears that chronic subcutaneous (s.c.) administration of ADM to rats at maximally-tolerated doses results in myocardial lesions with histological characteristics similar to those reported in humans, and the cardiotoxicity is delayed, progressive and frequently manifested by congestive heart failure[1,2]. We have used the above rat model for cardiotoxicity evaluation and incorporated ECGs to track evolving cardiotoxicity. A maximally-tolerated s.c. dose of ADM (2 mg/kg; N = 10) or vehicle was administered to rats once a week for 13 weeks followed by a 4-week recovery period. ECGs were obtained prior to drug administration and 1–2 times weekly during the drug administration and recovery periods. The general method of Zbinden and Brändle[3] was used to obtain the rat ECG and Fig. 1 is a flow chart for the rat ECG evaluation system used in our laboratories. A modification was used of the computer program for pattern recognition of ECGs[4]. The R wave amplitude was used as an estimate of QRS voltage and this parameter along with the QRS duration and ventricular rate were the major parameters evaluated although some observations were made on the PR and QT intervals. At the end of the 4-week recovery period portions of the left ventricular myocardium from ADM and vehicle-treated rats underwent histopathological examination using light microscopy and standard staining techniques.

Carminomycin (CARM), an anthracycline antitumor agent structurally related to ADM, was also evaluated for cardiac effects following chronic s.c. administration of a maximally-tolerated dose (1 mg/kg; N = 20) to rats. ECGs were taken for vehicle- and drug-treated rats in a manner similar to the ADM study but only at the end of the first and fifth week of the recovery period, since this is the time the major ECG effects of ADM are

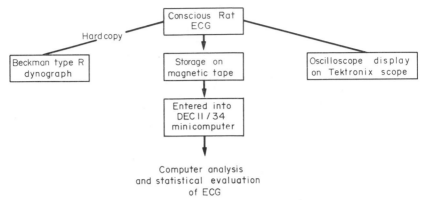

Fig. 1. Flow chart for rat ECG evaluation.

observed. At the end of the 6-week recovery period the hearts of the CARM and vehicle-treated rats were submitted for histopathological examination using light microscopy and standard staining techniques.

During the ADM treatment period a progressive reduction in QRS voltage occurred and at the end of the drug treatment period was reduced by $-28 \pm 4\%$ (mean $\pm$ 1 S.E.; $p < 0.01$) when compared to predrug values. During the 4 week recovery period a delayed further fall in QRS voltage occurred ($-45 \pm 11\%$; $p < 0.01$). Figure 2 is an unfiltered, computer printout of a rat ECG (1 mm/msec) prior to ADM treatment and Fig. 3 is an ECG from this same rat during the recovery period following ADM treatment. QRS voltage was reduced by about 50% in this rat with a slight prolongation of the QRS duration. In a separate group of 10 rats receiving vehicle in which the ECG was monitored over a similar period as the ADM-treated rats, QRS voltage showed a slight trend to increase with time. During the ADM treatment period there occurred relatively minimal

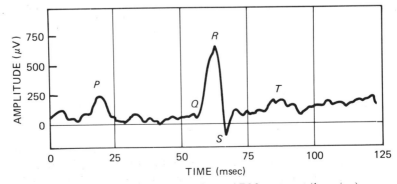

Fig. 2. Control ECG of Rat B-4 prior to ADM treatment (1 mm/sec).

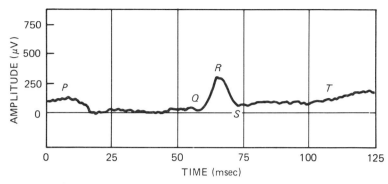

Fig. 3. ECG of Rat B-4 in the fourth week of the recovery period following 13 weeks of ADM treatment. Histopathological evaluation of the left ventricular myocardium showed diffuse myocyte vacuolation and degeneration with edema, fibrosis and fiber atrophy/myocytolysis.

reductions in ventricular rate. However, during the 4 week recovery period a delayed further fall in ventricular rate occurred (-143 ± 32 beats/min; $p < 0.01$). QRS duration showed a slight trend to increase by the end of the recovery period. No other important ECG changes were observed in the above studies.

Light microscopic examination of left ventricular myocardium of ADM-treated rats revealed a spectrum of alterations. Myofiber changes included vacuolation, degeneration, atrophy/myocytolysis, while interstitial alterations consisted of edema and fibrosis. Minimal, focal vacuolation of a few myocytes was occasionally observed in control hearts but there were no other changes associated with these vacuolated myofibers like those that occurred routinely in the ADM-treated rats. The CARM-treated rats showed no reduction in QRS voltage when compared to the vehicle-treated group nor were there clinically significant changes in other ECG parameters. Similarly, histopathological examination did not show ADM-like cardiac lesions.

Thus, these studies indicate that the rat ECG can be used in long-term studies to monitor the progress of cardiotoxicity due to the anthracycline antitumor agents, and to differentiate the cardiotoxic liabilities of these agents.

REFERENCES

1. Mettler, F. P., Young, D. M. and Ward, J. M. (1977) *Cancer Res.* **37**, 2705–2713.
2. Olson, H. M. and Capen, C. C. (1978) *Toxicol. Appl. Pharmacol.* **44**, 605–616.
3. Zbinden, G. and Brändle, E. (1975) *Cancer Chemother. Rep.* **59**, 707–715.
4. Wartak, J., Milliken, J. A. and Karchmar, J. (1970) *Computers and Biomed. Res.* **3**, 344–374.

The Anesthetized Rat as a Model for Investigating Early Post-ligation Dysrhythmias

K. A. KANE, F. M. McDONALD AND J. R. PARRATT

We have developed a model of coronary artery ligation in anaesthetized rats (Na pentobarbitone, 60 mg/kg i.p.) as a method of producing experimental dysrhythmias and consequently as a useful tool in the screening of compounds for antidysrhythmic activity. The experimental procedure is described in detail elsewhere (Clark et al., 1980).

Prior to ligation, heart rate was 451 ± 10 beats/min; P-wave 20 ± 1 ms; P–R interval 49 ± 1 ms; QRS 19 ± 0.5 ms and Q–T interval 63 ± 1.5 ms. Lead 1 ECG was chosen, as in our experience it best reflects the electrocardiographic changes occurring on ligation of the left coronary artery. Immediately after ligation, the marked electrocardiographic changes include an increase in R-wave amplitude. (The rat ECG has no true ST-segment; however the term "ST-segment" has been used here to describe the junction of the QRS and T waves.) This is accompanied by transient "ST-segment" elevation which proceeds to "ST-segment" depression. These changes occur in the first 1–2 min after ligation. Subsequently there is a gradual reduction in R-wave amplitude, slowly-developing, sustained "ST-segment" elevation and the appearance of Q-waves. At 30 min after ligation, heart rate, P-wave and P–R interval are unchanged. There is continued development of Q-waves, merging of the QRS and T-waves and prolongation of the Q–T interval to 96 ± 3 ms. These electrocardiographic changes are shown in Fig. 1.

In addition to these changes in sinus ECG, the animals display a period of considerable ventricular ectopic activity. These dysrhythmias occur mainly between 4 and 18 min post-ligation, and comprise isolated extrasystoles and bursts of ventricular tachycardia and ventricular fibrillation (VF). All untreated animals show extrasystoles (mean 1165 ± 135 over the initial 30 min post-ligation period) and tachycardia, and more than 50% of them exhibit VF. In the rat, VF will usually spontaneously revert to sinus rhythm, and the mortality in the control group was 16%. Figure 2 shows the effectiveness of lignocaine and propranolol in this model. Both drugs

235

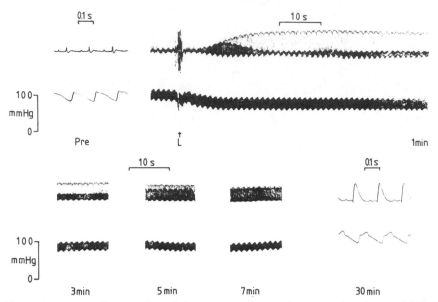

Fig. 1. A representative recording of the electrocardiogram (upper trace) and arterial blood pressure (lower trace) in an anaesthetized rat at various times after coronary artery ligation. L = coronary artery ligation.

reduced the number of extrasystoles and the incidence of VF. These drugs did not significantly alter mortality with the exception of lignocaine 5 mg/kg/h which increased mortality to 50% (P < 0.01). In about 60% of the animals, the extrasystoles seem to occur in two phases, the first having its peak at 5–7 min followed by an abrupt reduction in ectopic activity, and the peak of the second phase at 9–11 min post-ligation. VF is most likely to first occur towards the end of the initial phase, at 6–8 min post-ligation. Figure 3 shows the distribution of ventricular extrasystoles in a random group of 10 control animals and in those pretreated with lignocaine and propranolol.

We have examined several antidysrhythmic drugs in this model. It appears that membrane stabilizing drugs, e.g. lignocaine, are most effective in reducing the number of extrasystoles. A reduction in the incidence of VF requires higher doses of these drugs, yet doses that prevent VF do not completely inhibit ectopic activity. High doses of lignocaine seem to reduce dysrhythmias in the second phase preferentially. Whether this represents a true differential effect or merely a time shift is not yet clear.

We feel that this model fulfils a useful role in antidysrhythmic screening programmes, especially in the search for drugs to prevent early post-infarction ventricular fibrillation (sudden cardiac death).

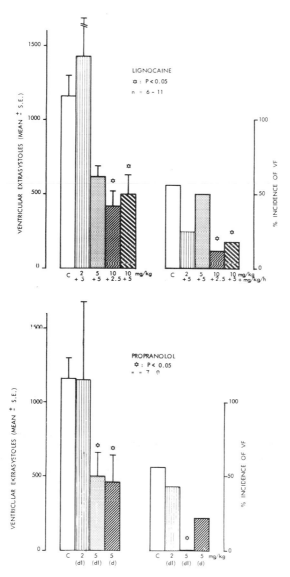

Fig. 2. Effects of lignocaine and d and dl propranolol against the ventricular extrasystoles and ventricular fibrillation occurring in the survivors during the first 30 min after coronary artery ligation. Lignocaine was administered as a bolus injection immediately followed by a continuous intravenous infusion, commencing 5 min before ligation. Propranolol was administered as a single intravenous injection 15 min before ligation.

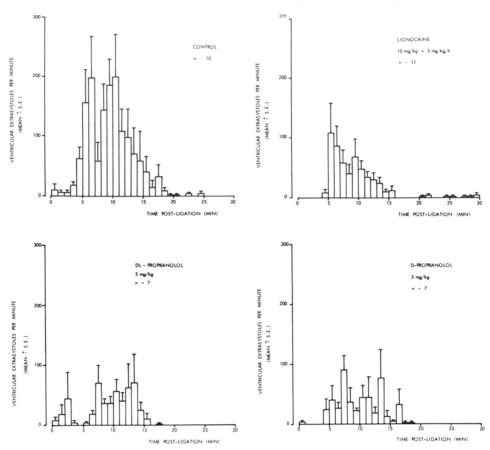

Fig. 3. Effects of lignocaine and propranolol on the distribution of ventricular extrasystoles in the first 30 min after coronary artery ligation. The mean total number of ventricular extrasystoles over this period was 1491 in the control group and 543, 502 and 462 in the lignocaine, dl-propranolol and d-propranolol groups respectively.

REFERENCE

Clark, C., Foreman, M. I., Kane, K. A., McDonald, F. M. and Parratt, J. R. (1980) Coronary artery ligation in anaesthetised rats as a method for the production of experimental dysrhythmias and for the determination of infarct size. *J. Pharmac. Methods* **3** (4), 357–368.

Ventricular Fibrillation following Coronary Artery Ligation in the Rat

T. ABRAHAMSSON AND O. ALMGREN

Experimental occlusion of the left coronary artery in the rat provides a relatively simple model for producing myocardial ischemia and for studying the concomitant acute arrhythmias (Kenedi and Losonci, 1973). Using this model we have studied the incidence of acute ventricular fibrillation (VF) following coronary occlusion with regard to effects of hypokalemia, seasonal variation and antiarrhythmic therapy.

Male Wistar rats (300–400 g) were anaesthetized with pentobarbitone sodium (60 mg/kg i.p.) and kept artificially ventilated. The chest was opened on the left side and the left coronary artery was ligated a few mm distal to its origin. Arterial blood pressure, heart rate and ECG were continuously recorded during 15 min following ligation. For the ECG

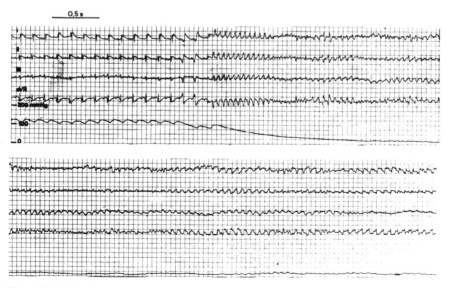

Fig. 1. ECG (leads I, II, III, aVR) and arterial blood pressure measured 5 min after left coronary artery ligation in a rat. During VF all ECG leads show chaotic activity and blood pressure decreases towards zero.

measurements, needles were inserted into the skin at the base of each limb and standard limb leads (I, II, III, aVR) were recorded using a mingograph ink jet recorder (Siemens–Elema). The criteria for the diagnosis of VF were determined as a total irregularity of the ECG for at least 5 s together with a decrease in arterial blood pressure towards zero level (Fig. 1). Hypokalemia was produced by furosemide (Lasix®) treatment (10 or 20 mg/kg i.p.) given twice daily 1 and 2 days before the experimental procedure. To some rats the antiarrhythmic agent tocainide (5 or 50 μmol/kg) was administered intravenously 15 min prior to the ligation.

The time of onset of arrhythmias following ligation of the left coronary artery was 4–5 min. In untreated rats (n = 8) the incidence of VF was 13% (1/8). Administration of furosemide (n = 7) decreased the plasma potassium concentration from 3.58 to 2.80 mmol/l and increased VF incidence to 86% (7/8). This high incidence of VF following furosemide treatment was found in three consecutive series of experiments performed during May to September. However, following coronary occlusions carried out in

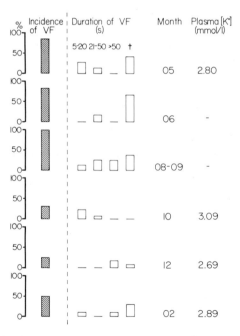

Fig. 2. Seasonal variation in VF incidence (i.e. the percentage of the experimental animals in which at least one period of VF occurred) following left coronary artery ligation in furosemide-treated rats. The experiments were carried out during a period from May (1979) to February (1980). The total duration of VF for each rat was quantified and grouped into one of four categories: 5–20 s, 21–50 s, >50 s and those who died in VF (†). Plasma [K⁺] in untreated control rats (May and October) = 3.46 ± 0.08 mmol/l (n = 13).

October, December and February the incidence of VF was lower (Fig. 2). Tocainide caused a reduction in the occurrence of VF in furosemide-treated rats from 100% in controls to 22% (2/9) (tocainide: 5 μmol/kg, n = 9) and 38% (3/8) (tocainide: 50 μmol/kg, n = 8).

It is concluded that hypokalemia, induced by furosemide treatment, is associated with a pronounced increase in the incidence of VF following left coronary occlusion in the rat. However, a marked seasonal variation in the occurrence of VF was noticed. The mechanism behind this variability is at present not known but may involve seasonal variations in hormonal, nervous (sympathetic) and metabolic activity which needs further studies. In this model, antiarrhythmic therapy with tocainide proved to be successful in decreasing the incidence of acute VF.

REFERENCE

Kenedi, I. and Losonci, A. (1973) *Acta Physiol. Acad. Sci. Hung.* **43**, 133–141.

ECG and Other Responses to Ligation of a Coronary Artery in the Conscious Rat

K. M. JOHNSTON, B. A. MacLEOD AND M. J. A. WALKER

ABSTRACT

A method is described in which the left anterior descending coronary artery is ligated in conscious unrestrained rats. Previous surgery allows a loose ligature to be placed around the artery together with the implantation of arterial and venous cannulae and permanent ECG electrodes in limbs and chest. After recovery (7 days), permanent ligation can be produced while continuously monitoring the animal. Ligation in conscious rats produces very small changes in blood pressure (fall of 3–10 mm Hg) and heart rate. Arrhythmias are consistently produced and these include PVC and episodes of ventricular tachycardia/flutter and fibrillation. Some animals recover spontaneously from such episodes while most of the others can be restored to sinus rhythm by precordial tapping. ECG changes with ligation are marked, they consist of an initial increase in QRS size, elevation of "S–T segments" and "Q-wave" appearance. All the above are associated with exclusion of dye to 20–30% of the ventricular mass and a 24-hr infarct of 20–30% as judged by red or blue tetrazolium staining. This preparation should be very useful for testing the effects of drugs, or other interventions, on the responses to ligation of a coronary artery.

INTRODUCTION

In studying myocardial ischaemia and infarction, and the action of drugs, there is a need for suitable test preparations (Fozzard, 1975). A good model should reflect all the responses that occur during heart attacks in humans but, as the aetiology of such attacks is probably mixed (Maseri *et al.*, 1978), no one model will ever suffice. In assessing the effect of drugs on the myocardial ischaemia-infarction sequence the following responses should be measured: occurrence of arrhythmias, changes in blood pressure, heart rate, cardiac output, temporary and permanent loss of cardiac tissue, morbidity and mortality.

For comparison with man, no species is ideal for studying the effects of drugs on the ischaemia-infarction sequence, for the human heart changes its vasculature during aging. While atheroma-free human hearts have few collaterals, old atheromatous hearts may rely heavily on collaterals (Crawford, 1977; Schaper, 1971). No single species meets these varying conditions. Furthermore, many models involve the complicating presence of recent surgery and of anaesthesia thus making extrapolation to conscious man even more difficult. The latter two complications are absent in conscious, unrestrained and chronically prepared animals.

Statistical verification of changes in an erratic response such as arrhythmias requires large experimental groups and, therefore, a model that allows large numbers of animals to be used is preferable.

To try and meet some of the above suggested requirements for a good model, we have ligated coronary arteries in healthy conscious rats. In such animals, blood pressure, ECG, heart rate and arrhythmias were monitored before and after ligation while the amount of ischaemic and infarcted myocardial tissue was measured along with morbidity and mortality. This allowed all changes associated with the induction of ischaemia and the subsequent development of infarction to be measured. The model was developed from one in which ligation was induced in anaesthetized rats (Au *et al.*, 1979a) in a development of a method first described by Selye *et al.* (1960).

METHODS

Surgical procedures for chronically preparing rats for ligation of the left anterior descending coronary artery (LAD) involved implanting occluder, venous and arterial lines and permanent ECG leads. Depending on the method for implanting an arterial cannula, surgery was in one or two stages. If an aortic cannula (Weeks, 1980) was used one operation (at which all surgery was done) was required, whereas, if a tail artery was cannulated, a second operation was performed the day before ligation (Au *et al.*, 1980).

Placement of Occluder

The rat was initially anaesthetized with halothane (4%) in a closed container and then intubated for positive pressure respiration; anaesthesia was maintained with 1% halothane in oxygen. Intubation was with a 14 gauge teflon catheter (Jelco) using an appropriately machined paediatric laryngoscope. Respiration was at a stroke volume of 10 ml/kg body weight and frequency of 60–80 per minute.

An incision (1.5–2.0 cm long) at the fourth intercostal space was made to allow medial retraction of the pectoralis muscle followed by lateral retraction of the rectus muscle. The pleura was punctured by blunt dissection to reveal the pericardium which was then carefully incised allowing retractors to be placed so as to form a pericardial sling. This approach revealed the left anterior descending coronary artery and its accompanying venous drainage.

The occluder consisted of a 5-0 polypropylene suture within a polythene guide (PE-10 or 20) which had a flared end. The suture was first passed through the tissue surrounding the LAD and accompanying veins with a 1/4 inch (0.6 cm) curved atraumatic needle and then passed through the flared end of the guide. Heat was applied to the suture to form a knot and hence a 1.0–1.5 cm loop around the LAD. The guide, containing the loose end of the suture, was then brought out of the thorax through a puncture wound and exteriorized in the neck region between the two scapula. The chest wound was closed under forced respiration to reduce the pneumothorax.

Venous (jugular) and arterial (aorta) cannulae were inserted according to the methods of Weeks (1980) in some animals. Alternatively, arterial cannulae were inserted in a tail artery the day before ligation (Au *et al.*, 1980). In a lightly halothane-anaesthetized animal a midline incision was made ventrally in the upper tail to allow the artery to be cannulated with a 22 gauge Jelco catheter. This was attached to a polythene cannula (20–25 cm long) whose end was exteriorized. Such cannulae remained patent for 2–3 days.

A variety of ECG leads were tried; the basic electrode consisted of stainless steel wire coated with insulating enamel (Enamel Type no. 304, wire size 63, Silver Harris Co., N.J.). The enamel was stripped for 1 cm at either end. To insert electrodes, the wire was threaded through a long (5–10 cm) 22 gauge needle until 3 mm protruded from the needle point and this protruding wire was bent back to form a hook. After penetrating the mid scapula skin the needle point was manipulated subdermally to the appropriate area and the electrode lodged in the surrounding tissue. A large number of such permanent electrodes can be inserted without apparent inconvenience to the rat. For the chest lead, an electrode was wound around that portion of rectus muscle overlying the left ventricle. The above electrode assembly was used for conventional limb or unipolar chest leads monitored on a Grass Polygraph at 0.5 mV/cm, 60 mm/sec paper speed with a low frequency time constant of 0.1 sec and high frequency 1/2 amp filter of 75 Hz (plus 60 Hz Grass line filter).

Production of Ligation

At least 6 days after its chest operation each rat was subjected to ligation. Two hours before ligation the rat was brought into the laboratory in its home cage and allowed free access to food and water. ECG and cannulae lines were connected, suspended by elastic bands, and the animal left for at least 30 min. During this control period it was periodically petted and stroked.

Ligation was produced (within 1–2 sec) by pulling on the suture while pushing on the guide. Traction was sufficient to result in tension between suture and guide and ensure full closure of the loop surrounding the LAD and its accompanying tissue. The ligature was completed by heat sealing suture to guide.

After continuous monitoring for 2–4 hr, cannulae were heat sealed and leads disconnected. Twenty-four hours after ligation, blood pressure and ECG were re-recorded, the rat killed by stunning and exsanguination, and its heart removed. The heart was perfused (Langendorff technique) with Krebs solutions (room temperature and 100 mmHg pressure) to clear all blood before giving a bolus (0.3 ml of 10 mg/ml in Krebs) of cardiac green to reveal perfused and unperfused (occluded zone) tissue. The unperfused tissue was dissected out and weighed before all tissue was sliced (2 mm) and incubated in one of two tetrazolium dyes (2,3,5,-Triphenyl Tetrazolium Chloride (T-413 Fischer) 10 mg/ml in 45 mM phosphate buffer pH 8.6 or Nitro blue tetrazolium (11350 Eastman) 0.5 mg/ml in 100 mM Sorensen's phosphate buffer (pH 7.4) for 30 min at 37°C. After incubation tissue was fixed in formaline (7 days) before the undyed (infarcted) tissue was dissected out (infarcted zone) and weighed.

Measured Responses

In addition to measurement of blood pressure ECG and heart rate, arrhythmias were detected from ECG and blood pressure traces. Morbidity (subjective scale), mortality, occluded and infarcted zones (% of ventricular weights) were also recorded.

ECG and Arrhythmia Measurement

All aspects of the ECG can be recorded but we noted:
(a) size of the QRS complex,
(b) "S–T segment"* elevation and
(c) the presence of "Q waves"**
For arrhythmias the number of premature ventricular contractions (PVC) were noted together with episodes of ventricular tachycardia/flutter (VT) (sharp fall in blood pressure with cyclic fluctuations on blood pressure and ECG traces) and fibrillation (VF) (precipitous blood pressure fall to less than 10 mmHg with typical ECG), their duration and reversibility. An

---

* "S–T segment" is the height of the complex above the isoelectric line (base of P to base of P) 10 msec after the peak of the R wave.
** "Q waves" are the first indication (greater than 0.025 mV) of a *sharp* negative deflection preceding the R wave.

attempt was made to reverse all episodes of ventricular tachycardia/flutter and fibrillation lasting longer than 10 sec. Reversion (95% successful) was achieved with rapid (2/sec) precordial taps. Episodes of VT or VF were recorded as being spontaneously reversible, non-spontaneously reversible or irreversible (death).

Arrhythmias were quantified as log PVC, incidence of VT/VF and number of episodes of VT/VF. In addition we have devised the normally distributed arrhythmia scoring scale, shown below:

Arrhythmia Scoring Scale

Score	Arrhythmia
0	0–50 PVC with no VT/VF.
1	50–500 PVC with no VT/VF.
2	More than 500 PVC or one episode of spontaneously reversible VT or VF irrespective of number of PVC.
3	More than one episode of spontaneously, or, one or more, episodes of non-spontaneously reversible VT or VF lasting less than 60 sec.
4	Spontaneously or non-spontaneously reversible episodes of VT or VF lasting 60–120 sec.
5	As in (4) but lasting longer than 120 sec.
6	Completely irreversible VT or VF.

Drugs, or other interventions can be administered in a variety of ways. Infusions can be continued for 8 or more hours when initiated before or after ligation while intravenous injections can be made before, after or during ligation. Animals can be treated for a number of days prior to ligation. Wherever possible experimental design is blind and random so as to remove observer bias.

We are using our preparation to test the effects of aspirin (a.s.a.) pretreatment and PGI_2, infusions (Harvie *et al.*, 1980) on the responses to ligation. The following data were obtained during the development of this method from our previous anaesthetized rat method (Au *et al.*, 1979a). The data are a base from which experiments can be initiated into the pathophysiology of the ischaemia-infarction sequence and the effects of drugs upon that sequence.

RESULTS

A typical response to ligation of the LAD in a conscious Wistar rat is shown in Fig. 1. A continuous record of this animal's blood pressure, ECG and heart rate was obtained before ligation and for 4 hr post-ligation. The

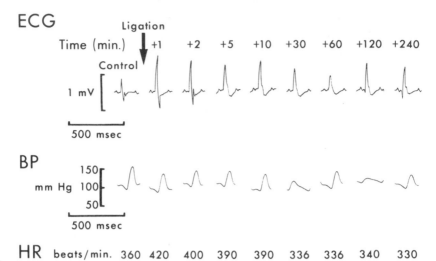

Fig. 1. Responses to ligation of the LAD coronary artery in the conscious rat. The rat was prepared as outlined in Methods and kept unrestricted in its home cage. Blood pressure was recorded by a Grass polygraph and the ECG from a unipolar chest lead. After control readings, the LAD coronary artery was rapidly ligated at time zero and the record subsequently sampled from the continuous record at the times indicated (in minutes). The sampling times, on an approximately logarithmic scale, are appropriate to the temporal pattern of changes induced by ligation. Note changes in the ECG signal size and the "S–T segment" changes with time post-ligation.

ligation was found, 24 hr later, to have produced a 32.4% occluded zone and 26.4% infarcted zone. The blood pressure of the animal was 155/95 mmHg prior to ligation and the heart rate was 360 beats/min. These values were stable prior to completing the ligation at zero time. Completion of the ligation produced a slight fall in blood pressure and increase in heart rate. The rat showed no subjective changes in behaviour with ligation and did not appear in pain. Throughout the 4-hr observation period no further major changes occurred in blood pressure and heart rate. Similar values were recorded 24 hr later.

The ECG changes after ligation are shown in greater detail in Fig. 2. In this figure the increase in ECG signal size that occurred very rapidly after ligation can be readily seen (Fig. 2A). Such rapid increases later fell toward control levels. The next change in the ECG was elevation of the "S–T segment" (Fig. 1, Fig. 2B) which developed over many minutes and persisted for hours. The last in the sequence of changes was the appearance of "Q waves" which appeared at least an hour after ligation (Fig. 2B). Figure 2C shows such typical arrhythmias as bigeminy, ventricular tachycardia/flutter and fibrillation. These patterns were typical of those seen in all rats.

Table 1 compares the blood pressure, heart rate, ECG, occluded and infarcted zone responses to ligation in two groups of rats. Both groups

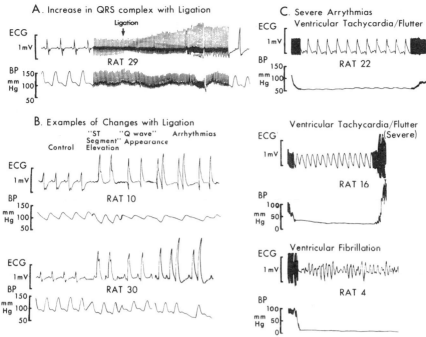

Fig. 2. Representative examples of ECG changes produced by ligation of the LAD coronary artery in a number of conscious rats. Each set of records in panels A, B and C were obtained in different rats. In each record the ECG (unipolar chest lead) is shown above the corresponding blood pressure. In A the effect of ligation, at the point indicated by the arrow, on ECG signal size and blood pressure is shown at slow and fast paper speeds. The records in B show typical examples of "S–T segment" elevation and "Q-wave" appearance in two different rats together with some simple arrhythmias (bigeminy). Examples of VT/VF are shown in C. In the cases of VT the upper record has a predominant pattern of tachycardia whereas in the lower record the pattern is of flutter.

were Wistar strain rats. Those in Group A were prepared and ligated by a different operator than those in Group B. Examination of the values obtained for all the responses measured showed no major differences between the two groups with regard to arrhythmias, although blood pressure was slightly higher, and heart rates slightly lower in Group B while mortality was not different in the two groups. Although occluded zones were the same in the two groups infarcted zones differed with the dye used. "S–T segment" elevation was greater in Group A while "Q-waves" appeared more rapidly. When the appearance of arrhythmias with time was plotted their time dependence (post-ligation) was easily seen (Fig. 3). Arrhythmia appearance, whether as PVC or VT/VF, was very time-dependent with at least two distinct phases: the first was within 5–15 min of ligation in which up to 50% of animals had VT/VF while the second

TABLE 1. RESPONSES TO LIGATION OF A CORONARY ARTERY IN TWO GROUPS OF CONSCIOUS CONTROL RATS

	Group A (n = 10)	Group B (n = 7)
Weight (grams ± s.e.m.)	339 ± 20	443 ± 12
	Mean B.P./H.R.	Mean B.P./H.R.
Control	104 ± 3/401 ± 15	112 ± 4/364 ± 15
+ 05 min post-ligation	97 ± 3/400 ± 40	106 ± 2/381 ± 10
+ 15 min post-ligation	91 ± 4/369 ± 36	102 ± 2/351 ± 10
+ 60 min post-ligation	91 ± 3/409 ± 18	104 ± 3/365 ± 9
+ 240 min post-ligation	94 ± 8/404 ± 41	99 ± 5/377 ± 20
ECG		
"S–T segment" elevation		
+ 60 min post-ligation (mV ± s.e.m.)	1.5 ± 0.6	0.4 ± 0.2
"Q-wave" appearance		
(min post-ligation ± s.e.m.)	55 ± 19	121 ± 21
Arrhythmias		
Arrhythmia Score ± s.e.m.	3.76 ± 0.63	4.28 ± 0.47
Mean log PVC ± s.e.m.	2.51 ± 0.26	2.81 ± 0.15
% Incidence VT/VF	90	100
Mortality (%)	30	14
Occluded Zone*	29.7 ± 2.3	26.2 ± 1.5
Infarcted Zone*	18.8 ± 3.3	28.8 ± 2.0

Table 1 compares all the responses to ligation in two groups of control Wistar rats. Rats in Group A were prepared and ligated by a different operator than those in Group B. For complete explanation of measured responses see Methods.
  * (as percentage of ventricular weight ± s.e.m.).

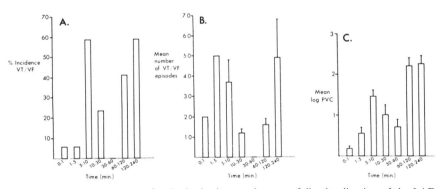

Fig. 3. Temporal appearance of arrhythmias in conscious rats following ligation of the LAD coronary artery. In Fig. 3A the incidence of VT/VF in control rats (groups A and B combined) is shown for the time intervals noted. The time intervals are chosen as they best reflect the times at which the events occurred. Incidence is the percentage of animals showing at least one episode of VT/VF in the time period shown. In B is shown the mean number of VT/VF episodes (± standard error of the mean), in those rats having such episodes, for the different time periods. Figure 3C shows the incidence of PVC (including bigeminy and trigeminy) in the different time periods. The total number of PVC for each rat in the appropriate time period was converted to $\log_{10}$ before the mean was taken. Log PVC show a more normal distribution than PVC.

appeared 2–4 hr postligation. The second phase was generally more severe and it was in this time period that irreversible fibrillation was most often encountered.

CONCLUSIONS

The method we have described is an extension and improvement of a technique due to Selye *et al.* (1960). Other workers (Kane *et al.*, 1980) have also improved on this basic procedure. The production of ischaemia followed by the development of infarction in the conscious rat produces fairly consistent responses in a number of different measurements. Blood pressure and heart rate responses to loss of 20–30% of the left ventricle were surprisingly small. Much greater responses are seen in anaesthetized rats which were acutely prepared (Au *et al.*, 1979a and b). In such animals the severity of cardiovascular responses to ligation depended on the anaesthetic agent used (Harvie *et al.*, 1979).

Arrhythmic responses to ligation in the conscious rat were very marked and all rats showed arrhythmias. Most control rats had at least one episode of ventricular tachycardia/flutter or fibrillation. The types of arrhythmias seen (PVC, ventricular tachycardia, flutter and fibrillation) and their temporal patterns of appearance give very good measures against which to test anti-arrhythmic and, more particularly, anti-fibrillatory drugs. Furthermore, the model exhibits early and late arrhythmias which may have different aetiologies (Wit and Bigger, 1977). The relative effectiveness of various anti-arrhythmics against these two patterns of arrhythmias may give insights into both the mechanisms of arrhythmias and those of the anti-arrhythmics.

Blood pressure and heart rate are also readily followed in time in this preparation and this fact, together with the low variability between animals, allows small drug, or other agent, induced changes to be accurately detected and measured.

In addition to the accurate and consistent measure of blood pressure, heart rate and arrhythmias the preparation also reveals ECG changes with ligation. The electrode assembly we used allows for the continuous monitoring of a high quality ECG. Our main findings of QRS complex increases, "S–T segment" changes and "Q-wave" appearance are consistently seen. Furthermore, the ECG signals were obtained in unrestrained animals and were uncomplicated by recent surgery or anaesthesia. Potentially a large number of ECG derivatives are obtainable from the ECG assembly we use providing adequate electronic and recording apparatus is used.

The initiating event of all of the above changes is, of course, the rapid interruption of blood supply by ligation giving an ischaemia which ultimately results in death of cardiac tissue. We attempt to measure both the amount of ischaemic and dead tissue. Estimates of the occluded zone appeared relatively consistent but the estimate of the infarcted zone, although accurate within a group, depended upon the type of tetrazolium used.

In conclusion, we have developed a method in which ligation is produced in conscious rats and in which the important responses to ligation are continuously monitored. In such a preparation it is possible to readily assess effects of drugs and procedures on ligation responses.

ACKNOWLEDGEMENTS

This research was funded by the British Columbia Heart Foundation.

REFERENCES

Au, T. L. S., Collins, G. A., Harvie, C. J. and Walker, M. J. A. (1979a) The actions of prostaglandins I_2 and E_2 on arrhythmias produced by coronary occlusion in the rat and dog. *Prostaglandins* **18** (5), 707–720.

Au, T. L. S., Collins, G. A., MacLeod, B. A. and Walker, M. J. A. (1979b) Actions of nitroglycerin (N) and propranolol (P) in rats. Abstract No. 680, *The Pharmacologist* **21** (3), 274. ,

Au, T. L. S., Collins, G. A., Harvie, C. J. and Walker, M. J. A. (1980) Actions of prostaglandin I_2 and E_2 on coronary occlusion-induced arrhythmias in the rat. In: *Advances in Prostaglandin and Thromboxane Research, Vol. 7*, (B. Samuelsson, P. W. Ramwell and R. Paoletti, eds). Raven Press, N.Y., pp. 647–649.

Crawford, T. (1977) *Pathology of Ischaemic Heart Disease*. Butterworths, London.

Fozzard, H. A. (1975) Validity of myocardial infarction models. *Circulation* **51, Suppl. III,** 131–138.

Harvie, C. J., Johnston, K. M., MacLeod, B. A. and Walker, M. J. A. (1980) The effect of prostaglandin infusions on arrhythmic and other responses to coronary artery ligation. *3rd. International Conference on Prostaglandins in the Cardiovascular System*. Halle, E. Germany, May 15–17, 1980.

Kane, K. A., Lepran, I., MacDonald, F. M., Parratt, J. R. and Szekeres, L. (1980) The effects of prolonged oral administration of a new antiarrhythmic drug (Org. 6001) on coronary artery ligation dysrhythmias in conscious and anaesthetized rats. *J. Cardiovasc. Pharmacol.* **2,** 411–423.

Maseri, A., L'Abbate, A., Baroldi, G., Chierchia, S., Marzilli, M., Ballestra, A., Severi, S., Parodi. O., Biagini, A., Distante, A. and Pesola, A. (1978) Coronary vasospasm as a possible cause of myocardial infarction *N.E.J.M.* **299** (23), 1271–1277.

Schaper, W. (1971) Comparative angiography of the collateral circulation. In: *The Collateral Circulation of the Heart*. (D. A. K. Black, ed.), North Holland, Amsterdam.

Selye, H., Bajusz, E., Grassos, S. and Mendell, P. (1960) Simple techniques for the surgical occlusion of coronary vessels in the rat. *Angiology* **11,** 398–407.

Weeks, J. R. (1980) Personal communication, letter of July 1980. Surgical Procedure—Aortic Cannulation in Rats. A full set of instructions are available on request to Dr. Weeks, Pharmacology Research, The Upjohn Company, Kalamazoo, Michigan 49001.

Wit, A. L. and Bigger, J. T. (1977) Treatment of arrythmias in the acute phase of myocardial infarction. *Postgrad. Med. J.* 53, 98–112.

A Rapid in vivo Technique for the Screening of Potential Anti-dysrhythmic Agents

P. G. DOLAMORE AND P. R. SAWYER

Aconitine exerts a dysrhythmogenic effect in cardiac tissues in a variety of species. The ability of anti-dysrhythmic drugs to influence aconitine-induced dysrhythmias has been utilized in a variety of screening tests (Vargaftig and Coignet, 1969, Dadkar and Bhattacharya, 1974; Nwangwu et al., 1977).

Using the artificially-respired anaesthetized rat we have developed a simple rapid technique for the intravenous or oral evaluation of potential anti-dysrhythmic agents depending on their ability to delay the occurrence of ventricular dysrhythmias induced by an infusion of aconitine. The test has been characterized using drugs of the four types described in the classification of Vaughan Williams (1970).

Rats weighing 250–300 g are anaesthetized with sodium pentobarbitone (50 mg kg^{-1}) via the tail vein. The trachea is cannulated to allow artificial respiration and the external jugular vein is cannulated for drug administration. Lead II electrocardiogram and heart rate are recorded on a Devices MX2 chart recorder and the ECG is also displayed on an oscilloscope. Drugs for intravenous evaluation are administered (1 ml kg^{-1} body weight) by slow infusion over 1 min into the jugular vein. Control rats receive 0.9% saline solution and each group consists of a minimum of 8 rats. Three minutes later aconitine (25 μg ml^{-1}) is infused slowly (0.2 ml min^{-1}) via the jugular vein using a peristaltic pump. Drugs for oral evaluation are administered (5 ml kg^{-1}) 1 hour before aconitine infusion. The end points recorded are:

(a) the time to onset of an uneven rhythm (Fig. 1) and

(b) the time to the appearance of ventricular tachycardia (Fig. 2) of at least 5 s duration.

These two times and the body weight for each rat are used to compute the dose of aconitine (μg kg^{-1}) required to produce each end point. Mean and median aconitine doses are calculated for each group and treated

253

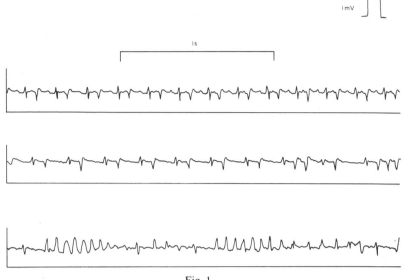

Fig. 1

groups are compared with controls using Wilcoxon's unpaired ranking test (Wilcoxon, 1945) and percentage changes.

Class I, II or III drugs used clinically in the management of ventricular dysrhythmias caused significant increases in the amount of aconitine

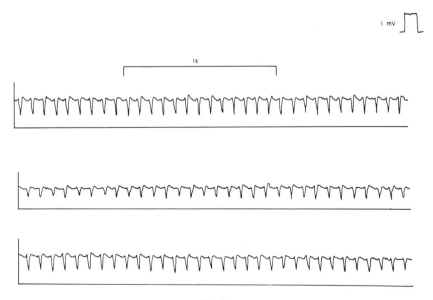

Fig. 2

TABLE 1

	Dose mg kg^{-1} i.v.	% increase in amount of aconitine required to elicit VT
Class I		
lignocaine	20	107*
disopyramide	5	94*
Class II		
atenolol	2.5	25*
Class III		
amiodarone	5	42*
Class IV		
verapamil	2.5	0

* $P' \leqslant 0.05$, Wilcoxon ranking test.

required to elicit VT. The calcium antagonist, verapamil, which is used in the treatment of atrial dysrhythmias had no effect. The test can also be adopted for the determination of relative potency estimates and duration of drug action after both intravenous and oral administration.

REFERENCES

Dadkar, N. K. and Bhattacharya, B. K. (1974) *Arch. Int. Pharmacodyn.* **212,** 297.
Nwangu, P. U., Holcslaw, T. L. and Stohs, S. J. (1977) *Arch Int. Pharmacodyn.* **229,** 219.
Vargaftig, B. and Coignet, J. L. (1969) *Eur. J. Pharmacol.* **6,** 49.
Vaughan Williams (1970) *Symposium on Cardiac Arrhythmias,* pp. 449 (Sandoe *et al.,* ed) A.B. Astra Sodertalje.
Wilcoxon, F. (1945) *Biometrics Bull.* **1,** 80.

Retardation of Aconitine-induced ECG-alterations in Rats as an Indication of Membrane-stabilizing Drug Effects

G. SCHOLTYSIK

ABSTRACT

Continuous intravenous infusion of aconitine in rats induces ECG changes which are characterized by ventricular extrasystoles, followed by ventricular tachycardia and cardiac arrest. These classical signs of aconitine intoxication are retarded dose-dependently by antiarrhythmics. The present experiments were designed to investigate whether the aconitine-antagonistic effects of antiarrhythmics correlate with their membrane-stabilizing effects.

In anaesthetized rats the protective effect of anti-arrhythmics against aconitine-induced ventricular extrasystoles was quantified by the determination of ED_{50}-values. In another set of experiments the membrane stabilizing drug effects were determined by measuring their prolonging effects on the functional refractory period in rat left atria. The rank order of potency was the same in both tests, namely: prajmalium > lorcainide > disopyramide > quinidine > mexiletine.

The close correlation between the aconitine-antagonistic activity *in vivo* and the prolongation of the functional refractory period in atria *in vitro* suggests that direct membrane-stabilizing effects of antiarrhythmics are responsible for their protective action against aconitine arrhythmia in rats.

INTRODUCTION

Intravenous treatment of rats with aconitine leads to typical ECG-alterations (Fekete and Borsy, 1964) which are characterized by ventricular extrasystoles, followed by ventricular tachycardia and cardiac arrest. These rhythm disturbances are prevented or reversed by antiarrhythmic agents. Therefore, the intravenous aconitine test on rats has been used for testing antiarrhythmic drugs (Szekeres, 1964; Szekeres and Papp, 1971).

The present experiments were performed to investigate the question, whether aconitine acts directly on the heart and whether the prevention of the cardiotoxic effects of aconitine by antiarrhythmic agents correlates with their membrane-stabilizing action.

Aconitine test on rats

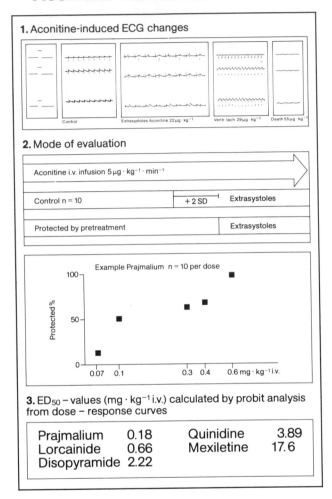

Fig. 1

METHODS

Aconitine test (Fig. 1)

Female rats of the strain OFA and body weight of 210–250 g were anaes-thetized with urethane, 1.5 g/kg i.p. The trachea and the jugular vein were cannulated. Needle electrodes were inserted subcutaneously on the limbs and the ECG was recorded on a three-channel Mingograph and displayed on an oscilloscope. Aconitine was infused intravenously at a rate of $5 \mu g/$ kg/min (0.1 ml/min) which induced arrhythmia in all animals. The arrhythmia induced by aconitine was observed in the ECG recordings. The dose of aconitine which produced extrasystoles, ventricular tachycardia and cardiac arrest persisting for at least 5 sec was determined.

Groups of 10 animals were pretreated with increasing doses of the test compound 5 min before the aconitine infusion was started. The control animals received physiological saline. For each animal, the aconitine dose for onset of arrhythmia was recorded as the endpoint. The endpoint doses in animals pretreated with antiarrhythmics were compared with the mean $+2\,SD$ of the control group. For each dose, an endpoint value greater than mean $+2\,SD$ of the corresponding control value was taken as a positive response (animal protected). The percent response was plotted against the log dose to construct a dose–response curve for antiarrhythmics. The percent response was also converted to a probit of response, and a dose–probit curve was constructed from which an ED_{50} value was calculated (Finney, 1971). The ED_{50} value is defined as the dose which protects 50% of the rats against aconitine arrhythmia. A similar test protocol has been described by Nwangwu *et al.* (1977) using mice.

Ten rats were pithed through one orbit under urethane anaesthesia (Scholtysik and Unda, 1971) and then treated with aconitine as described for the anaesthetized rats.

Functional Refractory Period (FRP) (Fig. 2)

The FRP of isolated rat left atria was determined by the paired stimulus method (Reuter *et al.*, 1971) as illustrated in Fig. 2. Female OFA rats weighing between 210 and 250 g were anaesthetized by exposure to CO_2, the hearts were rapidly excised and the atria separated. The left atria were attached to platinum iridium electrodes and suspended in an organ bath containing 100 ml oxygenated Krebs–Henseleit solution of the following composition: NaCl 6.95 g; $CaCl_2$ 0.37 g; KCl 0.36 g; $MgSO_4$ 0.29 g; $NaHCO_3$ 2.1 g; glucose 1.8 g; aqua dest. ad 1000 ml. All experiments were carried out at 31°C. The atria were connected to a Statham force transducer UC3 and contractions recorded on a Schwarzer polygraph. The organs were driven with a basic frequency of 60 beats per minute by suprathreshold square wave pulses of 3 msec duration delivered by an HSE stimulator. The FRP was measured by delivering a second stimulus (test stimulus), identical to the first, at increasing intervals following every third driving stimulus until a positive inotropic response was seen. Under these conditions the FRP is defined as the shortest interval between drive and test stimulus, at which a post extrasystolic potentiation of contractile force

Membrane stabilizing effects of antiarrhythmics in vitro

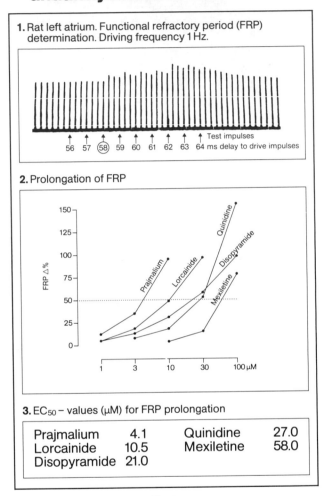

1. Rat left atrium. Functional refractory period (FRP) determination. Driving frequency 1 Hz.

56 57 (58) 59 60 61 62 63 64 ms delay to drive impulses

Test impulses

2. Prolongation of FRP

FRP $\triangle$ %

Prajmalium
Lorcainide
Quinidine
Disopyramide
Mexiletine

1   3   10   30   100 µM

3. EC$_{50}$ – values (µM) for FRP prolongation

Prajmalium	4.1	Quinidine	27.0
Lorcainide	10.5	Mexiletine	58.0
Disopyramide	21.0		

Fig. 2

appears. Following washout with fresh Krebs–Henseleit solution, measurements were made every 15 min during a 1 hour equilibration period. The drug solution was added cumulatively to the tissue bath every 15 min in geometrically increasing concentrations, and the FRP was determined 10 min later. The concentration inducing 50% prolongation of the FRP (EC$_{50}$) was determined graphically from the concentration–response curve.

TABLE 1. ARRHYTHMOGENIC DOSES OF ACONITINE IN ANAES-
THETIZED AND PITHED RATS. MEAN VALUES ± SEM FROM 10
EXPERIMENTS PER GROUP

	Aconitine μg/100 g i.v.	
	Extrasystoles	Ventricular tachycardia
Anaesthetized rats basic heart rate 347 ± 25 b.p.m.	2.56 ± 0.09	3.07 ± 0.06
Pithed rats basic heart rate 276 ± 12 b.p.m. (p < 0.001)	1.93 ± 0.08 (p < 0.001)	2.27 ± 0.14 (p < 0.001)

RESULTS

In a total of 50 control rats the doses of aconitine to induce extrasystoles, ventricular tachycardia and cardiac arrest were, respectively, 2.20 ± 0.04, 2.92 ± 0.06 and 6.68 ± 0.16 μg/100 g body weight (mean ± SEM).

In 10 pithed rats in which the heart rate was lowered by 20.4% in response to pithing, there was a statistically significant reduction in the doses of aconitine required to produce cardiac arrhythmias, compared with the control group (Table 1).

All results from experiments involving antiarrhythmic drug treatment are summarized in Fig. 1. Only the protective effects of antiarrhythmics against aconitine-induced extrasystoles have been evaluated for data presentation. The results for prajmalium are given as an example. Lorcainide, quinidine, disopyramide and mexiletine were tested under the same conditions. Their aconitine antagonistic potencies expressed as ED_{50} values, are given in Fig. 1.

In isolated rat left atria, the membrane-stabilizing activities of prajmalium, lorcainide, disopyramide, quinidine and mexiletine were determined by measuring their influence on the FRP. The results from these experiments are presented in Fig. 2. The rank order of potency judged on the basis of EC_{50} values for FRP prolongation is the same as in the rat aconitine test.

When the ED_{50} values from the *in vivo* test were plotted against the EC_{50} values from the *in vitro* test in a double-logarithmic scale a close correlation between these activities was found (Fig. 3).

Aconitine, added to the organ bath, caused irregular spontaneous contractions in the left driven atria from concentrations of 3×10^{-8} M. In the presence of 3×10^{-7} M, all organs were inexcitable by electrical stimulation (Table 2). Contractile force and FRP were hardly influenced by aconitine in concentrations up to 10^{-7} M.

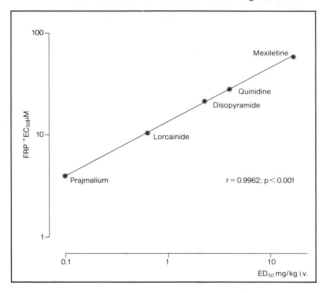

Fig. 3

DISCUSSION

Aconitine is a powerful membrane-depolarizer. Its effect has been ascribed to activation of the action potential Na^+ ionophore (Catterall, 1975). In rats aconitine induced typical and severe disturbances of cardiac rhythm when administered intravenously. Our results from anaesthetized rats are in good agreement with other findings relating to ECG signs of intoxication and aconitine doses (Eichbaum, 1973; Malinov *et al.*, 1955;

TABLE 2. EFFECTS OF ACONITINE ON DRIVEN RAT LEFT ATRIA *in vitro*

Aconitine concentration in the organ bath	FRP %	Contractile force in response to stimulation %	Incidence of arrhythmia
Control	100	100	0/6
1×10^{-8} M	107 ± 2	103 ± 6	0/6
3×10^{-8} M	103 ± 5	95 ± 5	2/6
1×10^{-7} M	107 ± 10	111 ± 6	3/6
3×10^{-7} M	—	—	6/6

Fekete and Borsy, 1964; Tripod, 1951; Scherf, 1947, 1948). From dog experiments, a central site of action of aconitine has been suggested (Bhargava *et al.*, 1969; Bhargava and Srivastava, 1972). However, the present results in pithed rats are not in accord with that suggestion. We have found that lower doses of aconitine are required to induce arrhythmia when the central nervous system has been destroyed by pithing. The present results show that the cardiotoxic effects of aconitine in rats are due to a direct peripheral action on the heart rather than to central actions. This view is supported by the spontaneous arrhythmic contractions of isolated guinea-pig left atria caused by aconitine in concentrations from 10^{-7} M.

The antiarrhythmics prajmalium, lorcainide, disopyramide, quinidine and mexiletine retarded the aconitine-induced arrhythmia in anaesthetized rats dose-dependently, continuing previous findings (Caillard and Louis, 1980). Our method is designed to quantify the aconitine-antagonistic action by the calculation of ED_{50} values for the correlation with the quantitative membrane-stabilizing effects *in vitro*.

The five antiarrhythmic agents investigated are membrane stabilizers and belong to the class I antiarrhythmics (Singh and Hauswirth, 1974). Their influence of FRP was investigated in rat left atria *in vitro*, prolongation of FRP having been shown to reflect membrane-stabilizing drug actions (Reuter *et al.*, 1971). From these experiments, the concentration which causes a 50% prolongation of the FRP (EC_{50}) was determined. The rank order of potency of the five antiarrhythmics was the same in the FRP test and in the aconitine test.

It is concluded from these results that the close correlation (Fig. 3) between the aconitine-antagonistic activity *in vivo* and the prolongation of the functional refractory period in atria *in vitro* suggests that direct membrane-stabilizing effects of antiarrhythmics are responsible for their protective action against aconitine arrhythmia in rats.

REFERENCES

Bhargava, K. P., Kohli, R. P., Sinha, J. N. and Tayal, G. (1969) Role of catecholamines in centrogenic cardiac arrhythmia by aconitine. *Br. J. Pharmacol.* **36**, 240–252.

Bhargava, K. P. and Srivastava, R. K. (1972) Analysis of the central receptors concerned in the cardiovascular response induced by intracerebroventricular aconitine. *Neuropharmacology* **11**, 123–135.

Caillard, C. G. and Louis, J. C. (1980) Assessment of antiarrhythmic drugs in experimental pharmacology. *Meth. and Find. Exptl. Clin. Pharmacol.* **2**(5), 223–252.

Catterall, W. A. (1975) Cooperative activation of action potential Na$^+$ ionophore by neurotoxins. *Proc. Nat. Acad. Sci. USA* **72**, No. 5, 1782–1786.

Eichbaum, F. W. (1973) Screening of heart-arrhythmic and antiarrhythmic drugs in the male albino rat. *Basic Res. Cardiol.* **68**, 73–79.

Fekete, M. and Borsy, J. (1964) On the antiarrhythmic effect of some thymoleptics: amitriptyline, imipramine, trimepropimine and desmethylimipramine. *Med. Exp.* **10**, 93–102.

Finney, D. J. (1971) *Probit Analysis*. 3rd edition, Cambridge University Press.

Malinow, M. R., Battle, F. F. and Malamud, B. (1955) The pharmacology of experimental ventricular arrhythmias in the rat. I. Antihistaminic drugs. *Arch. int. Pharmacodyn.* **102**, 55–64.

Nwangwu, P. U., Holcslaw, T. I. and Stohs, S. J. (1977) A rapid *in vivo* technique for preliminary screening of antiarrhythmic agents in mice. *Arch. int. Pharmacodyn.* **149**, 297–307.

Reuter, N., Heeg, E. and Haller, U. (1971) Beeinflussung der funktionellen Refraktärzeit und der Kontraktionskraft elektrisch gereizter Meerschweinchenvorhöfe durch Antiarrhythmica und Beta-Rezeptorenblocker. *Arch. Pharmacol.* **268**, 323–333.

Scherf, D. (1947) Studies on auricular tachycardia caused by aconitine administration. *Proc. Soc. Exp. Biol. Med.* **64**, 233–239.

Scherf, D. (1948) Effect of fagarine on auricular fibrillation. *Proc. Soc. Exp. Biol. Med.* **67**, 59–60.

Scholtysik, G. and Unda, R. (1971) A comparative study of the cardiovascular reactivity in various hypertensive and normotensive rats. *Arzneim.-Forsch. (Drug Res.)* **21**, 891–892.

Singh, B. N. and Hauswirth, O. (1974) Comparative mechanism of action of anti-arrhythmic drugs. *Am. Heart J.* **87**, 367–382.

Szekeres, L. (1964) Auswertung von flimmerwidrigen Substanzen. *Proceedings of the 2nd Hungarian Conference for Therapy and Pharmacological Research*. p. 165. Akadémiai Kiado, Budapest.

Szekeres, L. and Papp, J. Gy. (1971) *Experimental Cardiac Arrhythmias and Antiarrhythmic Drugs*. Akadémiai Kiado, Budapest.

Tripod, J. (1951) Fibrillation cardiaque et activité antifibrillante sur le coeur isolé de mammifère. *Arch. int. Pharmacodyn.* **85**, 121–128.

Bibliography of Papers on the Rat ECG

Abbott, C. P., Creech, O., Jr. and DeWitt, C. W. (1964) Histologic and electrocardiographic changes of the transplanted rat heart. *Surg. Forum.* **15**, 253–255.

Abbott, C. P., DeWitt, C. W. and Creech, O., Jr. (1965) The transplanted rat heart: Histologic and electrocardiographic changes. *Transplantation* **3**, 432–445.

Adolph, E. F. (1967) Ranges of heart rates and their regulations at various ages (rat). *Am. J. Physiol.* **212**, 595–602.

Agduhr, E. and Stenström, N. (1930) The appearance of the electrocardiogram in the heart lesions produced by cod liver oil treatment. *Acta Paediat.* (*Uppsala*) **9**, 280–306.

Allen, J. C. and Schwartz, A. (1969) A possible biochemical explanation for the insensitivity of the rat to cardiac glycosides. *J. Pharmacol. Exp. Ther.* **168**, 42–46.

Angelakos, E. T. and Bernardini, P. (1963) Frequency components and changes in electrocardiogram of the adult rat. *J. Appl. Physiol.* **18**, 261–263.

Arcasoy, M. M. and Smuckler, E. A. (1969) Acute effects of digoxin intoxication on rat hepatic and cardiac cells. *Lab. Invest.* **20**, 190–201.

Arrigo, L. and Dulio, C. (1964a) Sulla morfologia dell'elettrogramma intracellulare derivato dal curve di ratto *in situ. Boll. Soc. Ital. Biol. Sper.* **40** (11).

Arrigo, L. and Dulio, C. (1964b) Sull'elettrocardiogramme intracellulare in varie condizioni di vagotomia nel ratto. *Boll. Soc. Ital. Biol. Sper.* **40** (11).

Arrigo, L. and Dulio, C. (1964c) Modificazioni indotte dalla frequenza sulla morfologia dell'elettrogramme intracellulare del cuore di ratto *in situ. Boll. Soc. Ital. Biol. Sper.* (11).

Auclair, M. C., Mazzola, Ch. and Lechat, P. (1971) Potentialisation par l'asphyxie aigue des troubles electrocardiographiques provoqués par l'aconitine chez le rat. *Arch. int. Pharmacodyn.* **193**, 270–286.

Bachmann, E., Weber, E. and Zbinden, G. (1975) Effects of seven anthracycline antibiotics on electrocardiogram and mitochondrial function of rat hearts. *Agents and Actions* **4**, 383–393.

Bachmann, E., Zbinden, G. and Weber, E. (1975a) Anthracycline antibiotics: Correlations between cardiotoxicity, mitochondrial metabolism and drug levels in serum and heart of rats. In: *The Prediction of Chronic Toxicity from Short term Studies. Proc. Europ. Soc. Toxicol.* **17**, 309–314.

Badarau, G., Wasserman, L. and Dolinesco, S. (1969) Recherches sur les relations entre les modifications electrocardiographiques et les processus morphopathologiques au cours de l'évolution des myocardodystrophies expérimentales chez le rat. *Rev. Roum. Med. Int.* **2**, 121–130.

Balazs, T. (1973) Cardiotoxicity of sympathomimetic bronchodilator and vasodilating antihypertensive drugs in experimental animals. In: *Experimental Model Systems in Toxicology and their Significance in Man. Proc. Europ. Soc. Study Drug Toxicity* **15**, 71–79.

Barnard, R. J., Duncan, H. W. and Thorstensson, A. T. (1974) Heart rate responses of young and old rats to various levels of exercise. *J. Appl. Physiol.* **36** (4), 472–474.

Baur, H. R. and Pierach, C. A. (1979) Electrocardiographic changes after bilateral carotid sinus denervation in the rat. *Am. J. Physiol.* **237**, H475–H480.

Beinfield, W. H. and Lehr, D. (1956) Advantages of ventral position in recording electrocardiogram of the rat. *J. Appl. Physiol.* **9**, 153–156.

Beinfield, W. H. and Lehr, D. (1968a) QRS-T variations in the rat electrocardiogram. *Am. J. Physiol.* **214**, 197–204.

Beinfield, W. H. and Lehr, D. (1968b) P–R interval of the rat electrocardiogram. *Am. J. Physiol.* **213**, 205–211.

Berg, B. N. (1955) The electrocardiogram in aging rats. *J. Gerontol.* **10**, 420–423.

Bernard, G. and Gargouil, Y. M. (1970) Electrophysiologie.—Acquisitions successives, chez l'embryon de rat, des perméabilites specifiques de la membrane myocardique. *C.R. Acad. Sci.* **270**, 1495–1498.

Bianchetti, G., Bonaccorsi, A., Chiodaroli, A., Franco, R., Garattini, S., Gomeni, R. and Morselli, P. R. (1977) Plasma concentrations and cardiotoxic effects of desipramine and protriptyline in the rat. *Br. J. Pharmacol.* **60**, 11–19.

Bianchi, C., Sanna, G. P. and Turba, C. (1968) Anti-arrhythmic properties of 1,5-dimorpholino-3-(1-naphthyl)-pentane (DA 1686). *Arzneim. Forsch.* **18** (7), 845–850.

Blandon, R., Edgcomb, J. H., Guevara, J. F. and Johnson, C. M. (1974) Electrocardiographic changes in Panamanian *Rattus rattus* naturally infected by *Trypanosoma cruzi*. *Am. Heart J.* **88**, 758–764.

Buchanan, F. (1908) The frequency of the heart-beat in the mouse *J. Physiol.* **37**, lxxix–lxxx.

Buchanan, F. (1910) The frequency of the heart-beat in the sleeping and waking dormouse. *J. Physiol.* **40**, xlii–xliv.

Buchanan, F. (1911) Dissociation of auricles and ventricles in hibernating dormice. *J. Physiol.* **42**, xix–xx.

Budden, R. and Buschmann, G. (1979) Cardiovascular pharmacology: electrocardiographic studies. In: *Pharmacological Methods in Toxicology* (G. Zbinden and F. Gross, ed.) pp. 77–80. Oxford: Pergamon.

Caprino, L., Borrelli, F. and Falchetti, R. (1973) Effect of phosvitin on electrocardiographic changes produced by vasopressin in rats. *Experientia* **29**, 679–680.

Caprino, L., Borrelli, F., Falchetti, R., Biader, U. and Franchina, V. (1978) A new computerized system for automatic ECG analysis: an application to hypoxic rat ECGs. *Comput. Biomed. Res.* **11**, 195–207.

Cargill, C., Bachmann, E. and Zbinden, G. (1974) Effects of daunomycin and anthramycin on electrocardiogram and mitochondrial metabolism of the rat heart. *J. Natl. Cancer Inst.* **53**, 481–486.

Chalmers, D. V. and Levine, S. (1974) The development of heart rate responses to weak and strong shock in the preweaning rat. *Developm. Psychobiol.* **7** (6), 519–527.

Chau, T. T., Dewey, W. L. and Harris, L. S. (1973) Mechanism of the synergistic lethality between pentazocine and vasopressin in the rat. *J. Pharmacol. Exp. Ther.* **186**, 288–296.

Conrad, L. L. and Baxter, D. J. (1963) Effects of manganese on Q–T interval and distribution of calcium in rat heart. *Am. J. Physiol.* **205**, 1209–1212.

Conrad, L. L. and Baxter, D. J. (1966) Effect of calcium deficiency on Q–T interval and distribution of Ca^{45} in rat heart. *Am. J. Physiol.* **210**, 831–832.

Cooper, D. K. C. (1969) Electrocardiographic studies in the rat in physiological and pathological states. *Cardiovasc. Res.* **3**, 419–425.

Couch, J. R., West, T. C. and Hoff, H. E. (1969) Development of the action potential of the prenatal heart. *Circul. Res.* **24**, 19–31.

Crismon, J. M. (1944) Effect of hypothermia on the heart rate, the arterial pressure and the electrocardiogram of the rat. *Archiv. Intern. Med.* **74**, 235–243.

Cunningham, C. L., Fitzgerald, R. D. and Francisco, D. L. (1977) Excitatory and inhibitory consequences of explicitly unpaired and truly random conditioning procedures on heart rate in rats. *Animal Learning & Behavior* **5** (2), 135–142.

Davidson, W. J. (1977) Psychotropic drugs, stress, and cardiomyopathies. In: *Stress and the Heart* (D. Wheatley, ed.). pp. 63–85. Raven Press, New York.

Degwitz, R., Heushgem, C., Hollister, L. E., Jacob, J., Julou, L., Lambert, P. A., Marsboom, R., Meier-Ruge, W., Schaper, W. K. A. and Tuchmann-Duplessis, H. C. (1970) Toxicity and side effects in man and in the laboratory animal. In, Bobon, D. P., Janssen, P. A. J. and Bobon, J. (ed.): *Neuroleptics. Mod. Probl. Pharmacopsychiat.* **5**, 71–84.

Detweiler, D. K. (1967) Comparative pharmacology of cardiac glycosides. *Fed. Proc.* **26**, 1119–1124.

Detweiler, D. K. (1979) Spontaneous arrhythmias in normal miniature swine. Unpublished.

Detweiler, D. K. (1981) The use of electrocardiography in toxicological studies with Beagle dogs. In, Balazs, T. (ed.) *Cardiac Toxicology*. Boca Raton, Fla., CRC Press, Due.

Detweiler, D. K. and Patterson, D. F. (1965) The prevalence and types of cardiovascular disease in dogs. *Ann. N.Y. Acad. Sci.* **127**, 481–516.

Detweiler, D. K. and Spörri, H. (1957) Absence of "physiological" auricular fibrillation in the mole. *Cardiologia* **30**, 372–375.

Doherty, R. E. and Aviado, D. M. (1975) Toxicity of acrosol propellants in the respiratory and circulatory systems. VI. Influence of cardiac and pulmonary vascular lesions in the rat. *Toxicology* **3**, 213–224.

Dorato, M. A., Ward, C. O. and Sciarra, J. J. (1974) Evaluation of telemetry in determining toxicity of aerosol preparations. *J. Pharmaceutical Sci.* **63** (12), 1892–1896.

Driscoll, P. (1979) The electrocardiogram of Roman high- and low-avoidance rats under pentobarbital sodium anesthesia. *Arzneim.-Forsch.* **29**, 897–900.

Drury, A. N., Harris, J. J. and Maudsley, C. (1930) Vitamin B deficiency in the rat. Bradycardia as a distinctive feature. *Biochem. J.* **24**, 1632–1649.

Dunn, F. G., Pfeffer, M. A. and Frohlich, E. D. (1978) ECG alterations with progressive left ventricular hypertrophy in spontaneous hypertension. *Clin. exp. Hypertens.* **1**, 67–86.

Durakovic, Z., Stilinovic, L. and Bakran, I. (1976) Electrocardiographic changes in rats after inhalation of dichlorotetrafluorethane, arcton 114, $C_2 CL_2F_4$. *Jap. Heart J.* **17**, 753–759.

Eastwood, I., Forshaw, P. J., Jeyeratnam, J. and Magos, L. (1977) Cardiac sensitization induced by phenobartibone and prolonged by CS_2. *Arch. Toxicol.* **37**, 237–240.

Ensor, C. R. (1946) The electrocardiogram of rats on vitamin E deficiency. *Am. J. Physiol.* **147**, 477–480.

Everitt, A. V. (1958) The electrocardiogram of the ageing male rat. *Gerontol.* **2**, 204–212.

Fishburne, M. and Cunningham, B. (1938) Replacement therapy in thyroidectomized rats. *Endocrinol.* **22**, 122.

Fitzgerald, R. D. and Stainbrook, G. L. (1978) The influence of ethanol on learned and reflexive heart rate responses of rats during classical aversive conditioning. *J. Studies Alcohol*, **39**, No. 11, 1916–1930.

Franke, F. R. and Joshi, M. J. (1967) Digitoxin resistance of the rat as demonstrated by electrocardiograms *Expl Med. Surg.* **25**, 80–85.

Fraser, R. S., Harley, C. and Wiley, T. (1967) Electrocardiogram in normal rat. *J. Appl. Physiol.* **23**, 401–402.

Gargouil, Y. M. (1960) La sécrétion endocrinienne et l'activité cardiaque ventriculaire chez les mammiferes (activité électrique et mecanique). *J. Physiol.* **52**, 104–106.

Gargouil, Y. M., Trichoche, R. and Laplaud, J. (1960) Electrogramme intracellulaire électrocardiogramme et mecanogramme du coeur de rat hypophysectomise. *Compt. rend. Seances Acad. Sci.* **250**, 761–763.

Gargouil, Y. N., Tricoche, R. and Monnereau, H. (1961) Modification chez le rat, de l'electrocardiogramme et de l'electrogramme intracellulaire ventriculaire, par la surrenalectomie. *J. Physiol.* **53**, 346–347.

Gessler, U. and Kuner, E. (1959) Experimental contribution to the influence of ether and oxygen deficiency on the EKG of the white rat. *Z. Kreislaufforsch.* **48**, 870–877.

Godwin, K. O. (1965) Abnormal electrocardiograms in rats fed a low selenium diet. *Q. J. Exp. Physiol.* **50**, 282–288.

Godwin, K. O. and Fraser, F. J. (1965) Simultaneous recording of ECGs from disease-free rats using a cathode ray oscilloscope and a direct writing instrument. *J. Exp. Physiol.* **50**, 277–281.

Graf, E. and Leuschner, F. (1978) On the toxicity of dopamine. Toxicity acute and subacute and teratology (author's transl.) *Arzneim. Forsch.* **28**, 2208–2218.

Grauwiler, J. (1965) *Herz und Kreislauf der Säugetiere*. Birkhäuser Verlag, Basel und Stuttgart.

Grauwiler, J. and Spörri, H. Fehlen der ST-Strecke im Elektrokardiogramm von verschiedenen Säugetieren. *Helv. Physiol. Acta* **18**, C 77-C 78.

Grice, H. C., Heggtveit, H. A., Wiberg, G. S., Van Petten, G. and Willes, R. (1970) Experimental cobalt cardiomyopathy: correlation between electrocardiography and pathology. *Cardiovasc. Res.* **4**, 452–456.

Grünberg, H. and Hundt, H.-J. (1958) Ueber Typenwechsel im Elektrokardiogramm der Ratte bedingt durch die Körperhaltung. *Z. Kreislaufforsch.* **47,** 874–877.

Guideri, G., Barletta, M. A. and Lehr, D. (1974) Extraordinary potentiation of isoproterenol cardiotoxicity by corticoid pretreatment. *Cardiovasc. Res.* **8,** 775–786.

Guideri, G., Barletta, M., Chau, R., Green, M. and Lehr, D. (1975) Method for the production of severe ventricular dysrhythmias in small laboratory animals. In: *Recent Adv. Cardio. Structure and Metab.* (P. E. Roy and G. Rona, ed.). University Park Press, Baltimore, **10,** 661–679.

Hamlin, R. L. and Smith, C. R. (1965) Categorization of common domestic mammals based upon their ventricular activation process. *Ann. N.Y. Acad. Sci.* **127,** 195–203.

Hatton, D. C., Wilking, L. D., Francisco, D. L., Hoffman, J. W., Buchholz, R. A. and Fitzgerald, R. D. (1979) Heart rate responses of spontaneously hypertensive rats during aversive classical conditioning. *Behavioral and Neural Biol.* **27,** 107–114.

Hawley, P. L. and Kopp, S. J. (1975) Extension of PR interval in isolated rat heart by cadmium (39102). *Proc. Soc. Exp. Biol. Med.* **150,** 669–671.

Heering, H. (1970) Das Elektrokardiogramm der wachen und der narkotisierten Ratte. *Arch. int. Pharmacodyn.* **185,** 308–328.

Heering, H. (1970) Das EKG der Ratte bei Paraoxon-Intoxikation unter Einwirkung von Atropin und Pralidoxim (2-PAM). *Arch. int. Pharmacodyn.* **186,** 321–338.

Heerswynghels, J. V. and Thomas, J. (1945) Variations du glycogène et de l'acide pyruvique du coeur lors des modifications électrocardiographiques observées dans l'avitaminose B₁ chez le rat. Rôle de l'acide pyruvique. *Cardiology* **9,** 211–230.

Heethaar, R. M., Denier van der Gon, J. J. and Meijler, F. L. (1973a) A mathematical model of A–V conduction in the rat heart. *Cardiovasc. Res.* **7,** 106–115.

Heethaar, R. M., Burchart, R. M., Denier van der Gon, J. J. and Meijler, F. L. (1973b) A mathematical model of A–V conduction in the rat heart. II. Quantification of concealed conduction. *Cardiovasc. Res.* **7,** 542–556.

Heggtveit, H. A., Grice, H. C. and Wiberg, G. S. (1970) Cobalt cardiomyopathy. *Path. Microbiol.* **35,** 110–113.

Heise, E. and Kimbel, K. H. (1955) Das normale Elektrokardiogramm der Ratte. *Z. Kreislaufforsch.* **44,** 212–221.

Herman, E. H., Schein, P. and Farmar, R. M. (1969) Comparative cardiac toxicity of daunomycin in three rodent species. *Proc. Soc. Exp. Biol. Med.* **130,** 1098–1102.

Hill, J. D. (1968a) The electrocardiogram in dogs with standardized body and limb positions. *J. Electrocardiol.* **1,** 175–182.

Hill, J. D. (1968b) The significance of foreleg position in the interpretation of electrocardiograms and vectorcardiograms from research animals. *Am. Heart J.* **75,** 518–527.

Hill, R., Howard, A. N. and Gresham, G. A. (1960) The electrocardiographic appearances of myocardial infarction in the rat. *Br. J. Exp. Pathol.* **41,** 633–637.

Hillbom, M. E. and v. Boguslawsky, K. (1978) Effect of ethanol on cardiac function in rats genetically selected for their ethanol preference. *Pharmacol. Biochem. Behav.* **8,** 609–614.

Hoffman, B. F. and Cranefield, R. J. (1960) *Electrophysiology of the Heart.* McGraw–Hill, New York.

Hoffmann, J. W. and Fitzgerald, R. D. (1978) Classically conditioned heart rate and blood pressure in rats based on either electric shock or ammonia fumes reinforcement. *Physiology & Behavior.* **21,** 735–741.

Hoskins, R. G., Lee, M. O. and Durrant, E. P. (1927) The pulse rate of the normal rat. *Am. J. Physiol.* **82,** 621–629.

Hundley, J. M., Ashburn, L. L. and Sebrell, W. H. (1945) The electrocardiogram in chronic thiamine deficiency in rats. *Am. J. Physiol.* **144,** 404–414.

Hundt, H.-J. and Grünberg, H. (1960) Vergleichende Untersuchungen über das Ratten-EKG bei Sauerstoffmangelzuständen verschiedener Genese. *Z. Kreislaufforsch.* **49,** 769–780.

Hunsaker, W. G., Hulan, H. W., Kramer, J. K. G. and Corner, A. H. (1972) Electrocardiograms of male rats fed rapeseed oil. *Can. J. Physiol. Pharmacol.* **55,** 1116–1121.

Hunt, E. L. and Kimeldorf, D. J. (1960) Heart, respiration and temperature measurement in the rat during the sleep state. *J. Appl. Physiol.* **15,** 733–735.

Irmak, S. and Aykut, R. (1955) Vergleichende elektro-kardiographische Untersuchungen beim Menschen und bei den Laboratoriumstieren. *Münch. Med. Wschr.* **97**, 460–461.

Johansson, B. (1957) The electrocardiogram and phonocardiogram of the non-hibernating hedgehog. *Cardiology* **30**, 37–45.

Jones, D. C., Osborn, G. K. and Kimeldorf, D. J. (1967) Cardiac arrhythmia in the aging male rat. *Gerontologia* **13**, 211–218.

Juskowa, J. (1972) The effect of mercuric oxycyanide on the electrocardiographic curve in rat. *Acta Med. Pol.* **13**, 285–308.

Kayser, Ch. (1956) L'incrément thermique de la durée des différents accidents de l'électrocardiogramme chez le rat blanc, le hamster et le spermophile en hypithermie expérimentale. *Comp. rend. Seances Soc. Biol.* **7**, 1442–1445.

Kelly, J. J., Jr. and Hoffman, B. F. (1960) Mechanical activity of rat papillary muscle. *Am. J. Physiol.* **199**, 157–162.

Kenedi, I. (1968) The correct interpretation of the rat electrocardiogram. *Acta Physiol. Acad. Sci. Hung.* **34**, 29–35.

King, W. D. and Sebrell, W. H. (1946) Alterations in the cardiac conduction mechanism in experimental thiamine deficiency. *Pub. Hlth. Rep.* **61**, 410–414.

Kisch, B. (1953) The heart rate and the electrocardiogram of small animals. *Exptl. Med. Surg.* **11**, 117–130.

Klütsch, K., Wende, W., Braun, H. and Bohndorf, W. (1968) Das EKG der Ratte unter hochdosierter $_{60}$CO-Bestrahlung. *Arch. Kreislaufforsch.* **55**, 185–210.

Kopp, S. J. and Hawley, P. L. (1978) Cadmium feeding: Apparent depression of atrioventricular-His-Purkinje conduction system. *Acta Pharmacol. Toxicol.* **42**, 110–116.

Kowalczykowa, J., Gryglewski, R., Bigaj, M., Jaszcz, W., Kulig, A., Kostka-Trabka, E., Swies, J. and Ocetkiewicz, A. (1971) Dynamics of myocardial damage by isoprenaline in rats and an attempt to correlate the morphologic changes in the myocardium with electrocardiographic, biochemical and hematologic changes. *Acta Med. Pol.* **12**, 1–12.

Kruta, V. and Braveny, P. (1960) Potentiation of contractility in the heart muscle of the rat and some other mammals. *Nature* **187**, 327–328.

Lambert, G. A., Friedman, E., Buchweitz, E. and Gershon, S. (1978) Involvement of 5-hydroxytryptamine in the central control of respiration, blood pressure and heart rate in the anaesthetized rat. *Neuropharm.* **17**, 807–813.

Langer, G. A. (1978) Interspecies variation in myocardial physiology: the anomalous rat. *Environ. Hlth. Persp.* **26**, 175–179.

Langer, G. A., Brady, A. J., Tan, S. T. and Serena, S. D. (1975) Correlation of the glycoside response, the force staircase, and the action potential configuration in the neonatal rat heart. *Circul. Res.* **36**, 744–752.

Langslet, A. (1970) ECG-changes induced by phenothiazine drugs in the anaesthetized rat. *Acta Pharmacol. Toxicol.* **28**, 258–264.

Leblond, C. P. and Hoff, H. E. (1944) Comparison of cardiac and metabolic actions of thyroxine, thyroxine derivatives and dinitrophenol in thyroidectomized rats. *Am. J. Physiol.* **141**, 32–37.

Lepeschkin, E. (1951) *Modern Electrocardiography.* Williams and Wilkins, Baltimore.

Lepeschkin, E. (1965) The configuration of the T wave and the ventricular action potential in different species of mammals. *Ann N.Y. Acad. Sci.* **127**, 170–178.

Leszkovszky, G. P., Gal, G. and Tardos, L. (1967) Correlation between functional and morphological heart changes due to isoproterenol. *Experientia* **23** (2), 112–113.

Lisciani, R., Baldini, A., Benedetti, D., Campana, A. and Barcellona, P. S. (1978) Acute cardiovascular toxicity of trazodone, etoperidone and imipramine in rats. *Toxicology* **10**, 151–158.

Loiselle, D. S. and Gibbs, C. L. (1979) Species differences in cardiac energetics. *Am. J. Physiol., Heart Circ. Physiol.* **6** (1), H90–H98.

Lombard, E. A. (1952) Electrocardiograms of small mammals. *Am. J. Physiol.* **171**, 189–193.

Luisada, A. A., Sakai, A. and Feijen, L. (1970) Comparative electrocardiography and phonocardiography in six species of animals. *Am. J. Vet. Res.* **31**, 1695–1702.

Mainwood, G. W. and Lee, S. L. (1969) Rat heart papillary muscles: Action potentials and mechanical response to paired stimuli. *Science* **166**, 396–397.

Malinow, M. R. (1966) An electrocardiographic study of *Macaca mulatta. Folia Primat.* **4**, 51–65.

Manoach, M., Aygen, M. M., Netz, H. and Pauker, T. (1977) Q–T interval in young and old mammalian embryos. *Adv. Cardiol.* **19**, 52–54.

Marmo, E. (1969) Verhalten des EKG normaler, reserpinisierter oder emetinisierter Ratten, die mit verschiedenen Beta-Adrenolytika perfundiert wurden. *Arch. Kreislaufforsch.* **59**, 325–350.

Marmo, E. and Robertaccio, A. (1970) Analisi digli effetti sull'ECG del ratto di vari beta-adrenolitici. *Ann. Soc. Ital. Cardiol.* **30** (2), 221–222.

Marmo, E., De Giacomo, S. and Imperatore, A. (1969) Verhalten des Elektrokardiogramms normaler oder mit verschiedenen Pharmaka vorbehandelter und daraufhin mit Meto-chlopramid perfundierter Ratten. *Jpn. J. Pharmacol.* **19**, 551–562.

Mei, V., Fidanza, A. and Valora, N. (1964) Studio comparativo dell'elettrocardiogramma del neonato nel ratto, nel topino e nella cavia. *Boll. Soc. Ital. Sper.* **61**, 319–322.

Meinrath, M., Collins, P. and D'Amato, M. R. (1977) A nonobtrusive heart rate telemetry system for rats. *Behav. Res. Methods Instrument.* **9** (3), 253–246.

Meyer, A. E. and Yost, M. (1939) The stimulating action on metabolism and heart beat of various thyroid preparations, determined in the thyroidectomized rat. *Endocrinol.* **24**, 806–813.

Monnereau-Soustre, H. (1966) Electrocardiogramme du rat surrénalectomisé en hypothermie. *Compt. rend. Seances Soc. Biol.* **160**, 623–629.

Morvai, V., Hudak, A., Ungvary, Gy. and Varga, B. ECG changes in benzene, toluene and xylene poisoned rats. *Acta Med. Sci. Hung.* **33** (3).

Moses, L. E. (1946) Heart rate of the albino rat. *Proc. Soc. Exp. Biol. Med.* **63**, 58–62.

Mulvaney, D. A. and Seronde, J. (1979) Electrocardiographic changes in vitamin B_1 deficient rats. *Cardiovasc. Res.* **13**, 506–513.

Nadeau, R. and Champlain, J. (1973) Comparative effects of 6-hydroxy-dopamine and of reserpine on ouabain toxicity in the rat. *Life Sci.* **13**, 1753–1761.

Nemec, J. (1973) Cardiotoxic effects of tricyclic antipsychotics. Comparison of some newer derivatives from the 10,11-dihydrodibenzo/b,f/thiepin group with perphenazine and ami-triptyline. *J. Europ. Toxicol.* **4–5**, 224–231.

Noble, D. and Cohen, I. (1978) The interpretation of the T wave of the electrocardiogram. *Cardiovasc. Res.* **13**, 13–27.

Normann, S. J., Priest, R. E. and Benditt, E. P. (1961) Electrocardiogram in the normal rat and its alteration with experimental coronary occlusion. *Circul. Res.* **9**, 282–287.

Osborne, B. E. (1973) A restraining device facilitating electrocardiogram recording in rats. *Lab. Animals* **7**, 185–188.

Osborne, B. E. (1974) Uses and applications of electrocardiography in toxicology. In: *Experimental Model Systems in Toxicology and Their Significance in Man*, Vol. XV, pp. 85–97. Excerpta Medica, Amsterdam.

Petty, W. C. and Sulkowski, T. S. (1971) CO_2 narcosis in the rat: II. Effects on the ECG. *Aerospace Med.* **42** (5), 553–558.

v. Philipsborn, G. (1973) Zur Wirkung von N-Propyl-ajmalinium-hydrogentartrat (NPAB), Sparteinsulfat (Spartein) und NPAB + Spartein auf das Elektrokardiogramm und auf Akonitinarrhythmien von SIV-Ratten. *Arzneim. Forsch. Drug Res.* **23**, 1729–1733.

Rappaport, M. B. and Rappaport, I. (1943) Electrocardiographic considerations in small animal investigations. *Am. Heart J.* **26**, 662–680.

Repke, K., Est, M. and Portius, H. J. (1965) Ueber die Ursache der Speciesunterschiede in der Digitalisempfindlichkeit. *Biochem. Pharmacol.* **14**, 1785–1802.

Robb, J. S. (1965) *Comparative Basic Cardiology.* Grune and Stratton, New York.

Robertson, E. C. and Doyle, M. E. (1937) Difficulties in the use of bradycardia method of assaying vitamin B_1. *Proc. Soc. Exp. Biol.* **37**, 139–140.

Roshchevsky, M. P. (1978) *Elektrokardiologia Kopytnych Zivotnych.* Leningrad, Nauka.

Salako, L. A. and Durotoye, A. O. (1972) The electrocardiogram in acute dehydroemetine intoxication. *Cardiovasc. Res.* **6**, 150–154.

Sambhi, M. P. and White, F. N. (1960) The electrocardiogram of the normal and hypertensive rat. *Circul. Res.* **8**, 129–134.

Scheuer, J. and Stezoski, S. W. (1968a) Relationship of ATP to the electrocardiogram in the isolated rat heart. *J. Lab. Clin. Med.* **72**, 631–638.

Scheuer, J. and Stezoski, S. W. (1968b) Effects of high-energy phosphate depletion and repletion on the dynamics and electrocardiogram of isolated rat hearts. *Circul. Res.* **23**, 519–530.

Scheuer, J. and Stezoski, S. W. (1969) Discordance between the electrocardiogram and ATP levels in the isolated rat heart. *Amer. J. Med. Sci.* **257**, 218–227.

Schinzel, G. (1933) *Das Elektrokardiogramm der kleinen Laboratoriumstiere.* Inaug. Diss., München.

Siegfried, J. P. (1956) *Elektrokardiographische Untersuchungen an Zoo-Tieren.* Inaug. Diss., München.

Soato, G. G. and Krieger, E. M. (1974) Heart rate after acute hypertension in the rat. *Am. J. Physiol.* **227** (6), 1389–1393.

Spörri, H. (1944) Der Einfluss der Tuberkulose auf das Elektrokardiogramm. Untersuchungen an Meerschweinchen und Rindern. *Arch. Wiss. Prakt. Tierheilk.* **79**, 1–57.

Spörri, H. (1956) Starke Dissoziation zwischen dem Ende der elektrischen und mechanischen Systolendauer bei Känguruhs. *Cardiology* **28**, 278–284.

Staib, A. H. (1967) EKG-Veränderungen bei der Ratte nach chlorpromazin im Verlauf der postnatalen Entwicklung. *Arch. int. Pharmacodyn.* **166**, 11–19.

Stein, E. A. (1976) Morphine effects on the cardiovascular system of awake, freely behaving rats. *Arch. int. Pharmacodyn.* **223**, 54–63.

Stupfel, M. and Costagliola, D. (1979) Lifelong variations in heart rates in SPF Sprague–Dawley rats of both sexes. *Pflügers Arch.* **380**, 189–195.

Surawicz, B. (1966) Primary and secondary T wave changes. *Heart Bulletin* **15**, 31–35.

Surawicz, B. (1972) The Pathogenesis and Clinical Significance of Primary T-wave Abnormalities. In: *Advances in Electrocardiography* (R. C. Schlant and I. W. Hurst, eds.). New York, Grune and Stratton, pp. 377–421.

Tong, G. L., Cory, M., Lee, W. W., Henry, D. W. and Zbinden, G. (1978) Antitumor anthracycline antibiotics. Structure-activity and structure-cardiotoxicity relationships of rubidazone analogues. *J. Med. Chem.* **21**, 732–737.

Trautvetter, E., Detweiler, D. K. and Patterson, D. F. (1980) Evolution of the electrocardiogram in young dogs during the first 12 weeks of life. Submitted for publication. *J. Electrocardiol.*

Tricoche, R., Jallageas, M. and Gargouil, Y. M. (1963) Activité électrique comparée chez le rat noir (*Rattus rattus*) et chez le rat blanc (*Rattus norvegicus*). *Compt. rend. Seances Soc. Biol.* **157**, 1096–1099.

Tricoche, R., Monnereau, H., Galand, G. and Gargouil, Y. M. (1961) Electrocardiogramme, électrogramme intracellulaire et mécanogramme du rat surrénalectomisé. *Compt. rend. Seances Soc. Biol.* **155**, 1372–1375.

Valle, L. B. S., Oliveira-Filho, R. M., Arnomia, P. L., Nassif, M. and Saraceni, G. (1975) Sensitizing effect of lidocaine on bradycardia in the nadir of the final hypotension determined by serotonin in the rat. *Arch. Int. Physiol. Biochem.* **83**, 647–657.

Valora, N. and Mei, V. (1963) Studio delle modificazioni elettrocardiografiche indotte nel ratto dall'acetilcolina, dalla nor-adrenalina e da alcuni farmace ad azione elettiva sul cuore. *Quad. Nutrizione* **23**, 230, 291.

Van Petten, G. R., Evans, D. A. and Salem, F. A. (1970) A simple method for chronic measurement of the electrocardiogram and blood pressure in the conscious rat. *J. Pharm. Pharmacol.* **22**, 467–469.

Waller, R. K. and Charipper, H. A. (1945) Electrocardiographic observations in normal thyroidectomized and thiourea treated rats. *Am. J. Med. Sci.* **210**, 443–452.

Watanabe, T. and Aviado, D. M. (1975) Toxicity of aerosol propellants in the respiratory and circulatory systems. VII. Influence of pulmonary emphysema and anesthesia in the rat. *Toxicology* **3**, 225–240.

Werth, G. and Dadgar, P. (1965) Zum Elektrokardiogramm der Ratte mit und ohne Narkose, bei Beatmung mit Sauerstoffmangelgemischen, sowie bei Intoxikation mit Malachitgrün, unter gleichzeitiger Bestimmung des effektiven Sauerstoffverbrauches. *Arch. Kreislaufforsch.* **48**, 118–131.

Werth, G. and Wink, S. (1967) Das Elektrokardiogramm der normalen Ratte. *Arch. Kreis. Forschung* **54**, 272–308.

Wexler, B. C. and Greenberg, B. P. (1974) Effect of exercise on myocardial infarction in young vs. old male rats: electrocardiographic changes. *Am. Heart J.* **88**, 343–350.

Wexler, B. C., Willen, D. and Greenberg, B. P. (1973) Electrocardiographic differences between non-arteriosclerotic and arteriosclerotic rats. *Atherosclerosis* **18**, 129–140.

Wiester, M. J. (1975) Cardiovascular actions of palladium compounds in the unanesthetized rat. *Environ. Hlth Persp.* **12**, 41–44.

Wildt, S. and Nemec, J. (1976) Correlation of the duration of the PR and QT interval to the heart rate in small laboratory animals. *Physiol. bohemoslov.* **25**, 285.

Willard, P. W. and Horvath, S. M. (1959) Electrocardiographic studies on rats before and after cardiac arrest induced by hypothermia and asphyxia. *Am. J. Physiol.* **196**, 711–714.

Wright, G., Knecht, E. and Toraason, M. (1978) Cardiovascular effects of whole-body heating in spontaneously hypertensive rats. *J. Appl. Physiol.* **45** (4), 521–527.

Yamashita, S. (1971a) Effect of alcohol on thiamine deficient cardiac lesions. *Jap. Heart J.* **12** (4), 354–367.

Yamashito, S. (1971b) Effect of alcohol on normal rat's heart. *Jap. Heart J.* **12** (3), 242–250.

Yamori, Y., Ohtaka, M. and Nara, Y. (1976) Vectorcardiographic study on left ventricular hypertrophy in spontaneously hypertensive rats. *Jpn. Circ. J.* **40**, 1315–1329.

Zbinden, G. (1975) Inhibition of adriamycin cardiotoxicity by acetyldaunomycin. *Experientia* **31**, 1058–1060.

Zbinden, G. (1978) Méthodes pharmacologiques en toxicologie. *Actualités Pharmacologiques*, 30e Série, pp. 101–111. Masson et Cie., Paris.

Zbinden, G. Assessment of cardiotoxic effects in chronic rat toxicity studies. In: *Cardiac Toxicity* (T. Balazs, ed.). CRC Press Inc., Boxa Raton, FL, in press.

Zbinden, G. and Brändle, E. (1975) Toxicologic screening of daunorubicin (NSC-82151), adriamycin (NSC-123127), and their derivatives in rats. *Cancer Chemother. Rep.*, Part 1, **59**, 707–715.

Zbinden, G. and Rageth, B. (1978) Early changes of cardiac function in rats on a high-fat diet. *Fd. Cosmet. Toxicol.* **16**, 123–127.

Zbinden, G., Bachmann, E. and Bolliger, H. (1977) Study of coenzyme Q in toxicity of adriamycin. In: *Biomedical and Clinical Aspects of Coenzyme Q* (K. Folkers and Y. Yamamura, eds.) pp. 219–228. Elsevier/North-Holland Biomedical Press.

Zbinden, G., Bachmann, E. and Holderegger, Ch. (1978) Model systems for cardiotoxic effects of anthracyclines. *Antibiotics and Chemother.* **23**, 255–270.

Zbinden, G., Bachmann, E., Holderegger, Ch. and Elsner, J. (1978) Cardiotoxicity of tricyclic antidepressants and neuroleptic drugs. *Proc. First Internat. Congr. Toxicol.* pp. 285–308. Academic Press, Inc.

Zbinden, G., Brändle, E. and Pfister, M. (1977) Modification of adriamycin toxicity in rats fed a high fat diet. *Agents and Actions* **7**, 163–170.

Zbinden, G., Elsner, J. and Bolliger, H. (1977) Toxicological evaluation of imipramine in combination with adriamycin and strophanthin. *Agents and Actions* **7**, 341–346.

Zbinden, G., Kleinert, R. and Rageth, B. (1980) Assessment of emetine cardiotoxicity in a subacute toxicity experiment in rats. *J. Cardiovasc. Pharmacol.* **2**, 155–164.

Zbinden, G., Pfister, M. and Holderegger, Ch. (1978) Cardiotoxicity of N,N-dimethyladriamycin (NSC-261045) in rats. *Toxicol. Letters* **1**, 267–274.

Zoll, P. M. and Weiss, S. (1936) Electrocardiographic changes in rats deficient in vitamin B_1. *Proc. Soc. Exp. Biol.* **35**, 259–262.

Zuckermann, R. (1959) *Grundriss und Atlas der Elektrokardiographie.* Georg Thieme, Leipzig.